The Brain and Behavior

The Brain and Behavior

An Introduction to Behavioral Neuroanatomy

Third Edition

David L. Clark
Nash N. Boutros
Mario F. Mendez

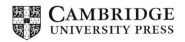

CAMBRIDGE
UNIVERSITY PRESS

CAMBRIDGE
UNIVERSITY PRESS

University Printing House, Cambridge CB2 8BS, United Kingdom

Cambridge University Press is part of the University of Cambridge.

It furthers the University's mission by disseminating knowledge in the pursuit of
education, learning and research at the highest international levels of excellence.

www.cambridge.org
Information on this title: www.cambridge.org/9780521142298

© D. Clark, N. Boutros, M. Mendez 2010

First published 2010
8th printing 2016

Printed in the United Kingdom by Print on Demand, World Wide

A catalogue record for this publication is available from the British Library

Library of Congress Cataloguing in Publication data
Clark, David L. (David Lee), 1939–
The brain and behavior : an introduction to behavioral neuroanatomy / David L. Clark,
Nash N. Boutros, Mario F. Mendez. –3rd ed.
  p. ; cm.
Includes bibliographical references and index.
ISBN 978-0-521-14229-8 (pbk.)
1. Brain–Anatomy. 2. Neuropsychology. I. Boutros, Nashaat N. II. Mendez, Mario F. III. Title.
[DNLM: 1. Brain–anatomy & histology. 2. Behavior. 3. Brain–physiology. WL 300 C592b 2010]
QM455.C55 2010
612.8'2–dc22   2010008743

ISBN 978-0-521-14229-8 Paperback

Contents

Preface to the second edition

The last ten years have witnessed an explosion in the understanding of the neurochemical and neurophysiological processes that underlie behavior. Our understanding of the pathophysiology of many psychiatric disorders has increased as well. Clinicians are now faced with the overwhelming challenge of the need to keep up with the flood of basic neuroscientific knowledge that appears monthly in scientific journals, as well as the need to assimilate it with an ever-increasing number of reports in the clinical journals that identify structural and biochemical abnormalities associated with clinical disorders. The gap that has always existed between the basic science of neuroanatomy and clinical behavioral science seems to be widening at an increasing rate.

Although the current level of knowledge of behavior and psychopathology does not necessitate a detailed understanding of all neuroanatomy, a basic level of some neuroanatomical knowledge is necessary. Familiarity with those brain regions that are heavily implicated in both normal and abnormal behavior will help the clinician assimilate new knowledge as the field evolves. As the clinician becomes more aware of the structure and function of the behaviorally sensitive regions of the brain, the concept that brain abnormalities can produce the symptomatology that is seen in the clinic becomes progressively more understandable.

Currently available neuroanatomy books are written with the neurologist in mind. Emphasis is placed on the neuroanatomy that is examined during a standard neurological exam. Areas that are known to be heavily involved in behavior such as the nucleus accumbens and the nucleus locus ceruleus receive only passing mention. We wrote this volume with the behavioral clinician in mind. It is meant to be an introduction rather than a comprehensive neuroanatomy text. We hope to be able to convey the immense complexity of the neuronal circuitry that subserves our cognitive and emotional lives. At the same time we hope to present the reader with a simplified view of the complexity of the neuroanatomy that underlies certain behaviors.

We will have accomplished our mission if we can convince the reader that the brain is an organ worthy of being the seat for the immensely complex function of behavior. Each chapter includes a list of suggested texts, as well as selected references for those who find the topic interesting and would like further details.

In preparing this volume many sources were utilized (textbooks and published articles). We encountered some discrepancies, particularly in the description of anatomical regions subserving behavior. We either elected to exclude that particular detail or chose the version compatible with the excellent and highly recommended *Principles of Neural Science*, by Kandel, Schwartz and Jessell, and its companion text, *Neuroanatomy: Text and Atlas*, by John Martin. One goal of our book is to provide a summary view of each topic. Every effort has been made to make that view as accurate as possible. Many details have been omitted because of the summary nature of the text. We hope the accuracy of the text has not been distorted by the process of summarization. Please contact us if you find errors in the material or in its interpretation (clark.32@osu.edu, nboutros@med.wayne.edu, mmendez@ucla.edu).

Cross chapter references are provided to help the reader link the related parts of the different chapters. Simplified diagrams are provided throughout the text. Selected material from clinical experience (N.N.B. and M.F.M.) is included to help relate the dry science of neuroanatomy to our everyday clinical encounters. Other clinical material is referenced. It is not the purpose of this book to present a complete picture of what is currently known about behavioral/anatomical relationships. This is the domain of clinical neuropsychiatry, for which many excellent textbooks are now available. Much ongoing research is aimed at defining the neuroanatomical bases of the various psychopathological states. A complete discussion of this research is beyond the scope of this introductory volume. Selected references regarding this fascinating research are included and may be used as starting points for readers who would like to obtain a more complete understanding of one specific area.

Two introductory chapters covering an overall view of the brain are included. Neuroanatomy has its own language. Such language tends to make reading neuroanatomy literature even more difficult. Chapter 1 includes definitions of the more commonly used neuroanatomy terms. Chapter 2 reviews some critical gross brain structures.

Many of the central nervous system (CNS) regions that are thought not to be central to behavior are mentioned only in passing in the two introductory chapters. It should be noted that as knowledge about brain and behavior increases such areas may attain more central positions. A chapter on histology includes an introduction to synaptic structure and to neurotransmission.

The book targets brain areas that are known to be heavily involved in behavior. Each chapter begins with a brief introduction. The majority of each chapter consists of anatomy and behavioral considerations. In some chapters further behavioral considerations are included before the select bibliography and references. We have allowed ourselves to speculate on the possible function of some of the CNS circuits for the purpose of stimulating the reader's interest. The speculative nature of such statements is clearly stated.

We suggest that the reader reads through the entire book at least once to develop an overview of the brain. Be sure to examine the orientation and terminology displayed in Figure 1.1. The reader can then return to individual chapters to develop a further understanding of a particular region.

References

Kandel, E.R., Schwartz, J.H., and Jessell, T.M. 2000. *Principles of Neural Science.* New York: Appleton and Lange.

Martin, J. 1996. *Neuroanatomy: Text and Atlas.* New York: Appleton and Lange.

Preface to the third edition

Our intent in this as well as earlier editions has been to provide the psychiatrist, psychologist, and others in the mental health field with a simple, easy-to-read introduction to clinically relevant brain anatomy from a functional perspective. The story of brain function continues to unfold, told through the continued publication of an impressive number of functional imaging studies. We have attempted to put the published results in simplified language while minimizing the distortion inherent in such an approach. The line drawings also reflect this perspective. The goal is to help the reader remember the basics. More cited references have been included in this edition to allow readers access to the original studies so that they may peruse the original publications at their leisure.

The results of published studies have dictated extensive revision of the chapters of the book dealing with the cortex. Updates are included in other chapters as well. Our knowledge of the anatomy of the parietal lobe has been advanced by studies revealing the function of its medial aspect and the intraparietal sulcus. These two areas have been infrequently explored until now and still receive little attention in basic neuroanatomy texts. Evaluation of the prefrontal lobes is now more complete with a somewhat better understanding of the function of the medial aspect of that portion of the cortex.

A number of networks have been introduced in Chapters 4, 5, and 6. A network may span several lobes and include subcortical structures with interconnecting white matter. The networks operate in support of various functions including attention, spatial orientation, threat recognition, and theory-of-mind, as well as mind-wandering. Several of the networks are related to clinical disorders such as schizophrenia and depression.

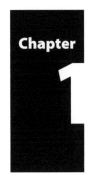

Chapter 1

Introduction

Human behavior is a direct reflection of the anatomy and physiology of the central nervous system. The goal of the behavioral neuroscientist is to uncover the neuro-anatomical substrates of behavior. Complex mental processes are represented in the brain by their elementary components. Elaborate mental functions consist of subfunctions and are constructed from both serial and parallel interconnections of several brain regions. Introduction to the nervous system covers general terminology and the ventricular system.

Major subdivisions

The nervous system is divided anatomically into the central nervous system (CNS) and the peripheral nervous system (PNS).

- The CNS is made up of the brain and spinal cord.
- The PNS consists of the cranial nerves and spinal nerves.

Physiologically, the nervous system can be divided into somatic and autonomic (visceral) divisions:

- The somatic nervous system deals with the contraction of striated muscle and the sensations of the skin (pain, touch, temperature), the innervation of muscles and joint capsules (proprioception), and the reception of sensations remote to the body by way of special senses. The somatic nervous system senses and controls our interaction with the environment external to the body.
- The autonomic nervous system controls the tone of the smooth muscles and the secretion of glands. It senses and controls the condition of the internal environment.

Common terms

The neuraxis is the long axis of the brain and spinal cord (Figure 1.1). A cross section (transverse section)

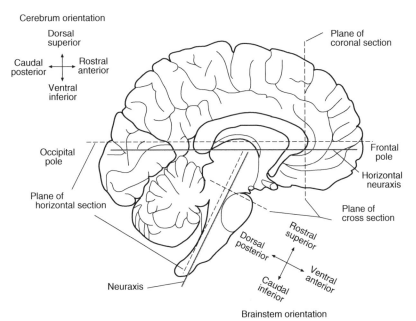

Figure 1.1. The neuraxis is the long axis of the spinal cord and brain. The neuraxis of the human brain changes at the junction of the midbrain and diencephalon. Caudal to this junction, orientation is as shown on the lower right (brainstem orientation). Rostral to this junction, orientation is as shown on the upper left (cerebrum orientation).

1

is a section taken at right angles to the neuraxis. The neuraxis in the human runs as an imaginary straight line through the center of the spinal cord and brainstem (Figure 1.1). At the level of the junction of the midbrain and diencephalon, however, the neuraxis changes orientation and extends from the occipital pole to the frontal pole (Figure 1.1). The neuraxis located above the midbrain is the neuraxis of the cerebrum and is sometimes called the horizontal neuraxis. A cross section taken perpendicular to the horizontal neuraxis is called a coronal (frontal) section.

With regard to the neuraxis of the spinal cord and brainstem:

- Dorsal (posterior) means toward the back.
- Ventral (anterior) means toward the abdomen.
- Rostral means toward the nose.
- Caudal means toward the tail.
- The sagittal (midsagittal) plane is the vertical plane that passes through the neuraxis. Figure 1.1 is cut in the sagittal plane.
- The parasagittal plane is parallel to the sagittal plane but to one side or the other of the midline.
- A horizontal section is a cut of tissue taken parallel to the neuraxis (Figure 9.1).
- A cross section (transverse section) is a cut taken perpendicular to the neuraxis (Figures 10.1, 10.2, 10.3, and 10.4).

With regard to the neuraxis of the cerebrum (horizontal neuraxis):

- Dorsal (superior) means toward the top (crown) of the skull.
- Ventral (inferior) means toward the base of the skull.
- Rostral (anterior) means toward the nose.
- Caudal (posterior) means toward the occipital bone of the skull.
- The sagittal (midsagittal) plane is the vertical plane that passes through the neuraxis.
- The parasagittal plane is parallel to the sagittal plane but to one side or the other of the midline.
- A horizontal section is a cut of tissue taken parallel to the horizon.
- A coronal section (transverse section) is a cut taken perpendicular to the neuraxis.

Other terms that relate to the CNS:

- Afferent means to or toward and is sometimes used to mean sensory.
- Efferent means away from and is sometimes used to mean motor.
- Ipsilateral refers to the same side; contralateral refers to the opposite side.

The CNS differentiates embryologically as a series of subdivisions called encephalons. Each encephalon can be identified in the adult brain. In many regions of the brain, the embryological terminology is applied to adult brain subdivisions:

- The prosencephalon is the most anterior of the embryonic subdivisions and consists of the telencephalon and diencephalon. The cerebrum of the adult corresponds with the prosencephalon.
  ‡ The telencephalon consists of the two cerebral hemispheres. These include the superficial gray matter of the cerebral cortex, the white matter beneath it, and the corpus striatum of the basal ganglia.
  ‡ The diencephalon is made up of the thalamus, the hypothalamus below it, and the epithalamus located above it (pineal and habenula; Figure 13.5).
- The brainstem lies caudal to the prosencephalon. It consists of the following:
  ‡ The mesencephalon (midbrain).
  ‡ The rhombencephalon, which is made up of:
    • The metencephalon, which contains the pons and cerebellum.
    • The myelencephalon (medulla oblongata).

Ventricular system

The central canal of the embryo differentiates into the ventricular system of the adult brain. The ventricular cavities are filled with cerebrospinal fluid (CSF), which is produced by vascular tufts called the choroid plexuses. The ventricular cavity of the telencephalon is represented by the lateral ventricles (Figure 1.2). The lateral ventricles are the first and second ventricles. They connect to the third ventricle of the diencephalon by the interventricular foramina (of Monro). Continuing caudally, the cerebral aqueduct of the midbrain opens into the fourth ventricle. The fourth ventricle occupies the space dorsal to the pons and medulla and ventral to the cerebellum. CSF flows from the fourth ventricle into the subarachnoid space through the median aperture (of Magendie) and the lateral apertures (of Luschka). Most of the CSF is produced by the choroid plexus of

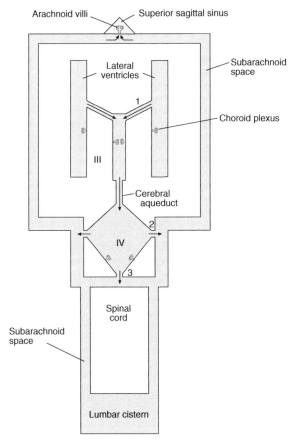

Figure 1.2. Cerebrospinal fluid (CSF) is produced by tufts of choroid plexus found in all four ventricles. CSF exits the lateral ventricles through the interventricular foramina (of Monro) (1). CSF exits the ventricular system through the lateral apertures (of Luschka) (2) and the median aperture (of Magendie) (3). CSF is reabsorbed into the blood by way of the arachnoid villi that project into the superior sagittal sinus.

the lateral ventricles, although tufts of choroid plexus are found in the third and fourth ventricles as well.

The lateral as well as the third ventricles have been noted to be enlarged in a number of psychiatric disorders, particularly schizophrenia (Daniel *et al.*, 1991; Elkis *et al.*, 1995). Enlargement of the ventricles usually reflects atrophy of the surrounding brain tissue. The term hydrocephalus is used to describe abnormal enlargement of the ventricles. In the condition known as normal-pressure hydrocephalus, the ventricles enlarge in the absence of brain atrophy or obvious obstruction to the flow of the CSF. Normal pressure hydrocephalus is classically characterized by progressive dementia, ataxia, and incontinence (Friedland, 1989). However, symptoms may range from apathy and anhedonia to aggressive or obsessive-compulsive behavior or both (Abbruzzese *et al.*, 1994).

References

Abbruzzese, M., Scarone, S., and Colombo, C. 1994. Obsessive-compulsive symptomatology in normal pressure hydrocephalus: A case report. *J. Psychiatr. Neurosci.* **19**:378–380.

Daniel, D.G., Goldberg., T.E., Gibbons, R.D., and Weinberger, D.R. 1991. Lack of a bimodal distribution of ventricular size in schizophrenia: A Gaussian mixture analysis of 1056 cases and controls. *Biol. Psychiatry* **30**:886–903.

Elkis, H., Friedman, L., Wise, A., and Meltzer, H.Y. 1995. Meta-analyses of studies of ventricular enlargement and cortical sulcal prominence in mood disorders. *Arch. Gen. Psychiatry* **52**:735–746.

Friedland, R.P. 1989. Normal-pressure hydrocephalus and the saga of the treatable dementias. *J.A.M.A.* **262**:2577–2593.

Clinical vignette

A 61-year-old man reported that his work performance was slipping. He was forgetting names and dates more than usual. Because of recent losses in his family, he assumed he was depressed. He saw a psychiatrist (his wife had a history of depression), who prescribed an antidepressant. Soon after this, the patient had an episode of urinary incontinence. A neurology consultation was obtained, which revealed gait problems. A computed tomographic scan showed enlarged ventricles without enlarged sulci (which would have indicated generalized brain atrophy). The diagnosis of normal pressure hydrocephalus was made. Progressive improvement in the patient's clinical condition was seen following the installation of a ventricular shunt.

Gross anatomy of the brain

Introduction

The brain is that portion of the central nervous system that lies within the skull. Three major subdivisions are recognized: the brainstem, the cerebellum, and the cerebrum. The cerebrum includes both the cerebral hemispheres and the diencephalon.

Brainstem

The brainstem is the rostral continuation of the spinal cord. The foramen magnum, the hole at the base of the skull, marks the junction of the spinal cord and the brainstem. The brainstem consists of three subdivisions: the medulla, the pons, and the midbrain (Figure 2.1).

Medulla

The caudal limit of the medulla lies at the foramen magnum. The central canal of the spinal cord expands in the region of the medulla to form the fourth ventricle (IV in Figure 1.2). The cranial nerves associated with the medulla are the hypoglossal, spinal accessory, vagus, and the glossopharyngeal.

Pons

The pons lies above (rostral to) the medulla (Figure 2.1). The bulk of the medulla is continuous with the pontine tegmentum. The tegmentum consists of nuclei and tracts that lie between the basilar pons and the floor of the fourth ventricle (IV in Figures 1.2 and 10.2). The basilar pons consists of tracts along with nuclei that are associated with the cerebellum. The fourth ventricle narrows at the rostral end of the pons to connect with the cerebral aqueduct of the midbrain (Figures 1.2, 10.2, 10.3, and 10.4). The cranial nerves associated with the pons are the vestibulocochlear (statoacoustic), facial, abducens, and trigeminal.

Midbrain

The dorsal surface of the midbrain is marked by four hillocks, the corpora quadrigemina (tectum). The caudal pair consists of the inferior colliculi (Figure 10.3; auditory system), and the cranial pair consists of the superior colliculi (Figure 10.4; visual system). The ventricular cavity of the midbrain is the cerebral aqueduct. Most nuclei and tracts found in the midbrain lie ventral to the cerebral aqueduct and together make up the midbrain tegmentum (Figure 2.1). The basilar midbrain contains the crus cerebri ("motor pathway" in Figures 10.3 and 10.4) and the substantia nigra, one of the basal ganglia. The cranial nerves associated with the midbrain are the trochlear and oculomotor.

Ischemia (particularly transient ischemia) of the midbrain tectum can result in visual hallucinations (peduncular hallucinosis). Auditory hallucinations have also been reported with lesions of the tegmentum of the pons and lower midbrain (Cascino and Adams, 1986). The sounds have the character of noise: buzzing and clanging. To one patient, the sounds reportedly had a musical character like chiming bells.

Cerebellum

The cerebellum arises embryologically from the dorsal pons. In the mature brain the cerebellum overlies the pons and medulla (Figure 2.2) and is connected with them by the three paired cerebellar peduncles (Figures 10.1 and 10.2). The cerebellum is separated from the pons and medulla by the cavity of the fourth ventricle. Like the cerebrum, it displays a highly convoluted surface. The cortex of the cerebellum is gray and a layer of white matter lies deep to it. Although it represents only about 10% of the brain, the cerebellum contains more than four times the number of neurons in the cerebral cortex (Andersen *et al.*, 1992).

Traditionally the cerebellum is thought to be involved in the control and integration of motor functions that subserve coordination, balance, and gait. It is usually divided into three functional/structural components: the flocculonodular lobe (archicerebellum), which is closely connected with the vestibular system and is involved in eye movements; the vermis and

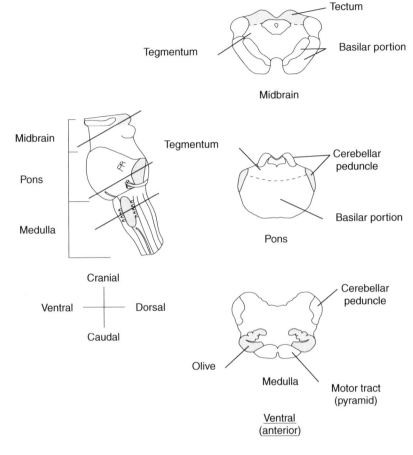

Dorsal
(posterior)

Tectum

Tegmentum

Basilar portion

Midbrain

Midbrain

Tegmentum

Cerebellar peduncle

Pons

Basilar portion

Pons

Medulla

Cranial

Ventral — Dorsal

Caudal

Cerebellar peduncle

Olive

Medulla

Motor tract (pyramid)

Ventral
(anterior)

Figure 2.1. The brainstem consists of the medulla, the pons, and the midbrain. A lateral view of the brainstem (left) is marked to indicate the level from which each of the cross sections (right) is taken. See Chapter 10 for significant structures found in each cross section. Cranial refers to the top of the head, and caudal refers to the spinal cord.

Clinical vignette

A 71-year-old man had no prior history of psychiatric or neurological problems. While at home with his two sons, daughter and wife, he suddenly experienced weakness in all four extremities and started seeing policemen entering the front door of his house. He became irritable and fearful that the police would take him away. He was brought to the emergency room (ER). A neurological examination was normal, and the hallucinations ceased. The patient was discharged with follow-up at the psychiatry clinic. Three days later he was brought to the ER completely comatose owing to a brainstem stroke. In retrospect, the patient was found to have had a brainstem transient ischemic attack (TIA), which caused him to experience peduncular hallucinosis.

paravermal area (spinocerebellum), which are related to the axial and paraxial musculature involved with walking; and the cerebellar hemispheres (neocerebellum), which are linked with the neocortex and function in the coordination of hand/arm movements and speech. The vermis is further divided into the classic lobules numbered from I to X, with I being most anterior/superior. Technical limits of imaging have produced a modified classification. The vermis is often reported to be subdivided into vermal regions V1–V4 (V1, lobules I–V; V2, lobules VI and VII; V3, lobule VIII; V4, lobules IX and X) (Sullivan *et al.*, 2000).

The cerebellum is generally credited with detecting and correcting errors in ongoing muscular activity (i.e., motor coordination). Accumulating evidence suggests that the cerebellum also plays a role in affective and higher cognitive functions. For example, stimulation of the fastigial nucleus, which relays signals from the flocculonodular lobe, has been shown to result in changes in blood pressure as well as changes in the nucleus accumbens and the hippocampus of the limbic system (Heath *et al.*, 1978; Andrezik *et al.*, 1984). The vermis has connections with limbic structures

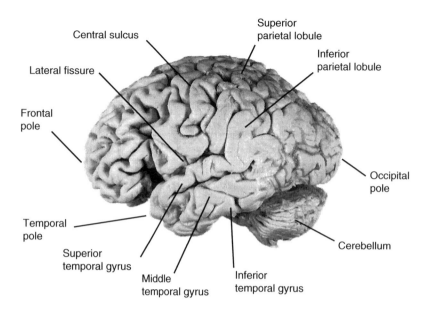

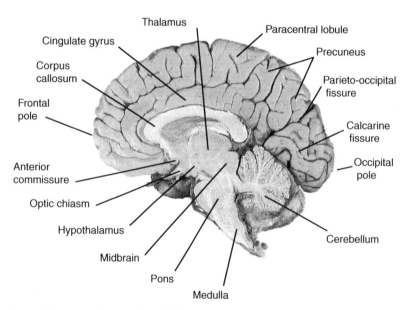

Figure 2.2. Lateral (above) and medial (below) views of the gross brain. Compare with Brodmann's areas, Figure 2.3.

(amygdala and hippocampus) as well as with the red nucleus (a motor nucleus). It is hypothesized that the vermis may affect emotional behavior through connections with the ventral tegmental area (Nestler and Carlezon, 2006). The lateral cerebellar lobes (including the dentate and emboliform nuclei) may be more involved with cognitive functions such as strategic planning, learning, memory, and language (Schmahmann, 1991; Roskies *et al.*, 2001). Activation of the cerebellar nuclear structures has been demonstrated during cognitive processing (Kim *et al.*, 1994). Abnormalities in cerebellar activity and size do not follow a particular pattern but relationships to neuropsychiatric disorders, including schizophrenia, have been summarized by Hoppenbrouwers *et al.* (2008) and Andreasen and Pierson (2008).

The cerebellar cognitive affective syndrome (CCAS) was described based on patients with cerebellar lesions. Symptoms may be motor and nonmotor. Among the nonmotor symptoms are anxiety, perseveration, anhedonia and aggression. In addition, visuospatial, linguistic dysfunction and impairments in working memory and planning have been reported (Schmahmann and Sherman, 1998). Other symptoms reported include lethargy, depression, and lack of empathy (Schmahmann *et al.*, 2007).

Abnormalities of the vermis are more frequently reported in behavioral disorders than in other portions of the cerebellum. Although observations in different studies vary, the vermis is generally smaller in autism spectrum disorders (vermal area V2) (Courchesne *et al.*, 1988, 1994a, 2001; Murakami *et al.*, 1989; Hashimoto *et al.*, 1995). In fact, V2 has been linked specifically with stereotyped behavior and reduced exploration (Pierce and Courchesne, 2001). Several studies have found a smaller vermis in several patients with schizophrenia (Sandyk *et al.*, 1991; Nopoulos *et al.*, 1999; Ichimiya *et al.*, 2001; Varnas *et al.*, 2007). A decrease in vermal volume has been reported in patients with bipolar disorder (V2 and V3), depression (Shah *et al.*, 1992; DelBello *et al.*, 1999; Mills *et al.*, 2005), and schizophrenia (Sandyk *et al.*, 1991; Nopoulos *et al.*, 1999; Ichimiya *et al.*, 2001; Varnas *et al.*, 2007). An increase in blood flow in the vermis has been observed in depression (Dolan *et al.*, 1992).

Courchesne *et al.* (2001), using head circumference, found that the total brain size in children with autism was normal at birth. However, 90% of 2–4-year-old autistic children had significantly larger (18%) brains compared with controls. Comparison of both groups as 5–15 year olds showed no difference. The authors hypothesized that the overgrowth is restricted to childhood followed by a period of slowed growth (Courchesne *et al.*, 2001; Sparks *et al.*, 2002).

Decreased cerebellar hemisphere size has been reported in autism (Murakami *et al.*, 1989) and schizophrenia (Bottmer *et al.*, 2005). A loss of cerebellar cortex granular cells has been reported in autism, and the same studies showed loss of Purkinje cells in both the vermis and the cerebellar hemispheres (Ritvo *et al.*, 1986; Kemper and Bauman, 1998). It was argued that these losses occurred before 30 weeks of gestation (Bauman and Kemper, 1985). An analysis of magnetic resonance imaging (MRI) of 50 subjects showed decreased vermal size in 86% but increased vermal size

in 12% (Courchesne *et al.*, 1994b). It is hypothesized that cerebellar abnormalities in autism may be responsible for deficits in shifting attention (Akshoomoff and Courchesne, 1992).

Higher blood flow to the cerebellum has been reported in patients with posttraumatic stress disorder (Bonne *et al.*, 2003) and reduced cerebellar size was described in attention-deficit hyperactivity disorder (Castellanos *et al.*, 2002; Valera *et al.*, 2007). A model has been proposed suggesting that abnormalities in connectivity within the cerebellum or between the cerebellum and other brain structures may be responsible for the "cognitive dysmetria" seen in schizophrenia (Andreasen *et al.*, 1998).

Cerebrum

The diencephalic portion of the cerebrum consists of the thalamus (Chapter 9), the hypothalamus, and the epithalamus (Chapter 8). The thalamus is an integrative center through which most sensory information must pass in order to reach the cerebral cortex (i.e., the level of consciousness). The hypothalamus serves as an integrative center for control of the body's internal environment by way of the autonomic nervous system (Figure 8.1). The pituitary gland (hypophysis) extends ventrally from the base of the hypothalamus. The epithalamus consists of the habenula and the pineal gland. The ventricular cavity of the diencephalon is the third ventricle (III in Figure 1.2). The optic nerve is associated with the diencephalon (dotted lines, Figure 8.3).

The cerebral hemispheres include the cerebral cortex and the underlying white matter, as well as a number of nuclei that lie deep to the white matter. Traditionally, these nuclei are referred to as the basal ganglia (Chapter 7). One of these forebrain nuclei, the amygdala (Figure 11.1), is now included as part of the limbic system (Chapters 11, 12, and 13). The surface of the cortex is marked by ridges (gyri) and grooves (sulci). Several of the sulci are quite deep, earning them the status of fissure. The most prominent fissure is the longitudinal cerebral fissure (sagittal or interhemispheric fissure), which is located in the midline and separates the two hemispheres. Each hemisphere is divided into four lobes: frontal, parietal, occipital, and temporal.

The frontal lobe lies rostral to the central sulcus and dorsal to the lateral fissure (Figures 2.2 and 2.3). An imaginary line drawn from the parieto-occipital sulcus to the preoccipital notch separates the occipital

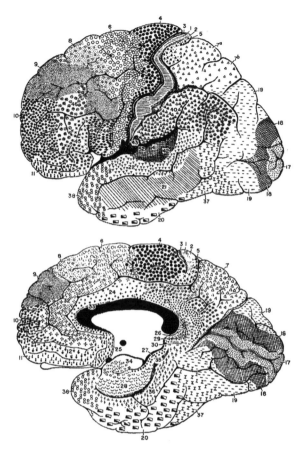

Figure 2.3. The cytoarchitectonic regions of the cortex as described by Brodmann. Compare with the surface of the brain, Figure 2.2.

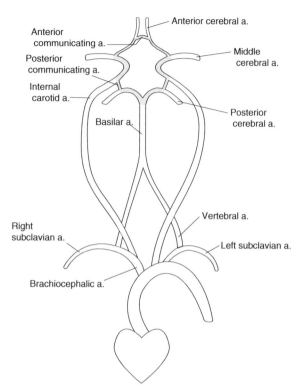

Figure 2.4. Principal arteries serving the brain. The shaded vessels make up the cerebral arterial circle (of Willis).

lobe from the rest of the brain (Figure 5.1). A second imaginary line, perpendicular to the first and continuing rostrally with the lateral fissure, divides the parietal lobe above from the temporal lobe below. Spreading the lips of the lateral fissure reveals the smaller insular region deep to the surface of the cortex.

The limbic system (limbic lobe) is made up of contributions from several areas. The parahippocampal gyrus and uncus can be seen on the ventromedial aspect of the temporal lobe (Figure 5.4). The hippocampus and amygdala lie deep to the ventral surface of the medial temporal lobe (Figure 11.1), and the cingulate gyrus lies along the deep medial aspect of the cortex (Figure 12.1). These structures are joined together by fiber bundles and form a crescent or limbus (Figure 13.1).

The basal ganglia represent an important motor control center.

- The neostriatum is made up of the caudate nucleus and putamen (Figure 7.1).
- The paleostriatum consists of the globus pallidus.
- Two additional nuclei that are included as basal ganglia are the subthalamic nucleus (subthalamus) and the substantia nigra.

The internal capsule is made up of fibers that interconnect the cerebral cortex with other subdivisions of the brain and spinal cord. The anterior and posterior commissures as well as the massive corpus callosum interconnect the left side with the right side of the cerebrum.

Vasculature

Two major systems supply blood to the brain (Figure 2.4). The vertebral arteries represent the posterior supply; they course along the ventral surface of the spinal cord, pass through the foramen magnum, and then merge medially to form the basilar artery on the ventral aspect of the medulla. The basilar artery splits at its rostral terminus to form the paired posterior cerebral arteries.

The internal carotid system represents the anterior supply and arises at the carotid bifurcation. Major branches of the internal carotid include the anterior

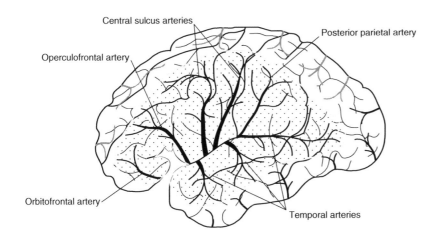

Figure 2.5. The stippled area represents the cortex served by the middle cerebral artery. The vessels emerging from the longitudinal cerebral fissure are the terminal branches of the anterior cerebral artery (after Waddington, 1974; compare with Figure 2.6).

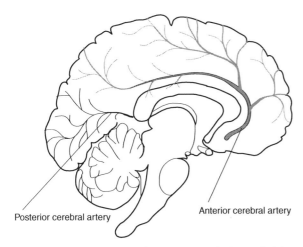

Figure 2.6. The distribution of the anterior cerebral artery (right) and the posterior cerebral artery (left) on the medial aspect of the brain.

cerebral and the middle cerebral arteries. The vertebral-basilar and the internal carotid systems join at the base of the brain to form the cerebral arterial circle (of Willis).

The cerebral cortex is served by the three major cerebral arteries (Figures 2.5 and 2.6):

- The anterior cerebral artery supplies the medial aspect of the frontal and parietal cortices, with terminal branches extending a short distance out of the sagittal fissure onto the lateral surface of the brain.
- The posterior cerebral artery serves the medial and most of the lateral aspect of the occipital lobe, as well as portions of the ventral aspect of the temporal lobe.

- The large middle cerebral artery serves the remainder of the cortex, including the majority of the lateral aspect of the frontal, parietal, and temporal cortices.

The blood–brain barrier is a physiological concept based on the observation that many substances, including many drugs, which may be in high concentrations in the blood, are not simultaneously found in the brain tissue. The location of the barrier coincides with the endothelial cells of the capillaries found in the brain. These endothelial cells, unlike those found in capillaries elsewhere in the body, are joined together by tight junctions. These tight junctions are recognized as the anatomical basis of the blood–brain barrier.

Sackeim *et al.* (1990) reported that blood flow to the brain was reduced in elderly patients diagnosed with major depressive disorder when compared with age-matched control subjects. Overall blood flow was reduced by 12%. The distribution of the effect was uneven, and there were brain regions in which the reduction was even greater.

Electroencephalogram

Electroencephalography uses large recording electrodes placed on the scalp (Figure 2.7). The activity seen on the electroencephalogram (EEG) represents the summated activity of large ensembles of neurons. More specifically, it is a reflection of the extracellular current flow associated with the summed activity of many individual neurons. Most EEG activity reflects activity in the cortex, but some (e.g., sleep spindles) represents activity in various subcortical structures. The record generated reflects spontaneous voltage fluctuations. Abnormalities in the brain can produce pathological synchronization of neural elements that

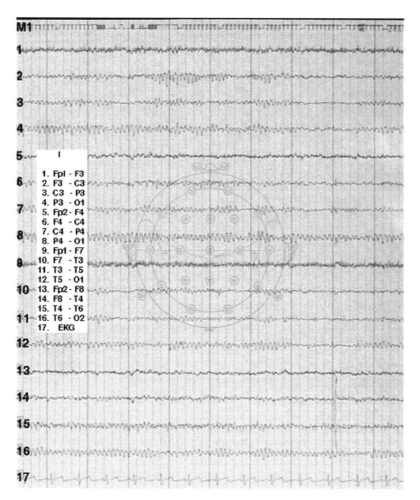

Figure 2.7. An example of a normal electroencephalogram (EEG). Metal sensors (electrodes) placed on various scalp locations are used to record the electrical activity of the brain. The actual brain electrical signal is amplified 10 000 times before it can be recorded for visual inspection. The various electrodes are electronically connected to form montages. The particular montage used for the example shown is listed on the left of the figure. Note that the rhythmic sinusoidal alpha activity is most developed on the occipital regions (electrodes 4, 8, 12, and 16).

1. Fpl - F3
2. F3 - C3
3. C3 - P3
4. P3 - O1
5. Fp2 - F4
6. F4 - C4
7. C4 - P4
8. P4 - O1
9. Fp1 - F7
10. F7 - T3
11. T3 - T5
12. T5 - O1
13. Fp2 - F8
14. F8 - T4
15. T4 - T6
16. T6 - O2
17. EKG

can be seen, for example, as spike discharges representing seizure activity. The detection of seizure activity is one of the most valuable assets of the EEG.

Meninges

The brain and spinal cord are surrounded by three meninges: the dura mater, the arachnoid, and the pia mater. Blood vessels as well as cranial and spinal nerves all pierce the meninges. The pia mater is intimate to the surface of the brain and spinal cord and envelops the blood vessels that course along its surface. The dura mater is a thick, heavy membrane that forms the internal periosteum of the skull. The dura is made up of two layers, and these layers separate at several locations to form the venous sinuses, such as the superior sagittal sinus (Figure 1.2). The epidural space and the subdural space are only potential spaces. The arachnoid lies between the pia mater and the dura mater and forms a very thin layer along the inner surface of the dura mater. The subarachnoid space is filled with cerebrospinal fluid.

Sexual dimorphism and aging

It has been found that men have significantly larger volumes of gray and white matter than women (7–10%) when controlling for weight (Allen *et al.*, 2003). This difference is also present in neonates (Gilmore *et al.*, 2007). In another study, women showed a higher proportion of gray matter than men (0.46 vs 0.45, respectively) and smaller ratio of white matter (0.29 vs 0.30, respectively), but the differences were not significant (Chen *et al.*, 2007). Regionally, men have been reported to have larger gray matter volume in the left parietal lobe and bilaterally in the frontal and temporal lobes (Carne *et al.*, 2006). Women have been shown to have larger gray matter volumes in the cingulate gyrus, inferior parietal lobe, and right dorsolateral temporal cortex (Van Laere and Dierckx, 2001). Women also have greater gyrification and fissuration of the brain surface than men (Luders *et al.*, 2004, 2006).

Gray matter volume begins to decrease at the end of the first decade whereas white matter volume begins to decrease at the end of the fourth decade (Courchesne *et al.*, 2000). A group of 662 individuals, controlled for age (63–75 years), were studied over four years. Brain tissue loss was observed to be 3.9 cm³/year. The largest rates of atrophy were seen in the primary auditory, somatosensory, visual, and motor cortices. The orbital prefrontal cortex and hippocampus also showed age-related reduction in volume (Salat *et al.*, 2004). The hippocampus loss appears to accelerate in the sixth decade (Raz *et al.*, 2004). Loss of white matter was much less than that of the gray matter and seen primarily in the corpus callosum. The pattern of age-related gray matter loss was not significantly different between men and women. However, a small, consistent, increased rate of loss was seen in women (Lemaître *et al.*, 2005). Others suggest the loss is greater in men (Coffey *et al.*, 1998). Age-related loss in white matter occurs in the anterior and posterior internal capsule, and the anterior corpus callosum (Hsu *et al.*, 2008).

References

Akshoomoff, N.A., and Courchesne, E. 1992. A new role for the cerebellum in cognitive operations. *Behav. Neurosci.* **106**:731–738.

Allen, J.S., Damasio, H., Grabowski, T.J., Bruss, J., and Zhange, W. 2003. Sexual dimorphism and asymmetries in the gray-white composition of the human cerebrum. *Neuroimage* **18**:880–894.

Andersen, B.B., Korbo, L., and Pakkenberg, B. 1992. A quantitative study of the human cerebellum with unbiased stereological techniques. *J. Comp. Neurol.* **326**:549–560.

Andreasen, N.C., and Pierson, R. 2008. The role of the cerebellum in schizophrenia. *Biol. Psychiatry* **64**:81–88.

Andreasen, N.C., Paradiso, S., and O'Leary, D.S. 1998. "Cognitive dysmetria" as an integrative theory of schizophrenia: A dysfunction in cortical-subcortical-cerebellar circuitry? *Schizophr. Bull.* **24**:203–218.

Andrezik, J.A., Dormer, K.J., Forman, R.D. and Person, R.J. 1984. Fastigial nucleus projections to the brain stem in beagles: Pathways for autonomic regulation. *Neuroscience* **11**:497–507.

Bauman, M., and Kemper, T.L. 1985. Histoanatomic observations of the brain in early infantile autism. *Neurol.* **35**:866–874.

Bonne, O., Gilboa, A., Louzoun, Y., Brandes, D., Yona, I., Lester, H., Barkai, G., Freedman, N., Chisin, R., and Shalev, A. 2003. Resting regional cerebral perfusion in recent posttraumatic stress disorder. *Biol. Psychiatry* **54**:1077–1086.

Bottmer, C., Bachmann, S., Pantel, J., Essig, M., Amann, M., Schad, LR, Magnotta, V., and Schröder, J. 2005. Reduced cerebellar volume and neurological soft signs in first-episode schizophrenia. *Psychiatry Res.* **140**:239–250.

Carne, R.P., Vogrin, S., Litewka, L., and Cook., M.J. 2006. Cerebral cortex: an MRI-based study of volume and variance with age and sex. *J. Clin. Neurosci.* **13**: 60–72.

Cascino, G.D., and Adams, R.D. 1986. Brainstem auditory hallucinosis. *Neurology* **36**:1042–1047.

Castellanos, F.X., Lee, P.P., Sharp, W., Jeffries, N.O., Greenstein, D.K., Clasen, L.S., Blumenthal, J.D., and James, R.S. 2002. Developmental trajectories of brain volume abnormalities in children and adolescents with attention-deficit/hyperactivity disorder. *J.A.M.A.* **288**:1740–1748.

Chen, X., Sachdev, P.S., Wen, W., and Anstey, K.J. 2007. Sex differences in regional gray matter in healthy individuals aged 44–48 years: A voxel-based morphometric study. *Neuroimage* **36**:691–699.

Coffey, C.E., Lucke, J.F., Saxon, J.A., Ratcliff, G., Unitas, L.J., Billig, B., and Bryan, R.N. 1998. Sex differences in brain aging: a quantitative magnetic resonance imaging study. *Arch. Neurol.* **55**:169–179.

Courchesne, E., Yeung-Courchesne, R., Press, G.A., Hesselink, J.R., and Jernigan, T.L. 1988. Hypoplasia of the cerebellar vermal lobules VI and VII in autism. *N. Engl. J. of Med.* **318**:1349–1354.

Courchesne, E., Saitoh, O., Yeung-Courchesne, R., Press, G.A., Lincoln, A.J., Haas, R.H., and Schreibman, L.1994a. Abnormality of cerebellar vermian lobules VI and VII in patients with infantile autism: Identification of hypoplastic and hyperplastic subgroups with MR imaging. *AJRAm. J. Roentgenol.***162**:123–130.

Courchesne, E., Townsend, J., and Saitoh, O.1994b. The brain in infantile autism: Posterior fossa structures are abnormal. *Neurology* **44**:214–223.

Courchesne, E., Chisum, H.J., Townsend, J., Cowles, A., Covington, J., Egass, B., Harwood, M., Hinds, S., and Press, G.A. 2000. Normal brain development and aging: quantitative analysis at in vivo MR imaging in healthy volunteers. *Radiology* **216**:672–682.

Courchesne, E., Karns, C.M., Davis, H.R., Ziccardi, R., Carper, R.A., Tigue, Z.D., Chisum, H.J., Moses, P., Pierce, K., Lord, C., Lincoln, A.J., Pizzo, S., Schreibman, L., Haas, R.H., Akshoomoff, N.A., and Courchesne, R.Y. 2001. Unusual brain growth patterns in early life in patients with autistic disorder: an MRI study. *Neurology* **57**:245–254.

DelBello, M.P., Strakowski, S.M., Zimmerman, M.E., Hawkins, J.M., and Sax, K.W. 1999. MRI analysis of the cerebellum in bipolar disorder: A pilot study. *Neuropsychopharmacology* **21**:63–68.

Dolan, R.J., Bench, C.J., Brown, R.G., Scott, L.C., Friston, K.J., and Frackowiak, R.S.J. 1992. Regional cerebral blood flow abnormalities in depressed patients with cognitive impairment. *J. Neurol. Neurosurg. Psychiatry* **55**:768–773.

Gilmore, J.H., Lin, W., Prastawa, M.W., Looney, C.B., Vetsa, Y.S.K., Knickmeyer, R.C., Evans, D.D., Smith, J.K., Hamer, R.M., Lieberman, J.A., and Gerig, G. 2007. Regional gray matter growth, sexual dimorphism, and cerebral asymmetry in the neonatal brain. *J. Neurosci.* **27**:1255–1260.

Hashimoto, T., Tayama, M., Murakawa, K., Yoshimoto, T., Miyazaki, M., Harada, M., and Kuroda, Y. 1995. Development of the brainstem and cerebellum in autistic patients. *J. Autism. Dev. Disord.* **25**:1–18.

Heath, R.G., Dempsey, C.W., Fontana, C.J. and Myers, W.A. 1978. Cerebellar stimulation: Effects on septal region, hippocampus, and amygdala of cats and rats. *Biol. Psychiatry* **13**:501–529.

Hoppenbrouwers, S.S., Schutter, D.J.L.G., Fitzgerald, P.B., Chen, R., and Daskalakis, Z.J. 2008. The role of the cerebellum in pathophysiology and treatment of neuropsychiatric disorders: A review. *Brain Res. Rev.* **59**:185–200.

Hsu, J-L., Leemans, A., Bai, C-H., Lee, C-H., Tsai, Y-F., Chiu, H-C., and Chen, W-H. 2008. Gender differences and age-related white matter changes of the human brain: A diffusion tensor imaging study. *Neuroimage* **39**:566–577.

Ichimiya, T., Okubo, Y., Suhara, T., Sudo, Y. 2001. Reduced volume of the cerebellar vermis in neuroleptic-naïve schizophrenia. *Biol. Psychiatry* **49**:20–27.

Kemper, T.L., and Bauman, M. 1998. Neuropathology of infantile autism. *J. Neuropathol. Exp. Neurol.* **57**:645–652.

Kim, S.-G., Ugurbil, K., and Strick, P.L. 1994. Activation of cerebellar output nucleus during cognitive processing. *Science* **265**:949.

Lemaître, H., Crivello, F., Grassiot, B., Alpérovitch, A., Tzourio, C., and Mazoyer, B. 2005. Age- and sex-related effects on the neuroanatomy of healthy elderly. *Neuroimage* **269**:900–911.

Luders, E., Narr, K.L., Thompson, P.M., Rex, D.E., Jancke, L., Steinmetz, H., and Toga, A.W. 2004. Gender differences in cortical complexity. *Nat. Neurosci.* **7**:799–800.

Luders, E., Narr, K.L, Thompson, P.M., Rex, D.E., Woods, R.P., Deluca, H., Jancke, L., and Toga, A.W., 2006. Gender effects on cortical thickness and the influences of scaling. *Hum. Brain Mapp.* **27**:314–324.

Mills, N.P., Delbello, M.P., Adler, C.M., and Strakowski, S.M. 2005. MRI analysis of cerebellar loops: Motor and cognitive circuits. *Brain Res. Rev.* **31**:1530–1532.

Murakami, J.W., Courchesne, E., Press, G.A., Yeung-Courchesne, R., and Hesselink, J.R. 1989. Reduced cerebellar hemisphere size and its relationship to vermal hypoplasia in autism. *Arch. Neurol.* **46**:689–694.

Nestler, E.J., and Carlezon Jr., W.A. 2006. The mesolimbic dopamine reward circuit in depression. *Biol. Psychiatry* **59**:1151–1159.

Nopoulos, P.C., Ceilley, J.W., Gailis, E.A., and Andreasen, N.C. 1999. An MRI study of cerebellar vermis morphology in patients with schizophrenia: Evidence in support of the cognitive dysmetria concept. *Biol. Psychiatry* **26**:703–711.

Pierce, K., and Courchesne, E. 2001. Evidence for a cerebellar role in reduced exploration and stereotyped behavior in autism. *Biol. Psychiatry* **49**:655–664.

Raz, N., Gunning-Dixon, F., Head, D., Rodrigue, K.M., Williamson, A., and Acker, J.D. 2004. Aging, sexual dimorphism, and hemispheric asymmetry of the cerebral cortex: replicability of regional differences in volume. *Neurobio. Aging* **25**:377–396.

Ritvo, E.R., Freeman, B.J., Scheibel, A.B., Duong, T., Robinson, H., Guthrie, D., and Ritvo, A. 1986. Lower Purkinje cell counts in the cerebella of four autistic subjects: Initial findings of the UCLA-NSAC autopsy research report. *Am. J. Psychiatry* **143**:862–866.

Roskies, A.l., Fiez, J.A., Balota, D.A., Raichle, M.E., and Petersen, S.E. 2001. Task-dependent modulation of regions in the left inferior frontal cortex during semantic processing. *J. Cogn. Neurosci.* **13**:829–843.

Sackeim, H.A., Prohovnik, I., Moeller, J.R., Brown, R.P., Apter, S., Prudic, J., Devanand, D.P., and Mukerjee, S. 1990. Regional cerebral blood flow in mood disorders. I. Comparison of major depressives and normal controls at rest. *Arch. Gen. Psychiatry* **47**:60–70.

Salat, D.H., Buckner, R.L., Snyder, A.Z., Grevel, D.N., Desikan, R.S.R., Busa, E., Morris, J.C., Dale, A.M., and Fischl, R. 2004. Thinning of the cerebral cortex in ageing. *Cereb. Cortex* **14**:721–730.

Sandyk, R., Kay, S.R., and Merriam, A.E. 1991. Atrophy of the cerebellar vermis: relevance to the symptoms of schizophrenia. *Int. J. Neurosci.* **57**:205–211.

Schmahmann, J.D. 1991. An emerging concept. The cerebellar contribution to higher function. *Arch. Neurol.* **48**:1178–1187.

Schmahmann, J.D., and Sherman, J.C. 1998. The cerebellar cognitive affective syndrome. *Brain* **121**:561–579.

Schmahmann, J.D., Weilburg, J.B., and Sherman, J.C. 2007. The neuropsychiatry of the cerebellum –insights from the clinic. *Cerebellum* **6**:254–267.

Shah, S.A., Doraiswamy, P.M., Husain, M.M., Escalona, P.R., Na, C., Figiel, G.S., Patterson, L.J., Ellinwood, E.H. Jr., McDonald, W.M., Boyko, O.B., Nemeroff, C.B., and Krishnan, K.R.R. 1992. Posterior fossa abnormalities in major depression: A controlled magnetic resonance imaging study. *Acta Psychiatr. Scand.* **85**:474–479.

Sullivan, E.V., Deshmukh, A., Desmond, J.E., Mathalon, D.H., Rosenbloom, M.J., Lim, K.O., and Adolf Pfefferbaum, A. 2000. Contribution of alcohol abuse to cerebellar volume deficits in men with schizophrenia. *Arch. Gen. Psychiatry* **57**:894–902.

Valera, E.M., Faraone, S.V., Murray, K.E., and Seidman, L.J. 2007. Meta-analysis of structural imaging findings in attention-deficit/hyperactivity disorder. *Biol. Psychiatry* **61**:1361–1369.

Van Laere, K.J. and Dierckx, R.A., 2001. Brain perfusion SPECT: age- and sex-related effects correlated with voxel-based morphometric findings in healthy adults. *Radiology* **221**:810–817.

Varnas, K., Okugawa, G., Hammarberg, A., Nesvag, R., Rimol, L.M., Franck, J., and Agartz, I. 2007. Cerebellar volumes in men with schizophrenia and alcohol dependence. *Psychiatry Clin. Neurosci.* **61**:326–329.

Waddington, M.M. 1974. *Atlas of Cerebral Angiography with Anatomic Correction.* Boston: Little, Brown.

Chapter 3

Histology

Introduction

The adult brain weighs between 1100 and 2000 g. It contains an estimated 100 billion neurons. The average neuron has up to 10 000 synapses. At least a third of this immensely complex system is dedicated to the function of behavior.

Two types of cells make up the nervous system: neurons and neuroglial cells (glia). Neurons are specialized to conduct bioelectrical messages, whereas the glial cells play an interactive and supportive role. Both are involved in the production and management of neurotransmitters.

The neuron

The neuron is the structural and functional unit of the nervous system. It is made up of four distinctive regions: the soma (nerve cell body), the dendrites, the axon, and the synapse (Figures 3.1 and 3.4). The soma is the metabolic center of the cell and contains the cell nucleus. The nucleus is centrally located in the soma, and the cytoplasm immediately surrounding the nucleus is called the perikaryon.

Most neurons have several dendrites, but each neuron has a single axon (Figure 3.2). The cytoplasm of the axon is called the axoplasm. The axon arises from a specialized region of the cell body called the axon hillock (Figure 3.1) that is specialized to facilitate the propagation of the all-or-none action potential.

Nissl substance (rough endoplasmic reticulum) and Golgi apparatus are restricted to the perikaryon and to the base of the dendrites. They synthesize proteins for use throughout the neuron. Three classes of proteins are produced. One of the classes produced in the perikaryon includes the neurotransmitters. Substances to be used in the axon for growth, for membrane repair, and for the neurotransmitters must be packaged into vesicles and transported along the axon to the presynaptic axon terminal. Therefore the axon and its synaptic terminal are dependent on the cell body for their normal function and survival.

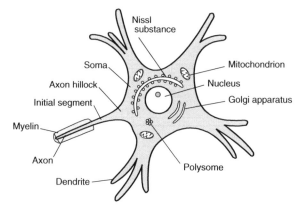

Figure 3.1. Major components of a typical neuron cell body. The cytoskeleton and lysosomes have been omitted.

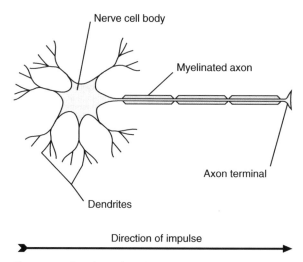

Figure 3.2. Signals pass from the dendrite to the cell body to the axon of the neuron.

Neuron cell membrane

There is a difference in electrical potential across the resting neuron cell membrane of about 70 millivolts (mV). This difference is due to an excess of negatively charged ions on the inside of the membrane relative to the outside. Three processes are responsible for this difference: an ion pump, simple diffusion, and electrostatic charge. Ion pumps move selected ions from one side of the cell membrane to the other. The sodium/potassium pump moves sodium ions to the outside and potassium ions to the inside. It is largely responsible for the membrane potential. The membrane is not freely permeable to ions, and ions can cross the membrane only through the transmembrane channels. The channels are controlled by transmembrane proteins. Different channels are specialized to allow only specific ions to pass. There are ion channels for potassium (K^+), sodium (Na^+) and chloride (Cl^-). Nongated channels are always open whereas gated channels only open or close in response to specific stimuli. The nongated channels restrict the rate of ion transfer and the pump normally is able to maintain the resting potential against the incoming tide of ions through the nongated channels. Gated channels may be voltage-gated or ligand-gated. Voltage-gated channels open in response to a change in membrane electrical potential. Ligand-gated channels open in response to the binding of a signal molecule (ligand), such as a neurotransmitter.

There are four specialized regions of the neuron cell membrane:

- The receptive region is represented by the dendrites and, to a lesser extent, the neuron cell body. When the dendrite membrane is depolarized, a wave of negativity passes down the dendrite toward the cell body cell membrane and the axon hillock. As the wave continues along the membrane of the dendrite and cell body, the amplitude of the voltage decreases due to the resistance inherent in the membrane.
- The trigger region for the generation of the all-or-none action potential is represented by the axon hillock. If the wave of negativity from the dendrite is of sufficient magnitude when it arrives at the axon hillock, an all-or-none action potential is produced in the initial segment of the axon.
- The conductance region of the neuron cell membrane is represented by the axon. Where the axon is myelinated, there are no sodium ion channels and the electrical signal must pass through the cytoplasm to the next node of Ranvier. The neuron cell membrane at the node contains many ion channels where the action potential is renewed.
- The output region of the neuron is represented by the axon terminal.

Dendrites

Dendrites are extensions of the cell body and expand the receptive surface of the cell. They branch repeatedly and, beginning a short distance from the cell body, are covered by cytoplasmic extensions called gemmules or dendritic spines. The spines further increase the receptive surface area of the dendrites.

Axon

The axon may be short but is typically depicted as being many times longer than the dendrites and, in fact, may extend up to a meter from the cell body. Microtubules and neurofilaments (microfilaments) are found throughout the cytoplasm of neurons and are of particular interest in the axon. Microtubules measure approximately 20–25 nm in diameter (a nanometer is one millionth of a millimeter), are hollow cylinders, and are made of the protein tubulin. They are the highways of the axon, that is, they are involved in the transport of macromolecules up and down the axon. Neurofilaments are approximately 10 nm in diameter and provide skeletal support for the neuron.

Substances produced in the soma must be transported along the axon to reach the cell membrane of the axon as well as the axon terminal (Figure 3.3). Substances are normally thought of as being transported from the soma to the axon terminal; however, transport from the axon terminal back to the soma also occurs.

- Anterograde (orthograde) axon transport carries substances from the soma to the axon terminal. Anterograde transport may be fast (3–4 cm/day) or slow (1–4 mm/day). Fast axon transport moves synaptic vesicles or their precursors via motor molecules along the external surface of the microtubules. Organelles, vesicles, and membrane glycoproteins are carried by fast axon transport. Slow axon transport reflects the movement of the entire axoplasm of the axon. Neurofilaments and components of microtubules are two elements that move by slow axon transport.
- Retrograde axon transport carries substances back from the axon terminal to the nerve cell body. Microtubules are involved in retrograde axon transport. The speed of retrograde transport is about half that of fast anterograde transport. Metabolic by-products and information about the condition of the axon terminal are sent back to the cell body by retrograde transport. Viruses (e.g.,

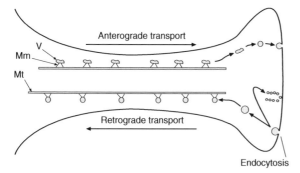

Figure 3.3. Microtubules are important in fast axon transport. Motor molecules (Mm) attach the vesicles (V) to the microtubules (Mt). Vesicles and mitochondria move at rates of up to 4 cm per day. Microtubules do not extend the entire length of the axon, and the vesicles can transfer across overlapping microtubules. Anterograde and retrograde transport can take place at the same time over a single microtubule.

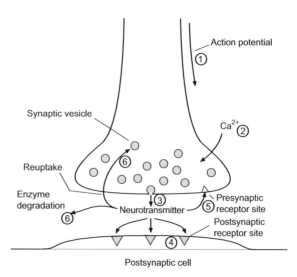

Figure 3.4. A chemical synapse. The arrival of the action potential at the synapse terminal (1) opens the calcium channels (2). The rise in intracellular Ca^{2+} releases neurotransmitter into the synaptic cleft (3). The neurotransmitter depolarizes the postsynaptic membrane (4) and sends an inhibitory feedback signal to the presynaptic cell (5). The neurotransmitter is metabolized or returns to the presynaptic terminal, or both (6).

herpes, rabies, polio) as well as toxic substances (e.g., tetanus toxin, cholera toxin) taken up by the nerve terminal may be transported back to the cell body by this same mechanism.

All the axon terminals of the same neuron contain the same neurotransmitters. However, there may be more than one transmitter found in a single neuron. When two or more neurotransmitters coexist within a single neuron, one is usually a small-molecule transmitter, whereas the second (or more) is usually a peptide.

Synapse

The synapse is the junctional complex between the presynaptic axon terminal and the postsynaptic tissue (Figure 3.4). There are two types of synapse: the electrical synapse and the chemical synapse. Electrical synapses provide for electrotonic coupling between neurons and are found at gap junctions between neurons. They permit bidirectional passage of ions directly from one cell to another. Electrical synapses are found in situations in which rapid stereotyped behavior is needed and are uncommon in the human nervous system.

One example of electrotonic coupling is found between axons of the neurons of the locus ceruleus (Chapter 10). It is proposed that these junctions help synchronize the discharge of a small grouping of closely related locus ceruleus neurons to optimize the regulation of tonic and phasic activity of the locus ceruleus and release of norepinephrine (Aston-Jones and Cohen, 2005).

A basic chemical synapse consists of a presynaptic element and a postsynaptic element separated by a synaptic cleft of 10–20 nm. Within the central nervous system (CNS), the postsynaptic tissue is usually another neuron. The presynaptic element is usually an axon terminal, although dendrites and even cell bodies can be a presynaptic element. The postsynaptic element is usually a receptor located on a dendrite or dendritic spine but also may be a receptor found on the cell body, or on the initial segment or terminal of an axon.

The chemical synapse can be identified in an electron micrograph by the large number of synaptic vesicles clustered in the axon terminal on the presynaptic side of the synaptic cleft (Figure 3.4). Each synaptic vesicle is filled with several thousand molecules of a chemical neurotransmitter. The arrival at the axon terminal of the action potential triggers an influx of calcium ions across the axon membrane into the axon terminal [(2) in Figure 3.4]. The influx of calcium ions causes synaptic vesicles located near the presynaptic membrane to fuse with the membrane and release the neurotransmitter into the synaptic cleft – a process called exocytosis [(3) in Figure 3.4].

Axon terminals can terminate on a dendrite (axodendritic), on the spine of a dendrite (axospinous), on the neuron cell body (axosomatic), or on another axon terminal producing an axoaxonic synapse. Axoaxonic arrangements allow for regulation of specific terminals of a neuron and not the whole neuron, as would, for example, the actions of an axodendritic synapse. Many axon terminals have receptor sites imbedded in their membrane sensitive to the neurotransmitter that they release. These are referred to as autoreceptors. Activation of an autoreceptor functions as part of a negative feedback loop to inhibit continued release of transmitter. Autoreceptors may also be located on the proximal axon or cell body. Most of these neurons have feedback axon collaterals or very short axons.

Synapses are associated with a number of specialized proteins that are asymmetrically distributed. For example, the presynaptic site contains specializations for transmitter release and the postsynaptic site contains receptors and ion channels for depolarization. Adhesion molecules are anchored in the membranes on both sides of the cleft and function to maintain a proper distance between the presynaptic and postsynaptic membranes. They are important in target recognition when new synapses are formed. Once the synapse is formed adhesion molecules promote mechanical security and help regulate proper function of the synapse (Yamagata *et al.*, 2003). Neurexins and neuroligins are proteins that represent a class of adhesion molecules, and like other adhesion molecules are important in forming and maintaining synapses. Genetic alterations that affect neurexins and neuroligins may play a role in autism (Sebat *et al.*, 2007).

Small (40 nm) vesicles are found in all presynaptic terminals. Large (100 nm) vesicles are found along with small vesicles in some terminals. Some of the small vesicles viewed with the electron microscope appear flattened and some appear dark. Some of the large vesicles have a dense core. The differences reflect the different neurotransmitter found in each. For example, clear and flattened vesicles are found in inhibitory axon terminals. Small molecule transmitters are found in small vesicles whereas neuropeptides are found in large vesicles. Some large vesicles contain both a neuropeptide and a small molecule transmitter.

Chemical transmission consists of two steps: the first is the transmitting step, in which the neurotransmitter is released into the synaptic cleft by the presynaptic cell, and the second is the receptive step in which the neurotransmitter becomes bound to the receptor site in the postsynaptic cell. Receptor sites located in the membrane of the postsynaptic cell are sensitive to and respond to the presence of a neurotransmitter. The action of an excitatory presynaptic terminal is to facilitate the entry of Ca^{2+}. This triggers depolarization of the postsynaptic membrane. Axon terminals located on the axon terminal of another axon are usually inhibitory. They inhibit the entry of Ca^{2+} into the presynaptic terminal and in this way can produce presynaptic inhibition. Neurotransmitters are potent and typically only two molecules of a neurotransmitter are required to open one postsynaptic ion channel. The response seen in the postsynaptic cell is dependent on the properties of the receptor rather than on the neurotransmitter, that is, the same neurotransmitter may excite one neuron and inhibit another.

Synapses located on distal dendrites and dendritic spines tend to be excitatory. For example, synapses of cortical neurons located on the distal dendrites and dendritic spines are glutamate-sensitive. Glutamate receptors are excitatory and the constant presence of glutamate tends to drive neurons continuously. Synapses located more proximally on the dendrites are γ-aminobutyric acid (GABA)-sensitive and are inhibitory. The GABA receptors function as "GABA-guards" to prevent overstimulation of the neuron by blocking discharges coming down the dendrite. Both excitatory and inhibitory synapses are found on the nerve cell body. Synapses found on axon terminals tend to be inhibitory in function.

Synapses change in response to stimuli. It is thought that some of these changes reflect a structural basis of learning. Within the cortex, the number of synapses appears to be stable within a given region, however, elements of individual synapses are subject to change. The number of vesicles physically docked to the presynaptic membrane (the readily releasable pool) may change as well as the number of vesicles held in reserve away from the membrane (the reserve pool). The presynaptic membrane may change in size and as a result be capable of releasing more neurotransmitter (Zucker, 1999). The presynaptic element may also change shape, including the size of the neck of the synaptic spine (Marrone *et al.*, 2005), the curvature of the cleft, and perforations in the presynaptic membrane (Marrone, 2007).

Receptors and receptor mechanisms

Receptors represent specialized regions of the neuron cell membrane. Channels through the membrane in these regions can be triggered to open (or close) and change the transmembrane electrical potential.

The fast-acting, ionotropic receptor consists of an ion channel that spans the neuron cell membrane.

The neurotransmitter receptor site is located on the extracellular surface of the wall of the ion channel itself. Some ion channels have an additional binding site for a regulator molecule. Anesthetics, alcohol, etc., are believed to have their effect on ionotropic receptors.

The slow-acting, metabotropic receptor has a different configuration. The receptor spans the neuron cell membrane just as does the ion channel of the ionotropic receptor, but it cannot open to allow the passage of ions (Figure 3.5). The slow receptor is linked by an intracellular protein to the ion channel that the receptor controls in an indirect manner. The linking protein is called a G-protein (guanine nucleotide-binding protein), and the receptors are called G-protein–linked receptors. G-protein receptors include α- and β-adrenergic, serotonin, dopamine, and muscarinic acetylcholine (ACh) receptors as well as receptors for neuropeptides. The G-protein is loosely associated with the inner layer of the neuron cell membrane and consists of three subunits. The subunits vary depending on the receptor with which they are affiliated and the effector enzyme with which they communicate and they also vary as to whether they excite or inhibit the effector enzyme.

When activated by a receptor, the subunit of the G-protein binds with a second messenger. Four major second messengers are recognized [calcium, cyclic nucleotides (cAMP and cGMP), inositol triphosphate, and diacylglycerol]. The second-messenger molecule may directly open (or close) an ion channel but more often initiates a cascade of enzymatic activity within the neuron cytoplasm. More than one second-messenger system may exist within a neuron, and cross talk can occur during the operation of two or more second-messenger systems. Amplification of the signal can occur with second messengers. More than one G-protein may be activated by a single receptor, and second messengers can diffuse to affect a distant part of the neuron. Second-messenger systems also can induce the synthesis of new proteins by altering gene expression, thus altering the long-term function of the neuron, including cell growth. Second-messenger, metabotropic systems operate relatively slowly, can interact with other transmitter systems within the neuron, and operate at some distance from the receptor site. The resulting action, which is relatively slow, is often described as one that modulates neuron activity. The neurotransmitter activating such a receptor is sometimes termed as neuromodulator.

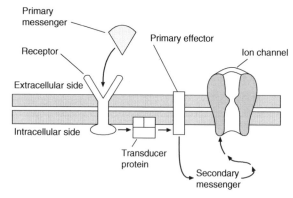

Figure 3.5. The opening of an indirect ion channel is a multistep process. The receptor, primary effector and ion channel span the cell membrane. The primary messenger is the neurotransmitter. The receptor activates a transducer protein, which excites primary effector enzymes to produce a secondary messenger. Secondary messengers may act directly on the ion channel or through several steps.

Neurotransmitter removal

Timely removal of neurotransmitters from the synaptic cleft prepares the synapse for continued usage. Four mechanisms are involved in transmitter removal:

- Active reuptake returns the transmitter substance into the presynaptic nerve terminal. This is the most common inactivation mechanism. Reuptake mechanisms have been described for norepinephrine, dopamine, serotonin, glutamate, GABA, and glycine.
- All neurotransmitters are passively removed to some degree by diffusion into the adjacent extracellular space.
- Enzyme systems break down neurotransmitters. For example, ACh is removed by the action of the enzyme acetylcholinesterase (AChE).
- Glial cells and astrocytes, in particular, play a role in transmitter removal.

Many drugs take advantage of neurotransmitter removal mechanisms: for example, monoamine oxidase inhibitors block the degradation of amine transmitters; cocaine blocks the reuptake of monoamines (norepinephrine, dopamine, and serotonin); tricyclic antidepressants block the reuptake of epinephrine and serotonin; and selective serotonin reuptake inhibitors (SSRIs) selectively block the reuptake of serotonin.

Neurotransmitters

To qualify as a neurotransmitter, a chemical must be recognized to be synthesized in the neuron, to be present in the presynaptic terminal, to depolarize the postsynaptic membrane and finally, must be removed from the synaptic cleft in a timely fashion. More than 100 substances have been recognized as neurotransmitters.

There are two general classes of neurotransmitters based on size: small-molecule neurotransmitters and neuropeptides. Small-molecule neurotransmitter precursors are synthesized in the soma. The precursors are transported to the axon terminal by way of rapid anterograde axon transport where they are assembled into neurotransmitters, which are stored in synaptic vesicles. Degraded (used) small-molecule neurotransmitters can be remanufactured within the axon terminal. Neuropeptide neurotransmitters are less well understood. They are short-chain amino acids consisting of three to 36 amino acids. They are supplied to the axon terminal in final form. They are also stored in vesicles in the synaptic terminal. Following exocytosis, however, neuropeptide neurotransmitters must be returned to the neuron cell body for remanufacture.

Four common small-molecule neurotransmitters are the amino acid neurotransmitters glutamate (GLU), aspartate (ASP), GABA, and glycine (GLY). Another group of small-molecule neurotransmitters consists of the biogenic amines including ACh, serotonin (5-HT), histamine, and the catecholamines dopamine (DA), epinephrine (EPI), and norepinephrine (NE).

Acetylcholine

Although better known as the neurotransmitter of spinal cord motor neurons, ACh is also a neurotransmitter within the CNS. Short-axon cholinergic interneurons are found in the striatum. Long axon cholinergic projection neurons are found primarily in the nucleus basalis (of Meynert), which is located in the substantia innominata of the basal forebrain. Fibers from the nucleus basalis project preferentially to the frontal and parietal lobes. A smaller number of cholinergic projection neurons are located in the nearby diagonal band (of Broca) and in the magnocellular preoptic nucleus of the hypothalamus. Brainstem cholinergic nuclei include the paramedian pontine tegmental nucleus and the laterodorsal (lateral and dorsal) tegmental nuclei.

There are two main classes of ACh receptor: nicotinic and muscarinic. Nicotinic receptors are fast-acting ionotropic receptors whereas muscarinic receptors are slow-acting metabotropic receptors. Nicotinic receptor subtypes include α and β. Muscarinic subtypes are M_1 and M_2. M_1 receptors are more common in the cortex and striatum whereas M_2 receptors are more common

in subcortical regions. Although ACh does not have a primary excitatory role, it increases excitability though the activation of muscarinic receptors.

Acetylcholine is associated with the control of cerebral blood flow (Sato et al., 2004), cortical activity (Lucas-Meunier et al., 2003), sleep–wake cycle (Lee et al., 2005), and cognitive function and cortical plasticity (McKinney, 2005). ACh is important in cognitive processes and damage to the basal forebrain cholinergic system produces cognitive deficits (McKinney, 2005). It plays a role in the formation of new synaptic contacts in the forebrain related to cognition (Berger-Sweeney, 2003).

Basal forebrain cholinergic neurons undergo moderate degenerative changes during normal aging and are related to the progressive memory decline of aging. Greater cell loss accompanies disorders such as Parkinson disease, Down syndrome, and Korsakoff syndrome, and Alzheimer disease, as well as following excessive chronic alcohol intake and head trauma (Bartus et al., 1982; Bohnen et al., 2003; Terry and Buccafusco, 2003; Toledano and Alvarez, 2004; Garcia-Alloza et al., 2005; Salmond et al., 2005; Schliebs and Arendt, 2006).

Postmortem studies of patients with schizophrenia have reported decreased muscarinic receptor density. The results are region-specific and include regions known to be affected in schizophrenia (e.g., frontal cortex, basal ganglia, and hippocampus). Whether the effects are primary or secondary is not known (Tandon, 1999; Raedler et al., 2007).

Glutamate

Glutamate is the workhorse excitatory neurotransmitter of the CNS. Nearly all CNS neurons are glutamatergic. GLU is regulated within the synaptic cleft by the rate of release and reuptake. Glial cells take up the majority of GLU, with neurons responsible for some reuptake (Shigeri et al., 2004). Reuptake is particularly important in preventing excitotoxicity resulting from high levels of GLU in the synaptic cleft. Reduced levels of glial cells in brain regions identified as abnormal in patients with mood disorders raises the question of the ability of glial cells in these areas to maintain normal GLU levels (Ullian et al., 2001). Indirect evidence links GLU and anxiety disorders and posttraumatic stress disorder (PTSD) (Cortese and Phan, 2005). N-methyl-D-aspartate (NMDA) receptor overactivity resulting in neuronal death is involved in neurodegenerative disorders, including Alzheimer disease, Huntington disease, and human immunodeficiency virus (HIV)-associated dementia (Lancelot and Beal, 1998; Kaul *et al.*, 2001).

Glutamate is synthesized in astrocytes and converted to glutamine that can be transferred to neurons, where it can be converted to glutamate. This forms the "glutamate–glutamine cycle." Disruption of the glutamate–glutamine cycle may play a role in schizophrenia. It has been shown that astrocytes in brains with schizophrenia are more vulnerable to mechanical damage than healthy brains (Niizato *et al.*, 2001). Evidence suggests that in schizophrenia, GLU is transferred normally from neurons to astrocytes but that it accumulates in abnormal amounts in the astrocytes, implying a disturbance of the glutamate–glutamine cycle. A decrease in GLU synthetase found in the brains of patients with schizophrenia lends further credence to this hypothesis (Burbaeva *et al.*, 2003).

There are a number of GLU receptor sites, many of which work in conjunction with other substances. The best known receptor is the NMDA ionotropic receptor. This receptor is critical for maintaining prolonged excitatory responses such as those seen in the wind-up of pain signals in the spinal cord substantia gelatinosa, long-term potentiation in the hippocampus, and epileptiform activity. There are at least five NMDA subtypes. Most glutamatergic synapses contain both NMDA and α-amino-5-hydroxy-3-methyl-4-isoxazole propionic acid (AMPA) receptors (see below).

Non-NMDA GLU receptors include AMPA, kainite, and metabotropic receptors. There are a number of subtypes of each. Synaptic currents produced by AMPA receptors are faster and shorter acting than those produced by NMDA receptors. Metabotropic receptors are least understood and several act in an inhibitory fashion.

Aspartate activates NMDA receptors weakly. Glycine and D-serine act on many NMDA receptors as co-agonists. Zinc (Zn^{2+}) is reported to co-localize with GLU in many cortical neurons, and zinc accumulation may play a role in excitotoxicity (Jeng and Sensi, 2005; Sekier *et al.*, 2007). Nitric oxide is a gas neurotransmitter that is activated by the calcium influx induced by activation of the GLU receptors. It is involved in excitotoxicity, synaptic plasticity, and long-term potentiation. Some anesthetics and recreational hallucinogenic drugs are NMDA receptor antagonists.

The NMDA receptor is important in memory and neuroprotection (Quiroz *et al.*, 2004). A reduction in density reflecting the glycine site of NMDA receptors has been reported in patients with bipolar disorder and depression (Nudmamud-Thanoi and Reynolds, 2004). Karolewicz *et al.* (2004) reported that nitric oxide synthetase, which is activated by NMDA stimulation, was reduced in patients with depression. Patients with unipolar major depression have been shown to have increased glutamate levels coupled with reduced GABA levels, suggesting a disruption in the normal glutamate:GABA ratio (Sanacora *et al.*, 2008). This disruption is speculated to be due to glial cell dysfunction (Kugaya and Sanacora, 2005). Healthy persons exhibiting anxiety as well as persons diagnosed with anxiety disorders have been reported to show increased levels of GLU in the frontal cortex and anterior cingulate cortex (Grachev and Apkarian, 2000; Phan *et al.*, 2005). GLU levels have also been found to be abnormal in the anterior cingulate cortex in adult patients with attention deficit/hyperactivity disorder (Perlov *et al.*, 2007).

Many genes associated with schizophrenia are known to play a role in synaptogenesis (Stephan *et al.*, 2006; Straub and Weinberger, 2006). Several of these target the NMDA receptor and control proteins that act to strengthen the synapse. Dysfunction of NMDA control proteins can result in hypofunction of the NMDA synapse: the NMDA receptor hypofunction hypothesis of schizophrenia (Stahl, 2007a). Weak synapses with AMPA receptors may be pruned, but this process takes time. In addition, synaptic pruning is very active during adolescence. This may explain why schizophrenia onset is associated with the adolescent period of life (Stahl, 2007b).

Evidence indicates a decreased production or release, or both, of GLU in the brains of patients with schizophrenia, especially in the hippocampal and dorsolateral prefrontal cortex. Reduced GLU is accompanied by an increase in GLU receptors and in receptor sensitivity (Tsai *et al.*, 1995). This, along with reports of alterations in dopamine in schizophrenia, has produced the "glutamate hypothesis of schizophrenia." This hypothesis describes a balance between dopamine and GLU in the cortex. These two neurotransmitters normally produce a balanced signal in the basal ganglia (striatum) that results in an optimal feedback from the basal ganglia and thalamus to the cortex. An increase in dopamine or a decrease in GLU would upset this balance and could result in psychosis (Tamminga, 1998; Carlsson *et al.*, 1999).

Glutamate may be involved in both the establishment and maintenance of addictive behavior. A greater number of GLU receptors are established in sensitive regions as cocaine addiction is established. It is proposed that increased levels of GLU in the amygdala mediate the craving experienced by cocaine addicts (Kalivas *et al.*, 1998).

AMPA receptors may be involved in depression. AMPA activation has been shown to increase levels of brain-derived neurotropic factor (BDNF) (Zafra *et al.*, 1990). BDNF promotes neuron proliferation and survival within the CNS as well as synapse formation. Levels of BDNF have been shown to increase in response to antidepressant drugs (Duman, 2004)). The time required to increase BDNF levels may be responsible for the delay in response to antidepressants (O'Neill and Witkin, 2007). In addition, evidence has been found of reduced AMPA receptor pathways in depressed suicide patients (Dwivedi *et al.*, 2001).

Glutamate NMDA synapses in the hippocampus of rats exposed to sensory stimuli (by stimulating only one whisker) have been shown to result in a change in synaptic strength (synaptic plasticity). The same stimulation continued over time resulted in further synaptic strengthening accompanied by the insertion of new GLU AMPA receptors into the synaptic membrane (Clem *et al.*, 2008). The different stages of synaptic strengthening may correspond with stages of memory formation.

γ-Aminobutyric acid

γ-Aminobutyric acid is the major inhibitory neurotransmitter in the brain, and it acts to hyperpolarize the postsynaptic membrane. GABA may activate receptors on the presynaptic or postsynaptic side of the synaptic cleft. It is found primarily in small, local circuit interneurons, and it is removed from the cleft by astrocytes and by reuptake into the GABAergic presynaptic neuron. There are three classes of GABA receptors: $GABA_A$, $GABA_B$, and $GABA_C$. $GABA_A$ receptors are the most common; they are directly linked to an ion channel and operate quickly (ionotropic). Three major $GABA_A$ receptor types are recognized (α, β, and γ-A). $GABA_B$ receptors are metabotropic; they use a second messenger and operate more slowly. $GABA_C$ receptors have been described almost exclusively as receptors on the horizontal cells of the retina. They are ionotropic receptors. More recent studies indicate they are also found in many areas the brain, where their function is unknown (Schmidt, 2008). Although GABA is an inhibitory neurotransmitter, GABAergic neurons may synapse on other GABAergic neurons and thus produce excitation through the process of disinhibition.

Neural networks in the cortex consist of two general types of neuron. Excitatory projection neurons are glutamatergic. The remainder consists of local circuit interneurons, which make up 20%–30% of all cortical neurons, most of which are GABAergic (Di Cristo, 2007). GABAergic neurons in the amygdala and possibly elsewhere have kainite glutamatergic endings located on their somatodendritic regions as well as axon terminals where they regulate GABA release. Norepinephrinergic endings on GABAergic neurons in the amygdala also regulate GABA output (Aroniadou-Anderjaska *et al.*, 2007).

The $GABA_A$ receptor is the target of benzodiazepines, anesthetics, barbiturates, and alcohol. These drugs operate at different sites but all function to increase the opening of the channel and increase postsynaptic inhibition. The $GABA_A$ receptor is involved in acute actions of alcohol as well as alcohol tolerance and dependence (Hanson and Czajkowski, 2008). Variations in the $GABA_A$ receptor genes may contribute to the vulnerability to alcoholism (Krystal, *et al.*, 2006).

Low GABA activity or low levels of GABA have been associated with anxiety (Nutt, 2006). Therapies effective in enhancing relaxation also result in increased levels of GABA (Streeter *et al.*, 2007). Studies suggest that GABA levels are decreased in individuals with depression (Krystal *et al.*, 2002; Brambilla *et al.*, 2003). GABA in physiological situations regulates cortical circuits and the plasticity of those circuits (Hensch and Stryker, 2004). GABAergic downregulation has been reported in the prefrontal cortex in psychosis and it is believed this is through regulatory action of glutamatergic neurons (Guidotti *et al.*, 2005).

GABA in the developing brain plays an excitatory role. This action appears to be instrumental in signaling and controlling proliferation, migration, and maturation of neurons. Once neuronal maturation is complete, GABA activity becomes inhibitory (Ben-Ari, 2002). This has implications of the effects of in utero exposure to drugs such as diazepam (Valium). It is suggested that alterations in GABA function during the prenatal period has a role in the formation of abnormal cortical circuits (Di Cristo, 2007).

Glycine

Glycine is an inhibitory neurotransmitter. Serine hydroxymethyltransferase (SHMT) is present in mitochondria of neurons and glial cells; SHMT converts L-serine to glycine. The GLY cleavage system (GCS), believed to be localized in astrocytes, is a four-enzyme complex that breaks down GLY. The serine resulting from the GCS is transported to nearby neurons, where it serves as the endogenous ligand for the glycine-binding site or is converted to GLY (Yang et al., 2003). The conversion of L-serine to GLY may operate much like the glutamine–glutamate cycle.

Glycine is found as a neurotransmitter primarily in the ventral spinal cord, where its action is inhibitory. In the brain GLY acts as a co-agonist at NMDA-type glutamate receptors and in this situation potentiates the effect of GLU, that is, it facilitates excitation rather than act as an inhibitor. Small levels of GLY added to antipsychotic drugs are reported to improve both negative and positive symptoms in patients with schizophrenia (Heresco-Levy and Javitt, 2004; Shim et al., 2008). Reduced levels of GLU and GLY have been found in patients with refractive unipolar and bipolar disorder, most of who were depressed at the time of the study (Frye et al., 2007). Another study found increased levels of GLY in the plasma of patients with bipolar disorder who were in the manic phase. The authors suggested that the changes in GLY levels are more critical than changes in those of GLU (Hoekstra et al., 2006).

Startle disease (hyperexplexia) is due to a mutation in chromosome 5 that results in a defect in the GLY receptor (Garg et al., 2008). This causes an exaggerated startle reflex because of the loss of normal inhibition.

Norepinephrine

Norepinephrine is produced primarily by neurons that make up the locus ceruleus, and it is also formed in some small nearby nuclei. NE is involved with arousal and alertness, and functions to help focus attention on salient stimuli. It is released in response to stress and has a role in stress-induced reinstatement of drug use as well as depression (Leri et al., 2002; Dunn et al., 2004). NE receptors make up two groups, α-adrenergic and β-adrenergic, both of which are metabotropic. Each group contains three subgroups. Fibers from the locus ceruleus descend to the spinal cord. There are two specific ascending pathways. The dorsal norepinephrinergic system arises from the locus ceruleus and projects to the hippocampus, cerebellum, and forebrain. The ventral norepinephrinergic system arises from a number of small nuclei in the lateral medulla and pons, and projects to the hypothalamus, midbrain, and extended amygdala (Moore and Bloom, 1979).

Norepinephrine released in the cortex inhibits the spontaneous, resting activity of cortical neurons.

At the same time these neurons become more sensitive to specific sensory inputs indicating that NE functions to increase the signal-to-noise ratio for sensory signals (Segal and Bloom, 1976). NE is associated with arousal, vigilance, and reward dependency (Cloninger, 1987; Menza et al., 1993). NE hyperactivity can lead to insomnia, weight loss, irritability, agitation, and a reduction in the pain threshold. Peripheral NE hyperactivity results in symptoms of anxiety (i.e., tachycardia, muscular cramps, and increased blood pressure). A decrease in NE activity is associated with some forms of depression, and an increase of NE is linked with mania (Schildkraut, 1965). Abnormal regulation of NE levels in the CNS is implicated in attention-deficit hyperactivity disorder (Pliszka, 2005).

Dopamine

Most of the dopaminergic neurons of the brain are found in the substantia nigra pars compacta (the A9 nucleus). A smaller concentration of DA neurons is found in the nearby ventral tegmental area (A10) and the retrorubral area (A8). There are four major DA systems in the brain:

- One extends from the substantia nigra and retrorubral area to the striatum (nigrostriatal system) and is associated with motor activity of the basal ganglia (Chapter 7).
- Two arise from cells located in the ventral tegmental area of the mesencephalon (Figure 10.3). One makes up the mesolimbic system and extends to the nucleus accumbens, which is involved with reward and reinforcement. The second is the mesocortical system and projects to the prefrontal cortex, where it acts in support of cognitive activity.
- One extends from the arcuate nucleus of the hypothalamus to the median eminence (tuberoinfundibular pathway), where DA inhibits the release of prolactin from the pituitary gland (Chapter 8).

There are five DA receptors, which make up two families; D_1-like and D_2-like. The D_1-like family consists of the D_1 and D_5 receptors, which are excitatory. D_2, D_3, and D_4 receptors make up the D_2-like family and are inhibitory. D_1 receptors are concentrated in the striatum, nucleus accumbens, and olfactory tubercle. D_2 receptors are also found in the striatum, nucleus accumbens, and olfactory tubercle, as well as on DA cell bodies, where they act as autoreceptors. D_3 receptors are fewer in number, with most found in the nucleus accumbens and olfactory tubercle. D_4 receptors are sparse and located in the frontal cortex, midbrain, and amygdala. There are up to 18 variants of the D_4 receptor type. The $D_{4.7}$ variant has been associated with ADHD (Bobb et al., 2005). The $D_{4.7}$ receptor gene may be associated with a milder form of ADHD (Gornick et al., 2007). D_5 receptors also appear to be fewer in number and are found in the hippocampus and hypothalamus.

D_1, D_2, and D_3 receptors are related to motivation and reward, whereas D_4 and D_5 receptors are more involved with behavioral inhibition. Activation of D_1 receptors correlates with stimulus reward (e.g., food, alcohol, cocaine), reward-related learning, and remodeling of neuron dendrites in the nucleus accumbens in response to cocaine (Wolf et al., 2004; Lee et al., 2006). Enhanced sensitivity of D_1 receptors may contribute to addiction (Goodman, 2008).

Dopamine in the cortex is described as acting as an amplifier, that is, its presence extends periods of quiescence in inactive glutamatergic neurons but increases and extends the periods of actively firing glutamatergic neurons (Kondziella et al., 2007). In contrast, the activity of DA neurons projecting to the cortex from the brainstem is regulated by cortical glutamatergic neurons either directly or via GABAergic interneurons, acting as accelerator and brakes, respectively (Carlsson et al., 2001). It is hypothesized that novel stimuli increase the level of DA production in the midbrain, which in turn increases the degree of synaptic plasticity in the striatum (Redgrave and Gurney, 2006).

Dopamine has an important role in the reward mechanisms. Amphetamines increase the concentration of DA in the synaptic cleft by accelerating its release from synaptic vesicles. Cocaine increases levels of DA in the synaptic cleft by blocking reuptake transporters. Prolonged use of cocaine may dysregulate brain dopaminergic systems and can result in persistent hypodopaminergia. The downregulation of dopaminergic pathways due to long-term cocaine abuse may underlie anhedonia and relapse in cocaine addicts (Majewska, 1996). Permanent changes are seen in the anterior cingulate cortex pyramidal cell dendrites in rabbits exposed prenatally to cocaine (Levitt et al., 1997).

The DA theory of schizophrenia proposes an excess of dopaminergic stimulation and is based on two observations (Snyder et al., 1974; Stone et al., 2007). First, there is a high correlation between the effective dose of traditional neuroleptics and the degree to which they block D_2 dopamine receptors. Second,

the paranoid psychosis that is often seen in amphetamine and cocaine addicts can be clinically indistinguishable from paranoid schizophrenia and appears to be due to DA activation (Manschreck et al., 1988). The DA hypothesis contends that negative and cognitive deficits of schizophrenia are primary and arise from DA insufficiency in the frontal lobe (Andreasen et al., 1999). Positive symptoms arise from secondary hyperfunction of DA in the striatum (Abi-Dargham and Moore, 2003). A dopamine–glutamate theory of schizophrenia has been proposed (Carlsson and Carlsson, 1990; Carlsson et al., 1999). It is now believed that DA may not be directly related to schizophrenia but may act in connection with glutamate. Abnormal modulation by DA may affect the signal-to-noise ratio in the prefrontal cortex (Rolls et al., 2008).

Reduced cortical DA function has been reported in schizophrenia and in Parkinson disease (Brozoski et al., 1979). Raising DA levels in these same groups improves performance on tests that examine working memory (Daniel et al., 1991; Lange et al., 1992). Low DA levels may be associated with dysfunctional eating patterns (Ericsson et al., 1997).

Evidence suggests that the D_1 receptor located in the dorsolateral prefrontal cortex may be particularly important in working memory and that an optimal level of DA is critical in facilitating working memory. Novelty-seeking behavior in humans and exploratory activity in animals are analogous (Cloninger, 1987) and may be related to the level of DA. Patients with Parkinson disease have reduced levels of DA and exhibit personality characteristics consistent with reduced novelty seeking that can be described as compulsive, industrious, rigidly moral, stoic, serious, and quiet (Menza et al., 1993).

These same D_1 receptors are found predominantly on the dendritic spines of pyramidal neurons, which place them in a position to directly affect corticothalamic, corticostriatal, and corticocortical projections. D_5 receptors are also associated with pyramidal neurons but are localized to the shafts of the dendrites. It is not surprising to find that a hyperactive DA system can result in increased motor activity, whereas a hypoactive DA system can result in decreased motoric activity (hypokinesia or akinesia) and a tendency to physical weariness. D_2 receptors appear to be on GABA-containing interneurons and on some pyramidal neurons (Goldman-Rakic and Selemon, 1997).

Clinically effective antipsychotic drugs are antagonists of D_2 receptors. For this reason, high levels of D_2

23

receptors or excessive DA-mediated neurotransmission was thought to underlie schizophrenia (Nestler, 1997). A comparison of drug-free schizophrenia patients with a control group showed no difference in the density of D_2 receptors in the striatum. No significant reduction in D_1 receptor density was seen in the prefrontal cortex of the patients with schizophrenia (Zakzanis and Hansen, 1998).

In another study, patients with schizophrenia showed greater amphetamine-induced release of DA in the striatum accompanied by an increase in positive (but not negative) symptoms (Abi-Dargham et al., 1998). The same increased DA release has been seen in individuals with schizotypal personality disorder but not with major depression or bipolar affective disorder (Anand et al., 2000; Parsey et al., 2001; Abi-Dargham et al., 2004). Negative symptoms are hypothesized to be a function of low levels of DA in the prefrontal cortex. There is some evidence to support this hypothesis (Abi-Dargham and Moore, 2003).

Dopamine is found in high concentrations in the retina, where it functions as a neurotransmitter and neuromodulator in conjunction with color vision. Patients recently withdrawn from cocaine show abnormalities in the electroretinogram accompanied by a significant loss of blue–yellow color vision (Desai et al., 1997). Abnormalities in retinal dopaminergic transmission in patients with seasonal affective disorder also have been suggested (Partonen, 1996) and that light exposure for treatment may operate through the retinal dopaminergic system (Gagné et al., 2007).

Decreased density of D_2 receptors in the ventral striatum is reported for alcoholics (Guardia et al., 2000) and obese individuals (Volkow and Wise, 2005). This indicates that reduced levels of D_2 receptors may predispose individuals to addiction. Individuals with higher levels of D_2 receptors reported a higher feeling of intoxication from a low dose of alcohol (Yoder et al., 2005). Most D_3 receptors which are located primarily in limbic regions are less studied but there are data indicating that D_3 receptors may also be involved in reward. D_3 hyposensitivity may also be associated with addiction (Goodman, 2008).

Serotonin (5-hydroxytryptamine)

Serotonin (or 5-HT) is produced in neuron cell bodies that make up the raphe nuclei. Axons of these neurons project caudally into the spinal cord as well as rostrally to all regions of the brain. At least 14 receptor subtypes are recognized. The 5-HT_1 class is inhibitory whereas the 5-HT_2 class is excitatory. Many of the effects of serotonin are through its modulation of DA and GABA neurons (Yan et al., 2004).

Selective serotonin reuptake inhibitors (SSRIs) slow the reuptake of serotonin, making it more available to the postsynaptic cell and prolonging its effect in the synaptic cleft. Low 5-HT levels can trigger high carbohydrate consumption and are associated with bulimia and carbohydrate preference in obese women (Bjorntorp, 1995; Brewerton, 1995; Steiger et al., 2001). In contrast, high levels of 5-HT or 5-HT turnover are associated with harm avoidance and compulsive behavior (Weyers et al., 1999). High levels of platelet serotonin is an early and consistent finding in autism (Cook and Leventhal, 1996).

Low levels of 5-HT turnover are associated with alcoholism, social isolation, and impaired social function and in similar behaviors in nonhuman primates (Heinz et al., 1998). 5-HT may also be altered in panic disorder (Maron and Shlik, 2006), in schizophrenia (Gurevich and Joyce, 1997), in aggressive behavior (Unis et al., 1997), and in borderline personality disorder (New and Siever, 2003). It has been hypothesized that obsessive-compulsive disorder (OCD) may involve brain regions that are modulated by normally functioning serotonin neurons. Drugs that affect 5-HT output improve symptoms of OCD by their actions in the involved brain regions (El Mansari and Blier, 2006). A significant decline in the number of 5-HT receptors in some parts of the brain has been reported with age. This decline may predispose elderly individuals to major depression (Meltzer et al., 1998).

Histamine

Histamine-producing neurons are found concentrated in the mammillary nucleus of the hypothalamus. Their axons project to almost all regions of the brain and spinal cord. There are three histamine receptors, H_1, H_2, and H_3, all of which are G-coupled. Histamine-producing neurons are related to the sleep–wake cycle, appetite control, learning, and memory (Yanai and Tashiro, 2007). Histamine also plays a role in the transmission of vestibular signals that can produce nausea and vomiting. Antihistamines that cross the blood–brain barrier interfere with histamine's role in arousal.

Adenosine

Adenosine triphosphate (ATP) is well known for its role in providing energy within cells. It is found in all synaptic vesicles and is co-released along with the resident neurotransmitter. Adenosine is a breakdown product of ATP. Both ATP and adenosine are known to function at the postsynaptic receptor sites located in diverse regions of the CNS. Adenosine is recognized as an important neuromodulator of synaptic activity.

Three classes of adenosine receptors are recognized. One is a ligand-gated ionotropic receptor. The other two are G-coupled metabotropic receptors. There are four adenosine receptor subtypes: A1, A2A, A2B, and A3.

Adenosine A1 receptors are found throughout the body. In the brain they are concentrated in the basal forebrain. The A1 receptor has an inhibitory function. It is believed to be a major contributor to the effect of deep brain stimulation. The A1 receptor is blocked by caffeine. It is thought that this is the mechanism by which caffeine has its effect to combat drowsiness and to exacerbate the tremors seen in essential tremor. A significant reduction in A1 receptor binding has been found in aged mice (26 months) compared with young mice (3 months). The reduction was restricted to a few sites. These included the hippocampus, cortex, basal ganglia, and, especially, the thalamus (Ekonomou *et al.*, 2000).

Adenosine acts as an anti-inflammatory agent at the A2A receptor. Following trauma, ischemia, or seizure activity adenosine levels increase and activation of the A2A evokes anti-inflammatory responses. A2A receptors are found in the periphery and in the brain are concentrated in the basal ganglia (Jacobson and Gao, 2006; Gao and Jacobson, 2007).

Neuroactive peptide neurotransmitters

More than 50 short peptides have been described as being neuroactive. Some of these are particularly important since they have relatively longlasting effects. Since these effects make them different from neurotransmitters, which by definition are short acting, this class of longlasting peptides is referred to as neuromodulators. There are five families of neuroactive peptides. The families of opioids, neurohypophyseal peptides, and tachykinins are better known. The opioids consist of the opiocortins, enkephalins, dynorphin, and FMRFamide. Neurohypophyseal peptides include vasopressin, oxytocin, and the neurophysins. Substance P is a tachykinin.

Among the neuropeptides, substance P and the enkephalins have been linked to the control of pain. Neuropeptide Y is a potent stimulator of food intake in rats (Sarika Arora, 2006). γ – Melanocyte–stimulating hormone, adrenocorticotropin, and β-endorphin regulate responses to stress. A neuropeptide may coexist with a small molecule transmitter within the same neuron.

Excitotoxicity

Excitotoxicity is the pathological process by which overactivity of a nerve cell produces damage and ultimately death of that neuron. This can occur when receptors for the excitatory neurotransmitter GLU are overactivated. Pathologically high levels of GLU in the synapse allow high levels of calcium ions to enter the cell accompanied by quantities of water. A cascade of events follows, including activation of enzymes that result in permanent destruction of the neuron.

Excitotoxicity is an important mechanism of neuron loss following hypoxia or ischemia. Ischemia for example, is believed to prevent reuptake of GLU, leaving pathological levels of the neurotransmitter in the synaptic cleft. Excitotoxicity has reported in the case of stroke, traumatic brain injury, and neurodegenerative diseases such as multiple sclerosis, Alzheimer disease, amyotrophic lateral sclerosis, Parkinson disease, and Huntington disease (Bedlack *et al.*, 2007; Carbonell and Rama, 2007; Olanow, 2007; Gonsette, 2008).

Excitotoxicity has been implicated in schizophrenia. Coyle and Puttfarcken (1993) suggested that GLU-stimulated intracellular oxidation in CNS neurons gradually produces neurotoxic damage and finally cell death. Olney and Farber (1995) proposed that acetylcholine overactivation secondary to reduced glutamatergic transmission can result in cell damage or death. GLU may be involved in both establishment and maintenance of addictive behavior. A greater number of GLU receptors are established in sensitive regions as cocaine addiction is established. Increased levels of GLU in the amygdala may mediate the craving experienced by cocaine addicts (Kalivas *et al.*, 1998).

Neuroglia

There are four neuroglial cells. Two of these produce myelin, which consists of multiple wrappings of the cell membrane of the myelin-producing cell around segments of axons. Myelin insulates the axon from the extracellular environment. As the myelin-producing cell wraps around a segment of an axon, the cytoplasm is squeezed out from between the layers of cell membrane of the myelin-producing cell. The cell membrane is a lipoprotein sheath and contains large amounts of lipid. The multiple wrappings produce a white, glistening appearance in the fresh state, accounting for the white matter of the brain and spinal cord. Myelin from one myelin-producing cell extends up to approximately a 1-cm segment along an axon. The segment of myelin does not overlap significantly with the next myelin segment. The discontinuity between myelin sheaths is called the node (of Ranvier). The myelin-covered length is called the internode and insulates the axon from the extracellular environment. The insulating effect of myelin is minimal at the node, where depolarization of the axon membrane occurs. Because the internodal distance is insulated, the action potential hops (saltates) along the axon from one node to the next.

Oligodendroglial cell

The oligodendroglial cell produces myelin in the CNS. The neurilemmal cell (of Schwann) produces myelin in the peripheral nervous system (PNS). After injury, neurilemmal cells (of Schwann) support the regeneration of PNS axons. However, within the CNS, axonal regrowth is insignificant following injury. The oligodendrocyte does not appear to provide the same support for regenerating CNS axons as does the neurilemmal cell for PNS axons. Other factors are also involved in the failure of a severed CNS axon to regenerate.

Astrocyte

Astrocytes are found only within the CNS and are of several types. In general, astrocytes provide structural and physiological support to neurons. Many astrocytes stretch between individual nerve cell bodies and capillaries. They have a characteristic perivascular end foot that is found in apposition to the capillary. The body of the same astrocyte embraces the body of the neuron, producing a bridge between the capillary and the neuron.

Astrocytes respond to nerve cell activity. They remove excess neurotransmitter from the synaptic cleft. Once inside the astrocyte the neurotransmitter is degraded into its precursor and then made available to the axon terminal for recycling. The astrocyte may play a role in directing growing axon terminals during development. Astrocytes provide a permissive substrate for developing axons and help direct neurite growth (Deumens et al., 2004). Astrocytes help maintain a balanced extracellular ion environment for the neurons.

The amyloid hypothesis of Alzheimer disease holds that amyloid β-peptides formed by neurons are the prime trigger for pathogenesis. Abnormalities of amyloid-β processing resulting in the overproduction of amyloid-β may be responsible for Alzheimer disease (Hardy and Selkoe, 2002). The excess is hypothesized to affect synaptic structure, disrupt neuronal function, and lead to cognitive impairment (Selkoe, 2002; Schliebs and Arendt, 2006; Haass and Selkoe, 2007). Amyloid-β may function as a biologically active peptide that acts on nicotinic acetylcholine receptors (Gamkrelidze et al., 2005). It is suggested that under normal conditions amyloid-β regulates synaptic plasticity, synaptic transmission, neuronal excitability, and neuron viability (Kamenetz, et al., 2003; Plant et al., 2003). Astrocytes act to clear and degrade amyloid-β and form a protective barrier between amyloid-β deposits and neurons (Rossner, et al., 2005).

Microglia

Microglial cells are the immune cells of the CNS and are normally found in a resting state along capillaries. The resting state is maintained in part by suppressive action of neurons. A glycoprotein, CD200, expressed on the surface of neurons reacts with a receptor site on microglia to maintain their quiescence (Hoek et al., 2000). Astrocytes may also help suppress microglial activation. Microglia are activated by the loss of inhibition and/or direct activation by neurons. If CNS tissue is damaged, microglial cells enlarge, migrate to the region of damage and become phagocytic. They are sensitive and respond to even small changes in ion homeostasis that precedes the pathological changes (Gehrmann et al., 1993). The inflammatory response with activation and cytokine activation may be neuroprotective in the early stages but may be damaging over time (Nagatsu and Sawada, 2005). Microglia may aggravate inflammation by releasing inflammatory cytokines as well as neurotoxins that recruit other cells and amplify the inflammatory response (Kim and Joh, 2006). When they act as phagocytes, microglial cells are called glitter cells.

Entry of HIV into the CNS is mediated by lymphocytes and monocytes that transfer the virus to perivascular macrophages and then to microglia (Lane et al., 1996). Microglia are also activated in multiple sclerosis (Raine, 1994) and Alzheimer disease (Kim and Joh, 2006). They secrete toxins that may result in neuron death (Liu et al., 2002). The substantia nigra has four to five times more microglia than other areas of the brain (Kim et al., 2000). Activation and an increase in microglia are seen in the substantia nigra prior to the loss of dopamine neurons following experimental axotomy in the medial forebrain bundle (Kim *et al.*, 2005). It is hypothesized that inflammation with the overactivation of microglia has a major role in the etiology of Parkinson disease (Whitton, 2007).

Other proteins

Cadherins

Cadherins (calcium-dependent adhesion molecules) are a group of transmembrane proteins that are dependent on calcium in order to function properly. They play an important role in keeping adjacent cells bound together, and in establishing and maintaining synapses. It has been speculated that mutations affecting cadherin function underlie some developmental disorders such as autism.

Cytokines

Cytokines are signaling molecules important in communication between cells. They act like hormones between cells and are produced by a number of cells including microglia. Cytokines are important in development. Their production can increase greatly following trauma or infection, and infection outside the brain can affect brain development. Genetic variation can have an effect on susceptibility to cytokine-related brain damage with implications for several psychiatric disorders (Kronfol and Remick, 2000; Dammann and O'Shea, 2008).

Select bibliography

Bohlen, O. and Halbach, R.D. *Neurotransmitters and Neuromodulators: Handbook of Receptors and Biological Effects.* (New York: John Wiley & Sons, Ltd., 2002.)

Cowan, M.W., Südhof, T.C. and Stevens, C.F. eds. *Synapses.* (Baltimore: Johns Hopkins University Press, 2001.)

Morgan, J.R., and Bloom, O. *Cells of the Nervous System.* (Philadelphia: Chelsea House Publishers, 2005.)

Schatzberg, A.F., and Nemeroff, C.B. *Textbook of Psychopharmacology.* (Washington, D.C.: American Psychiatric Press, 1995.)

Stanton, P.K., Bramhan, C., and Scharfman, H.E. eds. *Synaptic Plasticity and Transsynaptic Signaling.* (New York: Springer, 2005.)

Webster, R.A. ed. *Neurotransmitters, Drugs and Brain Function.* (New York, John Wiley & Sons, Ltd., 2001.)

References

Abi-Dargham, A., and Moore, H. 2003. Prefrontal DA transmission at D1 receptors and the pathology of schizophrenia. *Neuroscientist* 9:404–416.

Abi-Dargham, A., Gil, R., Krystal, J., Baldwin, R.M., Seibyl, J.P., Bowers, M., van Dyck, C.H., Charney, D.S., Innis, R.B., and Laruelle, M. 1998. Increased striatal dopamine transmission in schizophrenia: confirmation in a second cohort. *Am. J. Psychiatry* 155:761–767.

Abi-Dargham, A., Kegeles, L.S., Zea-Ponce, Y., Mawlawi, O., Martinez, D., Mitropoulou, V., O'Flynn, K., Koenisgsber, H.W., Van Heertum, R., Cooper, T., Laruelle, M., and Siever, L.J. 2004. Striatal amphetamine-induced dopamine release in patients with schizotypal personality disorder studied with single photon emission computed tomography and [123I]iodobenzamind. *Biol. Psychiatry* 55:1001–1006.

Anand, A., Verhoeff, P., Seneca, N., Zoghbi, S.S., Seibyl, J.P., Charney, D.S., and Innis, R.B. 2000. Brain SPECT imaging of amphetamine-induced dopamine release in euthymic bipolar disorder patients. *Am. J. Psychiatry* 157:1108–1114.

Andreasen, N. C., Nopoulos, P., O'Leary, D. S., Miller, D. D., Wassink, T., and Flaum, M. 1999. Defining the phenotype of schizophrenia: cognitive dysmetria and its neural mechanisms. *Biol. Psychiatry* 46:908–920.

Aroniadou-Anderjaska, V., Qashu, F., and Braga, M.F.M. 2007. Mechanisms regulating GABAergic inhibitory transmission in the basolateral amygdala: implications for epilepsy and anxiety disorders. *Amino Acids* 32:305–315.

Aston-Jones, G., and Cohen, J.D. 2005. An integrative theory of coeruleu-norepinephrine function: adaptive gain and optimal performance. *Annu. Rev. Neurosci.* 28:403–450.

Bartus, R.T., Dean, R.L., Beer, B., and Lippa, A.S. 1982. The cholinergic hypothesis of geriatric memory dysfunction. *Science* 21:408–417.

Bedlack, R.S., Traynor, B.J., and Cudkowicz, M.E. 2007. Emerging disease-modifying therapies for the treatment of motor neuron disease/amyotrophic lateral sclerosis. *Expert Opin. Emerg. Drugs* 12:229–252.

Ben-Ari, Y. 2002. Excitatory actions of GABA during development: The nature of the nurture. *Nat. Rev. Neurosci.* 3:728–739.

Berger-Sweeney, J. 2003. The cholinergic basal forebrain system during development and its influence on cognitive processes: important questions and potential answers. *Neurosci. Behav. Rev.* 27:401–411.

Bjorntorp, P. 1995. Neuroendocrine abnormalities in human obesity. *Metabolism* 44 (Suppl. 2):38–41.

Bobb, A.J., Castellanos, F.X., Addington, A.M., and Rapoport, J.L. 2005. Molecular genetic studies of ADHD: 1991 to 2004. *Am. J. Med. B Neuropsychiatr. Genet.* 132B:109–125.

Bohnen, N.I., Kaufer, K.I, Ivanco, L.S., Lopresti, B., Koeppe, R.A., Davis, J.G., Mathis, C.A., Moore, R.Y., and DeKosky, S.T. 2003. Cortical cholinergic function is more severely affected in Parkinsonian dementia than in Alzheimer's disease: an in vivo positron tomography study. *Arch. Neurol.* **60**:1745–1748.

Brambilla, P., Perez, J., Barale, F., Schettini, G., and Soares, J.C. 2003. GABAergic dysfunction in mood disorders. *Mol. Psychiatry* **8**:721–737.

Brewerton, T.D. 1995. Toward a unified theory of serotonin disturbances in eating and related disorders. *Psychoneuroimmunology* **20**:561–590.

Brozoski, T.J., Brown, R.M., Rosvold, H.E., and Goldman, P.S. 1979. Cognitive defect caused by regional depletion of dopamine in prefrontal cortex of rhesus monkey. *Science* **205**:929–932.

Burbaeva, G.S., Boksha, I.S., Turisheneva, M.S., Vorobyeva, E.A., Savushkina, O.K, and Tereshkina, E.B. 2003. Glutamine synthetase and glutamate dehydrogenase in the prefrontal cortex of patients with schizophrenia. *Prog. Neuropsychopharmacol. Biol. Psychiatry* **27**:675–680.

Carbonell, T., and Rama, R. 2007. Iron, oxidative stress and early neurological deterioration in ischemic stroke. *Curr. Med. Chem.* **14**:857–874.

Carlsson, A., Hansson, L.O., Waters, N., and Carlsson, M.L. 1999. A glutamatergic deficiency model of schizophrenia. *Br. J. Psychiatry* **174**(Suppl. 37):2–6.

Carlsson, A., Waters, N., Holm-Waters, S., Tedroff, J., Nilsson, M., and Carlsson, M.L. 2001. Interactions between monoamines, glutamate, and GABA in schizophrenia: new evidence. *Annu. Rev. Pharmacol. Toxicol.* **41**:237–260.

Carlsson, M., and Carlsson, A. 1990. Interactions between glutaminergic and monoaminergic systems within the basal ganglia – implications for schizophrenia and Parkinson's disease. *Trends Neurosci.* **13**:272–276.

Clem, R.L., Cilikel, T., and Barth, A.L. 2008. Ongoing in vivo experience triggers synaptic metaplasticity in the neocortex. *Science* **319**:101–104.

Cloninger, R.C. 1987. A systematic method for clinical description and classification of personality variants. *Arch. Gen. Psychiatry* **44**:573–588.

Cook, E.H.J., and Leventhal, B. 1996. The serotonin system in autism. *Curr. Opin. Pediatr.* **8**:348–354.

Cortese, B.M., and Phan, K.L. 2005. The role of glutamate in anxiety and related disorders. *CNS Spectrums* **10**:820–830.

Coyle, J.T., and Puttfarcken, P. 1993. Oxidative stress, glutamate, and neurodegenerative disorders. *Science* **262**:689–695.

Dammann, O., and O'Shea, T.M. 2008. Cytokines and perinatal brain damage. *Clin. Perinatol.* **35**:643–663.

Daniel, D.G., Weinberger, D.R., Jones, D.W., Zigun, J.R., Coppola, R., Handle, S., Bigelow, L.R., Goldberg, T.E., Berman, K.F., and Kelinman, J.E. 1991. The effect of amphetamine on regional blood flow during cognitive activation in schizophrenia. *J. Neurosci.* **11**:1907–1919.

Desai, P., Roy, M., Roy, A., Brown, S., and Smelson, D. 1997. Impaired color vision in cocaine-withdrawn patients. *Arch. Gen. Psychiatry* **54**:696–699.

Deumens, R., Koopmans, G.C., Den Bakker, C.G.J., Maquet, V., Blacher, S., Honig, W.M.M., Jerome, R., Pirard, J.-P., Steinbusch, H.W.M., and Joosten, E.A.J. 2004. Alignment of glial cells stimulates directional neurite growth of CNS neurons *in vitro*. *Neuroscience* **125**:591–604.

Di Cristo, G. 2007. Development of cortical GABAergic circuits and its implications for neurodevelopmental disorders. *Clin. Genet.* **72**:1–8.

Duman, R.S. 2004. Depression: A case of neuronal life and death? *Biol. Psychiatry* **56**:140–145.

Dunn, A.J., Swiergiel, A.H., and Palamarchouk, V. 2004. Brain circuits involved in corticotrophin-releasing factor – norepinephrine interactions during stress. *Ann. N. Y. Acad. Sci.* **1018**:25–34.

Dwivedi, Y., Rizavi, H.S., Roberts, R.C., Conley, R.C., Taminga, C.A., and Pandey, F.N. 2001. Reduced activation and expression of ERK1/2 MAP kinase in the post-mortem brain of depressed suicide subjects. *J. Neurochem.* **77**:916–928.

Ekonomou, A., Pagonopoulou, O., and Angleatau, F. 2000. Age-dependent changes in adenosine A1 receptor and uptake site binding in the mouse brain: An autoradiographic study. *J. Neurosci. Res.* **60**:257–265.

El Mansari, M., and Blier, P. 2006. Mechanisms of action of current and potential pharmacotherapies of obsessive-compulsive disorder. *Prog. Neuropsychopharmacol. Biol. Psychiatry* **30**:362–373.

Ericsson, M., Poston, W.S.C. II, and Foreyt, J.P. 1997. Common biological pathways in eating disorders and obesity. *Addict. Behav.* **21**:733–743.

Frye, M.A., Tsai, G.E., Gouchuan, E.T., Huggins, T., Coyle, J.T., and Post, R.M. 2007. Low cerebrospinal fluid glutamate and glycine in refractory affective disorder. *Biol. Psychiatry* **61**:162–166.

Gagné, A-M., Gagné, P., and Hébert, M. 2007. Impact of light therapy on rod and cone functions in healthy subjects. *Psychiatry Res.* **151**:259–263.

Gamkrelidze, G., Yun, S.H., and Trommer, B.L. 2005. Amyloid-β as a biologically active peptide in CNS. In: P.K.Stanton, C.Bramham, and H.E.Scharfman (eds.) *Synaptic Plasticity and Transsynaptic Signaling*. New York: Springer, pp. 529–538.

Gao, Z.G., and Jacobson, K.A. 2007. Emerging adenosine receptor agonists. *Expert Opin. Emerg. Drugs* **12**:479–492.

Garcia-Alloza, M., Gil-Bea, F.J., Diez-Ariza, M., Chen, C.P.L.-H., Francis, P.T., Lasheras, B., and Ramirez, M.J. 2005. Cholinergic-serotonergic imbalance contributes to cognitive and behavioral symptoms in Alzheimer's disease. *Neuropsychologia* **43**:442–449.

Garg, R., Ramachandran, R., and Sharma, P. 2008. Anaesthetic implications of hyperekplexia – "startle disease." *Anaesth. Intensive Care* **36**:254–256.

Gehrmann, J., Banati, R.B., and Kreutzberg, G.W. 1993. Microglia in the immune surveillance of the brain: human microglia constitutively express HLA-DR molecules. *J. Neuroimmunol.* **48**:189–198.

Goldman-Rakic, P.S., and Selemon, L.D. 1997. Functional and anatomical aspects of prefrontal pathology in schizophrenia. *Schizophr. Bull.* **23**:437–458.

Gonsette, R.E. 2008. Oxidative stress and excitotoxicity: a therapeutic issue in multiple sclerosis? *Mult. Scler.* **14**:22–34.

Goodman, A. 2008. Neurobiology of addiction. An integrative review. *Biochem. Pharmacol.* **75**:266–322.

Gornick, M.C., Addington, A., Shaw, P., Bobb, A.J., Sharp, W., Greenstein, D., Arepalli, S., Castellanos, F.X., and Rapoport, J. L. 2007. Association of the dopamine receptor D4 (DRD4) gene 7-repeat allele with children with attention-deficit/hyperactivity disorder (ADHD): An update. *Am. J. Med. Genet. B Neuropsychiatr. Genet.* **144B**:379–382.

Grachev, I.D., and Apkarian, A.V. 2000. Chemical mapping of anxiety in the brain of healthy human: an in-vivo 1H-MRS study on the effects of sex, age, and brain region. *Hum. Brain Mapp.* **11**:261–272.

Guardia, J., Catagau, A.M., Batile, F., Martin, J.C., Segura, L., Gonzalvo, B., Prat, G., Carrio, I., and Casas, M. 2000. Striatal dopaminergic D(2) receptor density measured by [(123)I]iodobenzamide SPECT in the prediction of treatment outcome of alcohol-dependent patients. *Am. J. Psychiatry* **157**:127–129.

Guidotti, A., Auta, J., Davis, J.M., Dong, E., Grayson, D.R., Veldic, M., Zhang, X., and Costa, E. 2005. GABAergic dysfunction in schizophrenia: new treatment strategies on the horizon. *Pysychopharmacology* **180**:191–205.

Gurevich, E.V., and Joyce, J.N. 1997. Alterations in the cortical serotonergic system in schizophrenia: A postmortem study. *Biol. Psychiatry* **42**:529–545.

Haass, C., and Selkoe, D.J. 2007. Soluble protein oligomers in neurodegeneration: lessons from the Alzheimer's amyloid β–peptide. *Nat. Rev. Mol. Cell Biol.* **8**:101–312.

Hanson, S.M., and Czajkowski, C. 2008. Structural mechanisms underlying benzodiazepine modulation of the GABAA receptor. *J. Neurosci.* **28**:3490–3499.

Hardy, J., and Selkoe, D.J. 2002. The amyloid hypothesis of Alzheimer's disease: progress and problems on the road to therapeutics. *Science* **297**:353–356.

Heinz, A., Higley, J.D., Gorey, J.G., Saunders, R.C., Jones, D.W., Hommer, D., Zajicek, K., Suomi, S.J., Lesch, K.-P., Weinberger, D.R., and Linnoila, M. 1998. In vivo association between alcohol intoxication, aggression, and serotonin transporter availability in nonhuman primates. *Am. J. Psychiatry* **155**:1023–1028.

Hensch, T.K., and Stryker, M.P. 2004. Columnar architecture sculpted by GABA circuits in developing cat visual cortex. *Science* **303**:1678–1681.

Heresco-Levy, U., and Javitt, D.C. 2004. Comparative effects of glycine and D-cycloserine on persistent negative symptoms in schizophrenia: a retrospective analysis. *Schizophr. Res.* **66**:89–96.

Hoek, R.M., Ruuls, S.R., Murphy, C.A., Wright, G.J., Goddard, R., Zurawski, S.M., Blom, B., Homola, M.E., Streit, W.J., Brown, M.H., Barclay, A.N., and Sedgwick, J.D. 2000. Down-regulation of the macrophage lineage through interaction with OX2 (CD200). *Science* **290**:1768–1771.

Hoekstra, R., Fekkes, D., Loonen, A.J.M., Pepplinkhuizen, L., Tuineier, S., and Verhoeven, W.M.A. 2006. Bipolar mania and plasma amino acids: increased levels of glycine. *Eur. Neuropsychopharmacol.* **16**:71–77.

Jacobson, K.A., and Gao, Z.G. 2006. Adenosine receptors as therapeutic targets. *Nat. Rev. Drug Discov.* **5**:247–264.

Jeng, J-M., and Sensi, S.L. 2005. In: P.K.Stanton, C.Bramham, and H.E.Scharfman (eds.), *Synaptic Plasticity and Transsynaptic Signaling*. New York, Springer, pp. 139–157.

Kalivas, P.W., Pierce, R.C., Cornish, J., and Sorg, B.A. 1998. A role for sensitization in craving and relapse in cocaine addiction. *J. Psychopharmacol.* **12**:49–53.

Kamenetz, R., Tomita, T., Hsieh, H., Seabrook, G., Borchelt, D., Iwatsubo, T., Sisodia, S., and Malinow, R. 2003. APP processing and synaptic function. *Neuron* **37**:925–937.

Karolewicz, B., Szebeni, K., Stockmeier, C.A., Konick, L., Overholser, J.C., Jurjus, G., Roth, B.L., and Ordway, G.A. 2004. Low nNOS protein in the locus ceruleus in major depression. *J. Neurochem.* **91**:1057–1066.

Kaul, M., Garden, G.A., and Lipton, S.A. 2001. Pathways to neuronal injury and apoptosis in HIV-associated dementia. *Nature* **410**:988–994.

Kim, W.G., Mohney, R.P., Wilson, B., Jeohn, G.H., Liu, B., and Hong, J.S. 2000. Regional difference in susceptibility to lipopolysacchride-induced neurotoxicity in the rat brain: role of microglia. *J. Neurosci.* **20**:6309–6316.

Kim, Y.S., and Joh, T.H. 2006. Microglia, major player in the brain inflammation: their roles in the pathogenesis of Parkinson's disease. *Exp. Mol. Med.* **38**:333–347.

Kim, Y.S., Kim, S.S., Cho, J.J., Choi, D.H., Hwang, O., Shin, D.H., Chun, H.S., Beal, M.F., and Joh, T.H. 2005. Matrix metalloproteinase-3: a novel signaling proteinase from apoptotic neuronal cells that activates microglia. *J. Neurosci.* **25**:3701–3711.

Kondziella, D., Brenner, E., Eyjolfsson, E.M., and Sonnewald, U. 2007. How do glial-neuronal interactions fit into current neurotransmitter hypotheses of schizophrenia? *Neurochem. Int.* **50**:291–301.

Kronfol, Z., and Remick, D.G. 2000. Cytokines and the brain: Implications for clinical psychiatry. *Am. J. Psychiatry* **157**:683–694.

Krystal, J.H., Sanacora, G., Blumberg, H., Anand, A., Charney, D.S., Marek, G., Epperson, C.N., Goddard, A., and Mason, G.F. 2002. Glutamate and GABA systems as targets for novel antidepressant and mood stabilizing treatments. *Mol. Psychiatry* **7**:S71–S80.

Krystal, J.H., Staley, J., Mason, G., Petrakis, I.L., Kaufman, J., Harris, R.A., Gelernter, J., and Lappalainen, J. 2006. γ-Aminobutyric acid type A receptors and alcoholism. *Arch. Gen. Psychiatry* **63**:957–968.

Kugaya, A., and Sanacora, G. 2005. Beyond monoamines: glutamatergic function in mood disorders. *CNS Spectrums* **10**:808–819.

Lancelot, E., and Beal, M.F. 1998. Glutamate toxicity in chronic neurodegenerative disease. *Prog. Brain Res.* **116**:331–347.

Lane, J.H., Sasseville, V.G., Smith, M.O., Vogel, P., Pauley, D.R., Heyes, M.P., and Lackner, A.A. 1996. Neuroinvasion by simian immuno deficiency virus coincides with increased numbers of perivascular macrophages/microglia and intrathecal immune activation. *J. Neurovirol.* **2**:423–432.

Lange, K.W., Robbins, T.W., Marsden, C.D., James, M., Owen, A.M., and Paul, G.M. 1992. L-dopa withdrawal in Parkinson's disease selectively impairs cognitive performance in tests sensitive to frontal lobe dysfunction. *Psychopharmacology* **107**:395–404.

Lee, K-W., Kim, Y., Kim, A.M., Helmin, K., Nairn, A.C., and Greengard, P. 2006. Cocaine-induced dendritic spine formation in D1 and D2 dopamine receptor-containing medium spiny neurons in nucleus accumbens. *Proc. Natl. Acad. Sci. U. S. A.* **103**:3399–3404.

Lee, M.G., Hassani, O.K., Alonso, A., and Jones, B.E. 2005. Cholinergic basal forebrain neuron burst with theta during waking and paradoxical sleep. *J. Neurosci.* **25**:4365–4369.

Leri, F., Flores, J., Rodaros, D., and Stewart, J. 2002. Blockade of stress-induced but not cocaine-induced reinstatement by infusion of noradrenergic antagonists into the bed nucleus of the stria terminalis or the central nucleus of the amygdala. *J. Neurosci.* **22**:5713–5718.

Levitt, P., Harvey, J.A., Friedman, E., Simansky, K., and Murphy, E.H. 1997. New evidence for neurotransmitter influences on brain development. *Trends Neurosci.* **20**:269–274.

Liu, B., Gao, H.M., Wang, J.Y., Jeohn, G.H., Cooper, C.L., and Hong, J.S. 2002. Role of nitric oxide in inflammation-mediated neurodegeneration. *Ann. N. Y. Acad. Sci.* **962**:318–331.

Lucas-Meunier, E., Fossier, P., Baux, G., and Amar, M. 2003. Cholinergic modulation of the cortical neuronal network. *Plugers Arch.* **446**:17–29.

Majewska, M.D. 1996. Cocaine addiction as a neurological disorder: Implications for treatment. In: M.D.Majewska (ed.) *Neurotoxicity and Neuropathology Associated with Cocaine Abuse; NIDA Research Monograph 163*. Rockville, MD: National Institute on Drug Abuse.

Manschreck, T.C., Laughery, J.A., Weisstein, C.C., Allen, D., Humblestone, B., Neville, M., Podlewski, H., and Mitra, N. 1988. Characteristics of freebase cocaine psychosis. *Yale J. Biol. Med.* **61**:115–122.

Maron, E., and Shlik, J. 2006. Serotonin function in panic disorder: important, but why?*Neuropsychopharmacology* **31**:1–11.

Marrone, D.F. 2007. Ultrastructural plasticity associated with hippocampal-dependent learning: a meta-analysis. *Neurobiol. Learn. Mem.* **87**:361–371.

Marrone, D.F., LeBoutillier, J.C., and Petit, T.L. 2005. In: P.K.Stanton, C.Bramham, and H.E.Scharfman (eds.) *Synaptic Plasticity and Transsynaptic Signaling*. New York: Springer, pp. 495–517.

McKinney, M. 2005. Brain cholinergic vulnerability: relevance to behavior and disease. *Biochem. Pharmacol.* **70**:1115– 1124.

Meltzer, C.C., Smith, G., DeKosky, S.T., Pollock, B.G., Mathis, C.A., Moore, R.Y., Kupfer, D.J., and Reynolds, C.F. 3rd. 1998. Serotonin in aging, late-life depression, and Alzheimer's disease: The emerging role of functional imaging. *Neuropsychopharmacology* **18**:407–430.

Menza, M.A., Golve, L.I., Cody, R.A., and Forman, N.E. 1993. Dopamine-related personality traits in Parkinson's disease. *Neurology* **43**:505–508.

Moore, R.Y., and Bloom, F.E. 1979. Central catecholamine neuron systems: anatomy and physiology of the norepinephrine and epinephrine systems. *Ann. Rev. Neurosci.* **2**:113–168.

Nagatsu, T., and Sawada, M. 2005. Inflammatory process in Parkinson's disease: role for cytokines. *Curr. Pharm. Des.* **11**:999–1016.

Nestler, E.J. 1997. An emerging pathophysiology. *Nature* **385**:578–589.

New, A.S., and Siever, L.J. 2003. Biochemical endophenotypes in personality disorders. *Methods Mol. Med.* **77**:199–213.

Niizato, K., Iritani, S., Ikeda, K., and Arai, H. 2001. Astroglial function of schizophrenic brain: a study using lobotomized brain. *Clin. Neurosci. Neuropathol.* **12**: 1457–1460.

Nudmamud-Thanoi, S., and Reynolds, G.P. 2004. The NR1 subunit of the glutamate/NMDA receptor in the superior temporal cortex in schizophrenia and affective disorders. *Neurosci. Lett.* **372**:173–177.

Nutt, D., 2006. GABAAreceptors: subtypes, regional distribution, and function. *J. Clin. Sleep Med.* **2**:S7–S11.

O ' Neill, M.J., and Witkin, J.M. 2007. AMPA receptor potentiators: application for depression and Parkinson's disease. *Curr. Drug Targets* **8**:603–620.

Olanow, C.W. 2007. The pathogenesis of cell death in Parkinson's disease – 2007. *Mov. Disord.* **22**(Suppl. 17):S335–342.

Olney, J.W., and Farber, N.B. 1995. Glutamate receptor dysfunction and schizophrenia. *Arch. Gen. Psychiatry* **52**:998–1007.

Parsey, R.V., Oquendo, M.A., Zea-Ponce, Y., Rodenhiser, J., Kegeles, L.S., Pratap, M., Cooper, T.B., Van Heertum, R., Mann, J.J., and Laruelle, M. 2001. Dopamine D(2) receptor availability and amphetamine-induced dopamine release in unipolar depression. *Biol. Psychiatry* **50**:313–322.

Partonen, T. 1996. Dopamine and circadian rhythms in seasonal affective disorder. *Med. Hypotheses* **47**:191–192.

Perlov, E., Philipsen, A., Hesslinger, B., Buechert, M., Ahrendts, J., Feige, B., Bubl, E., Hennig, J., Ebert., D., Tebartz van Elst, L. 2007. Reduced cingulate glutamate/glutamine-to-creatine ratios in adult patients with attention deficit/hyperactivity disorder – a magnet resonance spectroscopy study. *J. Psychiatr. Res.* **41**:934–941.

Phan, K.L., Fitzgerald, D.A., Corteses, B.M., Seraji-Bozorgzad, N., Tancer, M.E., and Moore, G.J. 2005. Anterior cingulate neurochemistry in social anxiety disorder: 1H-MRS at 4 Tesla. *Neuroreport* **16**:183–186.

Plant, L.D., Boyle, J.P., Smith, I.F., Peers, C., and Pearson, H.A. 2003. The production of amyloid beta peptide is a critical requirement for the viability of central neurons. *J. Neurosci.* **23**:5531–5535.

Pliszka, S.R. 2005. The neuropsychopharmacology of attention-deficit/hyperactivity disorder. *Biol. Psychiatry* **57**:1385–1390.

Quiroz, J.A., Singh, J., Gould, T.D., Denicoff, K.D., Zarate, C.lA., and Manji, H.K., 2004. Emerging experimental therapeutics for bipolar disorder: clues from the molecular pathophysiology. *Mol. Psychiatry* **9**:756–776.

Raedler, T.J., Bymaster, F.P, Tandon, R., Copolov, D., and Dean, B. 2007. Towards a muscarinic hypothesis of schizophrenia. *Mol. Psychiatry* **12**:232–246.

Raine, C.S. 1994. Multiple sclerosis: immune system molecule expression in the central nervous system. *J. Neuropathol. Exp. Neurol.* **53**:328–337.

Redgrave, P., and Gurney, K. 2006. The short-latency dopamine signal: a role in discovering novel actions?*Nat. Rev. Neurosci.* 7:967–975.

Rolls, E.T., Loh, M., Deco, G., and Winterer, G. 2008. Computational models of schizophrenia and dopamine modulation in the prefrontal cortex. *Nat. Rev. Neurosci.* **9**:696–709.

Rossner, S., Schultz, I., Zeitschel, U., Schliebs, R., Bigl, V., and Denmuth, H.V. 2005. Brain propyl endopeptidase expression in aging, APP transgenic mice and Alzheimer's disease. *Neurochem. Res.* **30**:695–702.

Salmond, C.H., Chatfield, D.A., Menon, D.K., Pickard, J.D., and Sahakian, B.J. 2005. Cognitive sequelae of head injury: involvement of basal forebrain and associated structures. *Brain* **128**:189–200.

Sanacora, G., Zarate, C.A., Krystal, J.H., and Manji, H.K. 2008. Targeting the glutamatergic system to develop novel, improved therapeutics for mood disorders. *Nat. Rev. Drug Discov.*7:426–437.

Sarika Arora, A. 2006. Role of neuropeptides in appetite regulation and obesity – A review. *Neuropeptides* **40**:375–401.

Sato, A., Sato, Y., and Uchida, S. 2004. Activation of the intracerebral cholinergic nerve fibers originating in the basal forebrain increases regional cerebral blood flow in the rat's cortex and hippocampus. *Neurosci. Lett.*361:90–93.

Schildkraut, J.J. 1965. The catecholamine hypothesis of affective disorders: a review of supporting evidence. *Am. J. Psychiatry* **122**:509–522.

Schliebs, R., and Arendt, T. 2006. The significance of the cholinergic system in the brain during aging and in Alzheimer's disease. *J. Neural. Transm.* **113**:1625–1644.

Schmidt, M. 2008. GABA(C) receptors in retina and brain. *Results Probl. Cell Differ.* **44**:49–67.

Sebat, J., Lakshmi, B., Malhotra, D., Troge, J., Lese-Martin, C., Walsh, T., Yamrom, B., Yoon, S., Krasnitz, A., Kendall, J., Leotta, A., Pai, D., Zhang, R., Lee, Y-H., James Hicks, J., Spence, S.J., Lee, A.T., Puura, K., Lehtimäki, T., Ledbetter, D., Gregersen, P.K., Bregman, J., Sutcliffe, J.S., Jobanputra, V., Chung, W., Warburton, D., King, M-C., Skuse, D., Daniel H. Geschwind, D.H., Gilliam, T.C., Ye, K., and Wigler, M. 2007. Strong association of de novo copy number mutations with autism. *Science* **316**:445–449.

Segal, M., and Bloom, F.E. 1976. The action of norepinephrine in the rat hippocampus. IV. The effects of locus coeruleus stimulation on evoked hippocampal unit activity. *Brain Res.* **107**:513–525.

Sekier, I., Sensi, S.L., Hershfinkel, M., and Silverman, W.F. 2007. Mechanism and regulation of cellular zinc transport. *Mol. Med.*13:337–343.

Selkoe, D.J. 2002. Alzheimer's disease is a synaptic failure. *Science* **298**:789–791.

Shigeri, Y., Seal, R.P., and Shimamoto, K. 2004. Molecular pharmacology of glutamate transporters, EAATs and VGLUTs. *Brain Res. Rev.* **45**:250–265.

Shim, S.S., Hammonds, M.D., and Kee, B.S., 2008. Potentiation of the NMDA receptor in the treatment of schizophrenia: focused on the glycine site. *Eur. Arch. Psychiatry Clin. Neurosci.* **258**:16–27.

Snyder, S.H., Bannerjee, S., Yamamura, H., and Greenberg, D. 1974. Drugs, neurotransmitters and schizophrenia: Phenothiazines, amphetamine and enzymes synthesizing psychotomimetic drugs and schizophrenia research. *Science* **243**:398–400.

Stahl, S.M.2007a. Beyond the dopamine hypothesis to the NMDA glutamate hypofunction hypothesis of schizophrenia. *CNS Spectrums* **12**:265–268.

2007b. The genetics of schizophrenia converge upon the NMDA glutamate receptor. *CNS Spectrums* **12**:583–588.

Steiger, H., Koerner, N., Engelberg, M.J., Israel, M., Ng Ying Kin, N.M., and Young, S.N. 2001. Self-destructiveness and serotonin function in bulimia nervosa. *Psychiatry Res.* **103**:15–26.

Stephan, K.E., Baldeweg, T., and Friston, K.J. 2006. Synaptic plasticity and disconnection in schizophrenia. *Biol. Psychiatry* **59**:929–939.

Stone, J.M., Morrison, P.D., and Pilowsky, L.S. 2007. Glutamate and dopamine dysregulation in schizophrenia – a synthesis and selective review. *J. Psychopharmacol.* **21**:440–452.

Straub, R.E., and Weinberger, D.R. 2006. Schizophrenia genes: famine to feast. *Biol. Psychiatry* **60**:81–83.

Streeter, C.E., Jensen, J.E., Perlmutter, R.M., Cabral, H.J., Tian, H., Terhune, D.B., Ciraulo, D.A., and Renshaw, P.F. 2007. Yoga asana sessions increase brain GABA levels: a pilot study. *J. Altern. Complement. Med.* **13**:419–426.

Tamminga, C.A. 1998. Schizophrenia and glutamatergic transmission. *Crit. Rev. Neurobiol.* **12**:21–36.

Tandon, R. 1999. Cholinergic aspects of schizophrenia. *Br. J. Psychiatry* **174**(Suppl. 37):7–11.

Terry, R.D., and Buccafusco, J.J. 2003. The cholinergic hypothesis of age and Alzheimer's disease-related cognitive deficits: recent challenges and their implications for novel drug development. *J. Pharmacol. Exp. Ther.* **306**:821–827.

Toledano, A., and Alvarez, M.I. 2004. Lesions and dysfunctions of the nucleus basalis as Alzheimer's disease models: general and critical overview and analysis of the long-term changes in several excitotoxic models. *Curr. Alzheimer Res.***1**:189–214.

Tsai, G., Passani, L.A., Slusher, B.S., Carter, R., Baer, L., Kleinman, J.E., and Coyle, J.T. 1995. Abnormal excitatory neurotransmitter metabolism in schizophrenic brains. *Arch. Gen. Psychiatry* **52**:829–836.

Ullian, E.M., Sapperstein, S.K., Christopherson, K.S., and Barres, B.A. 2001. Control of synapse number by glia. *Science* **291**:657–661.

Unis, A.S., Cook, E.H., Vincent, J.G., Gjerde, D.K., Perry, B.D., Mason, C., and Mitchell, J. 1997. Platelet serotonin measures in adolescents with conduct disorder. *Biol. Psychiatry* **42**:553–559.

Volkow, N.D., and Wise, R.A. 2005. How can drug addiction help us understand obesity? *Nat. Neurosci.* **8**:555–560.

Weyers, P., Krebs, H., and Janke, W. 1999. Harm avoidance and serotonin. *Biol. Psychol.* **51**:77–81.

Whitton, P.S. 2007. Inflammation as a causative factor in the aetiology of Parkinson's disease. *Br. J. Pharmacol.***150**:963–976.

Wolf, M.E., Sun, X., Mangiavacchi, S., and Chao, S.Z. 2004. Psychomotor stimulants and neuronal plasticity. *Neuropharmacology* **47**:61–79.

Yamagata, M., Sanes, J.R., and Weiner, J.A. 2003. Synaptic adhesion molecules. *Curr. Opin. Cell Biol.* **15**: 621–632.

Yan, Q.S., Zheng, S.Z., and Yan, S.E. 2004. Involvement of 5-HT1B receptors within the ventral tegmental area in regulation of mesolimbic dopaminergic neuronal activity via GABA mechanisms: a study with dual-probe microdialysis. *Brain Res.* **1021**:82–91.

Yanai, K., and Tashiro, M. 2007. The physiological and pathophysiological roles of neuronal histamine: an insight from human positron emission tomography studies. *Pharmacol. Ther.* **113**:1–15.

Yang, Y., Ge, W., Chen, Y., Zhang, Z., Shen, W., Wu, C., Poo, M., and Duan, S. 2003. Contribution of astrocytes to hippocampal long-term potentiation through release of D-serine. *Proc. Natl. Acad. Sci. U. S. A.***100**:15194–15199.

Yoder, K.K., Kareken, D.A., Seyoum, R.A., O'Connor, S.J., Wang, C., Zheng, Q-H., Mock, B., and Morris, E.D. 2005. Dopamine D2 receptor availability is associated with subjective responses to alcohol. *Alcohol Clin. Exp. Res.* **29**:965–970.

Zafra, F., Hengerer, B., Leibrock, J., Thoenen, H, and Lindholm, D. 1990. Activity dependent regulation of BDNF and NGF mRNSs in the rat hippocampus is mediated by non-NMDA glutamate receptors. *EMBO J.* **9**:3545–3550.

Zakzanis, K.K. and Hansen, K.T. 1998. Dopamine D2 densities and the schizophrenic brain. *Schizophr. Res.* **32**:201–206.

Zucker, R.S. 1999. Calcium- and activity-dependent synaptic plasticity. *Curr. Opin. Neurobiol.* **9**:305–313.

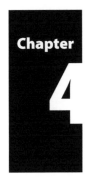

Occipital and parietal lobes

Occipital lobe

Functional anatomy

The occipital lobe is clearly demarcated from the parietal lobe on the medial surface by the parieto-occipital sulcus and the anterior limb of the calcarine fissure (Figure 4.1). The short section of parieto-occipital sulcus on the dorsolateral surface is used as an anchor for an imaginary line that extends ventrally to the preoccipital notch (Figure 5.1). This imaginary line is the border between the occipital and parietal lobes as well as the temporal lobe on the lateral cortical surface. The border between the occipital lobe and temporal lobe on the ventral surface is less distinct (Figure 5.4). Some authors include all of the lingual (medial occipitotemporal) gyrus and fusiform (lateral occipitotemporal) gyrus with the temporal lobe; others assign the posterior portions of these gyri to the occipital lobe.

The entire cortex of the occipital lobe is dedicated to vision and consists of Brodmann's areas 17, 18, and 19 (Figures 2.2, 2.3, 4.1, and 4.2). Brodmann's area (BA) 17 is the primary visual cortex (striate cortex) and occupies a large portion of the medial aspect of the occipital lobe. Much of the primary visual cortex lies within the calcarine fissure, which extends approximately 2.5 cm deep into the occipital lobe. A portion of BA 17 curves posteriorly around onto the posterolateral surface of the occipital lobe. Brodmann's areas 18 and 19 are recognized as secondary and tertiary visual areas, respectively, and represent the visual association area of the occipital lobe.

Many direct and indirect connections exist between the occipital lobe and other cortical regions. The superior occipitofrontal (subcallosal) fasciculus links the occipital, parietal, and temporal cortices with the insular and frontal regions. The superior occipitofrontal fasciculus is joined by the arcuate fasciculus in its anterior

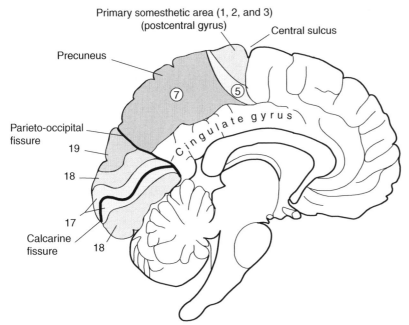

Figure 4.1. The primary visual cortex (BA 17) is largely buried within the calcarine fissure. A greater portion of the superior parietal lobule (BA 5 and 7) lies along the midline (compare with Figure 4.2).

Primary somesthetic area (1, 2, and 3) (postcentral gyrus)

Central sulcus

Precuneus

Parieto-occipital fissure

Cingulate gyrus

19

18

17

Calcarine fissure

18

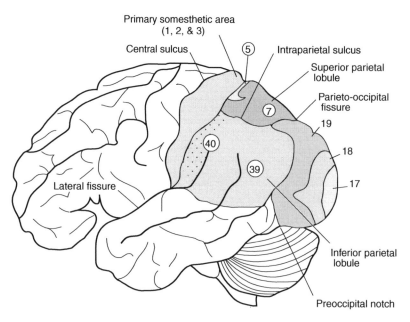

Primary somesthetic area
(1, 2, & 3)

Central sulcus

⑤

Intraparietal sulcus

Superior parietal
lobule

Parieto-occipital
fissure

19

40

18

39

17

Lateral fissure

Inferior parietal
lobule

Preoccipital notch

Figure 4.2. The secondary (BA 18) and tertiary (BA 19) visual cortex is better appreciated from the lateral view. The primary somesthetic cortex coincides with BA 1, 2 and 3. The superior parietal lobule coincides with BA 5 and 7 and the inferior parietal lobule coincides with BA 39 (angular gyrus) and 40 (supramarginal gyrus). Stippling indicates approximate location of parietal lobe mirror neurons.

flow at the junction of the parietal and temporal lobes. The arcuate fasciculus is important in speech. The inferior occipitofrontal fasciculus interconnects the occipital cortex with the lateral and ventrolateral parts of the frontal lobes. Two transverse occipital fasciculi have been described. Together they interconnect the primary visual cortex on the medial aspect with the lateral occipital cortex and the inferior occipitotemporal cortex.

Primary visual cortex (BA 17; V1; striate cortex)
Fibers that originate from nerve cell bodies located in the lateral geniculate body (thalamus) project to the V1, where they terminate in an orderly fashion to produce a retinal map. Macular areas of the retina are represented close to the occipital pole and occupy a relatively large area of the visual cortex. Peripheral vision is represented more anteriorly.

Small spots of light are very effective in exciting the cells of the retina and the lateral geniculate body. In contrast, cells of the primary visual cortex respond only to visual images that have linear properties (lines and edges). The neurons of the primary visual cortex interpret contours and boundaries of a visual target in terms of line segments.

A lesion of V1 will produce an area of blindness (scotoma) in the contralateral visual field. Loss of an area as large as an entire quadrant of vision may go unnoticed by the patient. A lesion of the entire primary visual cortex on both sides results in cortical blindness.

An 84-year-old woman underwent craniotomy 17 years previously for the removal of a right occipital meningioma (Nagaratnam *et al*, 1996). She presented at this time with a three-year history of formed hallucinations, the ringing of bells, and the monotonous repetition of the same Christmas carol. The hallucinations had increased in frequency and intensity in the past few months. She reported people standing to her left, and, to her annoyance, some of them stroked her face. She had been observed brushing away imaginary objects. A computed tomography scan revealed a 5-cm diameter mass superior to the tentorium in the right occipital region. She was treated with steroids for an unrelated cardiac condition. The musical hallucinations continued unabated until her death from left ventricular failure.

Secondary and tertiary visual cortex (BA 18 and BA 19)
Brodmann's areas 18 and 19 are often referred to as the extrastriate visual cortex. Recent studies show that areas of both the temporal and parietal cortices are also involved in visual processing. BA 18 (V2; prestriate cortex) receives binocular input and allows for the appreciation of three dimensions (stereopsis). Target distance is coded by some neurons. Some neurons of BA 19 integrate visual with auditory and tactile signals.

Area V3 is located dorsal and anterior to V2 on both the medial and lateral surfaces of the occipital lobe. Area V4 is represented by the cortex of the lingual and fusiform gyri, located on the inferior surface of the brain, and is important in color perception. It also responds to moving visual targets regardless of the direction of movement. Area MT of the monkey is comparable with area V5 of the human and like V2, it is important in stereopsis. Area V5/MT of the human is located just posterior to the junction of the ascending limb of the inferior temporal sulcus with the lateral occipital sulcus. It extends over a small part of the posterior BA 37 as well as a small part of the anterior BA 19. Area MT contains neurons that respond selectively to the direction of moving visual objects and determines target velocity in space. There appear to be two regions of MT: one region responds to visual targets in a retinotopic frame of reference and the second appears to use a spatiotopic frame of reference (d'Avossa et al., 2006). Area V5/MT in the human (sometimes referred to as the MT+ complex) may correspond to areas MT and MST in the monkey (Becker et al., 2009). This area is important in planning smooth pursuit eye movements (Ono and Mustari, 2006; Nuding et al., 2008).

Clinical vignette

A 47-year-old right-handed woman (DF) had a severe form of agnosia as a result of carbon monoxide poisoning and was incapable of discriminating even the simplest geometric forms. She could not recognize objects but was able to use information about location, size, shape, and orientation to reach out and grasp the object. She could not copy objects but was able to draw them from memory. She was better able to recognize objects based on surface information than on outline. She could correctly identify objects with colored or gray-scale surfaces but performed poorly with line drawings. Her primary visual cortex appeared to be largely intact. The ventral stream pathway ("what") seemed to be defective (Figure 4.3). The dorsal stream pathway ("where") proved to be intact.

Parallel visual pathways

Two parallel pathways from the retina process visual images simultaneously. The magnocellular (magno) pathway arises from large, parasol retinal ganglion cells concentrated near the periphery of the retina and terminates on cells in the magnocellular layer of the lateral geniculate body. The magnocellular pathway carries signals related to object motion and location. The parvocellular (parvo) pathway arises from small,

midget retinal ganglion cells that serve mainly cones associated with the macula of the retina and terminates on cells in the parvocellular layer of the lateral geniculate body. The parvocellular pathway carries signals related to color and form. These two continue as separate parallel pathways to V1 of the occipital cortex. A third pathway arises from small cells in the lateral geniculate body that make up the koniocellular layer. The koniocellular layer receives color information from the retina as well as input from the superior colliculus (Hendry and Reid, 2000). There is considerable mixing of all three pathways in V1.

Two cortical visual streams arise from V1. They appear to diverge within V3 with the dorsal stream represented in dorsal V3 and the ventral stream in ventral V3. The ventral visual stream represents foveal vision. It leaves V1 and passes through V2, ventral V3, and on to V4. The ventral stream is sometimes called the "What Pathway" and is associated with object recognition (Himmelbach and Karnath, 2005; Karnath and Perenin, 2005). Signals pass to the extrastriate body area located bilaterally in the lateral occipito-temporal cortex (Downing et al., 2001). The extrastriate body area is sensitive to static and dynamic human and nonhuman bodies, and body parts exclusive of the face. Activation of the extrastriate body area (more so on the right) is increased to images of bodies or body parts presented from an external (allocentric) perspective (i.e., another person) as opposed to one's self (Saxe et al., 2005). The extrastriate body area is believed to be important in reasoning about others' actions since activation here is a first step in recognizing the presence of another's body or body part (Saxe, 2006). It is also activated during goal-directed hand and foot movements of the observer and may function to distinguish between the consequence on one's own and another's behavior (Astafiev et al., 2005; David et al., 2007). It also receives input from the right posterior superior temporal sulcus where body movements are evaluated in terms of their goals (Pelphrey et al., 2004). A lesion of the occipital lobe extrastriate body area results in body form and body action agnosia (Moro et al., 2008).

A region of the striate cortex in the inferior occipital gyrus is sensitive to faces (face-responsive occipital region). This appears to be an initial screening area for face recognition since the signals from this area project to the fusiform gyrus on the ventral surface of the brain –the fusiform face area. The occipital face region is bilateral and is sensitive to physical differences

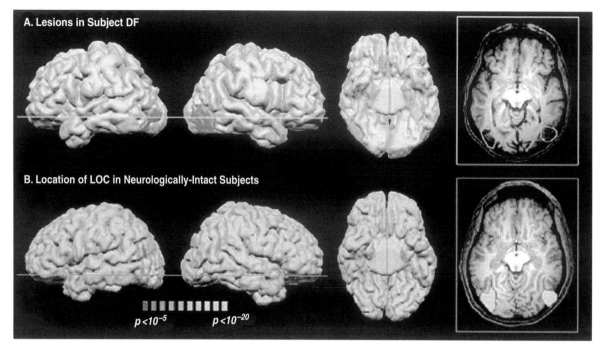

Figure 4.3. A, B. The ventral visual stream lesions in a patient with visual agnosia (subject DF) are compared with the expected region (lateral occipital complex) for object recognition. A. Lesions in subject DF. Her lesions were traced on slices that indicated tissue damage and rendered on the pial surface in pale blue (see color plate). Lateral views of the left and right hemispheres are shown, as is a ventral view of the underside of the brain. B. The expected location of the lateral occipital complex based on functional magnetic resonance imaging date from seven neurologically intact participants. The activation of the slice is shown in orange in panel A in the color plate for comparison with the lesions in patient DF's brain. (Reproduced with permission from Oxford University Press from James *et al.*, 2003.) See also color plate.

between faces and between faces and objects, but it does not extract face identity.

The dorsal visual stream deals with location and motion and represents peripheral vision. Dorsal stream signals from V1 pass through V2, dorsal V3 and on to V5/MT. The dorsal stream terminates in the posterior parietal cortex. Area V5/MT is retinotopic, and is particularly sensitive to the direction of moving visual targets. The dorsal stream is sometimes called the "where pathway" and is responsible for the registration of location, movement, and spatial relationships (Figures 4.5 and 6.10).

The cortical area in the human representing the medial superior temporal area (MST) of the monkey is not completely clear. Area MST in the human is believed to include a portion of the occipitotemporoparietal cortex just anterior to V5/MT. It includes a portion of the inferior parietal lobule (IPL) as well as the posterior superior and middle temporal gyri. The MST is further divided into a dorsal (MSTd) and ventral region (MSTv). The ventral region is more involved

Clinical vignette

A 58-year-old right-handed woman (DF) had a three- to four-year history of progressive difficulty "seeing" objects. Her visual acuity and visual fields were intact, but she could not draw simple geometrical figures, such as a triangle or a square. Even more distressing to her was the presence of visual agnosia, or the inability to recognize objects by sight despite intact basic vision. She could not visually recognize common objects such as a cork, a thimble, or a pipe, especially if they appeared in unusual views, angles, or lighting. When she touched the objects, however, she was immediately able to identify and name them. Her performance on photographs and drawings of objects was similarly impaired. The patient had a progressive visual agnosia from disease affecting her ventromedial occipital cortex (see Figure 4.4). Her slowly progressive history and positron emission tomography scan were consistent with the syndrome of posterior cortical atrophy. At autopsy, this syndrome has usually been a variant of Alzheimer disease with a shift of the characteristic pathology into visual areas of the brain.

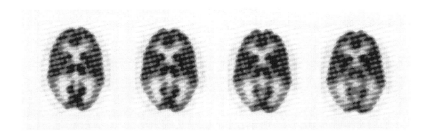

Figure 4.4. The patient's 18-fluor-odeoxyglucose positron emission tomography image revealed bilateral hypometabolism in the secondary and tertiary visual cortex (posterior, lateral light areas), while sparing the primary visual cortex (posterior, mesial dark area). (Reprinted with permission from Mendez, 2001.)

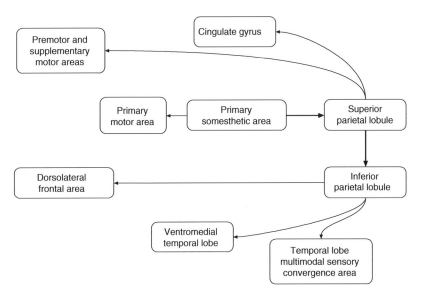

Figure 4.5. A schematic outline of the projections of the parietal lobe. The superior parietal lobule projects to the premotor and supplementary motor areas of the frontal lobe. The inferior lobule projects to the multimodal region of the temporal lobe as well as to the ventromedial temporal lobe. Inferior lobule projections include those to the dorsolateral prefrontal area.

with analysis of visual target direction and velocity, and the generation of pursuit eye movements. Neurons in MSTd are activated in response to radial motion, rotation and translation related to optic flow (Orban, 2008). Optic flow is defined as the perceived visual motion of stationary objects as the observer moves relative to them. Input to MSTd includes V5/MT as well as signals reflecting smooth pursuit commands (Ono and Mustari, 2006). The MST works in conjunction with the ventral intraparietal area to combine signals from visual, vestibular, auditory, and tactile input to plot and guide movement through the environment (Britten, 2008).

Behavioral considerations

Schizophrenia

V1, along with BA 9 in the frontal lobe, has been found to be decreased in thickness in the brains of patients with schizophrenia. This decrease in V1 was not statistically significant but was consistent and was accompanied by a 10% increase in neuronal density. It was speculated that the decrease in neuronal density in the visual cortex is related to poor eye tracking (Selemon et al., 1995). A group of patients with schizophrenia regardless of medication status exhibited visual defects when tested for contrast sensitivity and form discrimination (O'Donnell et al., 2006). Patients with schizophrenia exhibiting reduced gray matter in the occipital lobe were found to have a poor outcome compared with patients with reduced gray matter in more anterior regions (Mitelman and Buchsbaum, 2007).

Hallucinations

Four general categories of visual hallucinations are elementary, complex, and illusions and distortions. Elementary hallucinations include static or moving spots, line segments or simple geometric shapes. Complex hallucinations include objects, faces and scenes. Illusions and distortions are alternations in perception of the external world, commonly alterations in shape, color, size, or movement. It has been suggested that elementary hallucinations reflect activity in primary visual areas or even precortical structures. Complex hallucinations reflect activity in the ventral visual stream. Distortions reflect the dorsal visual stream (Santhouse *et al.*, 2000).

Stimulation of V1 produces elementary hallucinations in the contralateral visual field. These hallucinations include sparks and flashes of color or bright light. Hallucinations of object fragments (e.g., lines, corners, patterns) have been reported following a stroke in the occipital cortex (Anderson and Rizzo, 1994). Parekh *et al.* (1995) reported an increase in the cerebral blood flow to the occipital cortex in patients who experienced procaine-induced visual hallucinations. Blood flow also was increased in limbic structures and in the lateral frontal lobe.

Electrical stimulation of BA 18 and BA 19 can produce complex visual hallucinations. Objects may become disproportionately large (macropsia) or distorted in shape. Images of people, animals, and various geometrical shapes have been reported. Many complex hallucinations appear real to the patient (Hecaen and Albert, 1978). Complex hallucinations occur more frequently after right-sided lesions. A complete bilateral lesion of all visual cortices which can result from occlusion of both posterior cerebral arteries may produce denial of blindness (Anton syndrome; Redlich and Dorsey, 1945).

The migraine visual aura typically consists of simple positive and/or negative (scotoma) components. They may occur up to an hour before the onset of a migraine headache. The positive component often includes bright, white, silver, or colored line segments, patterns or geometrical shapes. The auras usually last only a few seconds followed by other, more severe manifestations of the aura. The hallucinations are often seen as dots, spots or disks that may flicker, pulsate, or move. More complex hallucinations, including faces, may be seen (Panayiotopoulos, 1999). Activity corresponding with the aura usually begins near the fovea and then spreads across the visual field. The blindness that usually follows may persist for several minutes. The aura begins in a restricted area of the occipital lobe representing the fovea then migrates as a form of spreading depression across the cortex representing the peripheral retina (Hadjikhani *et al.*, 2001; Wilkinson, 2004).

Infarction of the left posterior cerebral artery involving the medial occipital lobe (Figure 2.6) is sufficient to produce a confusional state, including disorientation, distractibility, irritability, and paranoia. Confusion and agitation may alternate with mutism. The acute confusional state presented by the patient may be misdiagnosed as a psychiatric illness (Devinsky *et al.*, 1988).

Visual agnosia

Visual agnosia sometimes occurs after lesions in the ventromedial occipital lobe. The objects are seen but cannot be named, and the patient does not know what the object can be used for (Critchley, 1964). Loss of the ability to recognize the faces of known people (prosopagnosia) may follow unilateral or bilateral lesions of the ventromedial occipital lobe that extend into the ventral temporal lobe and include the fusiform gyrus. Color naming may also be impaired, especially with right-sided lesions (DeRenzi and Spinnler, 1967). It is hypothesized that visual agnosia results from disconnection of the visual cortex from the temporal lobe rather than from destruction of occipital lobe tissue (Joseph, 1996). Lesions restricted to BA 19 may result in loss of only color vision (achromatopsia), leaving shape detection relatively intact.

Blindsight

Activity in V1 is believed to be required for visual stimuli to be perceived. V1 acts as the gatekeeper of visual awareness (Silvanto, 2008). Loss of the V1 renders the patient blind according to conventional clinical tests (Rees, 2007). However, when confronted with forced-choice testing some patients show residual capacity in the blind visual field. This residual capacity is called blindsight (Rees, 2008). The patient retains a sense of the presence of a nearby object. Some can accurately guess the location or identity of objects presented in their blind hemifield (Weiskrantz, 2004). The retained vision favors the dorsal visual stream with the retention of a sense of motion, flicker, and contrast more often than object recognition. The probable neuroanatomical basis has been identified with the discovery of direct ipsilateral connections from the lateral geniculate body of the thalamus to the middle temporal area (MT/V5) in the monkey (Sincich *et al.*, 2004). This pathway has been confirmed in the human (Behrens *et al.*, 2003). Blindsight subject GY, who has been extensively studied and has been blind since an auto accident at age 8, has been shown to have responses to visual input in area MT/V5 (Morland *et al.*, 2004). Evidence indicates

Figure 4.6. Subjects (N =14) with phobias (snakes and spiders) were examined during exposure to videotapes of spiders and during exposure to videotapes of a neutral park scene. The positron emission tomographic image data were subtracted. Blood flow is increased to the visual association area (right panel) and decreased to the orbital prefrontal cortex (left panel) during exposure to phobia-provocative visual stimuli. rCBF, relative cerebral blood flow. (Reproduced by permission from Fredrickson, M., Fischer, H., and Wik, G. 1997. Cerebral blood flow during anxiety provocation. *J. Clin. Psychiatry* 48 (Suppl. 16):16–21.)

the presence in GY of a right lateral geniculate to left MT/V5 pathway as well as strengthened transcallosal connections (Bridge *et al.*, 2008).

The emotional valence of facial images can be detected by way of a separate subcortical pathway involving the colliculus, pulvinar, and amygdala (Williams *et al.*, 2006). This pathway does not pass through the occipital lobe and allows for the nonconscious recognition of fearful as well as happy expressions in sighted individuals. If retained in blind patients it is called affective blindsight (Tamietto and de Gelder, 2007).

Anxiety disorder

Increased blood flow has been reported in the occipital region in patients with generalized anxiety disorder (Buchsbaum *et al.*, 1987) and with obsessive-compulsive disorder (Zohar *et al.*, 1989). Wik *et al.* (1992) found that blood flow to the secondary visual cortex (BA 18 and BA 19) in subjects with snake phobia was increased over control levels when they viewed images of snakes. The relative blood flow increase seen during visually induced anxiety is limited to BA 18 and 19 (Fredrikson *et al.*, 1997). The increase seen in the visual association area is coupled with a decrease in blood flow to the prefrontal areas (Figure 4.6). The authors propose that the increased activity reflects an externally directed vigilance function. The secondary visual area may take control of limbic areas during visually elicited defense reactions (Fredrikson *et al.*, 1997).

Charles Bonnet syndrome

The Charles Bonnet syndrome is characterized by visual hallucinations following loss of vision, often due to cataracts, glaucoma, or age-related macular degeneration. The hallucinations may be simple or complex and are experienced as amusing or sometimes disturbing but are not emotionally laden events (Wilkinson, 2004). Hallucinations involving color activate the posterior fusiform area; faces the left middle fusiform area, objects the right middle fusiform area, and textures the cortex bordering the collateral sulcus (ffytche *et al.*, 1998).

Other behavioral considerations

Visual objects compete for attention, and it is believed that emotional aspects can operate in a top-down fashion to direct attention to a specific target while simultaneously suppressing attention to peripheral targets (Kastner and Ungerleider, 2001; Pessoa *et al.*, 2002). Signals conveying emotional bias from areas such as the prefrontal cortex and amygdala can alert the occipital lobe to anticipate specific emotion-provoking stimuli, such as looking for a familiar face in a crowd. Pourtois *et al.* (2004) showed that activity in the primary visual cortex was enhanced when viewing fearful faces, suggesting the ability of other areas such as the amygdala to enhance attention to emotional stimuli in a top-down manner.

Age affects visual processing. Davis *et al.* (2008) found that compared with 20-year olds, activity in the occipital region was decreased but increased in the frontal region of 60-year olds, as measured by fMRI. The shift in activity from occipital to frontal lobe was independent of task or degree of difficulty. The authors suggested the shift is a compensation for age-related declines in occipital processing. Chronic alcohol consumption also has an effect. A group of nine detoxified male alcohol-dependent patients showed significantly lower bilateral occipital lobe activation than controls (Hermann *et al.*, 2007).

Parietal lobe

Since the masterful volume by Macdonald Critchley was published in 1953, the parietal lobe has come to be recognized as being heavily involved in the higher cognitive functions of the brain. The parietal lobe receives incoming somatosensory signals, but, unlike the occipital lobe, is involved in far more than processing a single sensory modality. The parietal lobe is integral to the perception of external space, body image, and attention. The complex and fascinating cognitive disturbances that can occur with parietal lobe lesions may at first be mistaken for hysteria. Information perceived and elaborated by the parietal lobe is submitted to the frontal association areas. One may speculate that if the information received by the frontal lobes is inaccurate, delusional perception or ideas could develop.

Functional anatomy

The parietal lobe underlies the parietal bone of the skull. Its anterior border on the lateral aspect is marked by the central sulcus and its posterior border by the parieto-occipital fissure (Figures 2.2, 4.1, 4.2 and 5.1). On the medial aspect it extends inferiorly to the cingulate gyrus, anteriorly to the central sulcus, and posteriorly to the parieto-occipital sulcus. The parietal lobe consists of the primary somatosensory (somesthetic) cortex (BA 1, BA 2, and BA 3), the superior parietal lobule (SPL; BA 5 and BA 7), and the inferior parietal lobule (IPL; BA 39 and BA 40). It makes up about a fifth of the total neocortex.

The anterior parietal lobe, made up of the postcentral gyrus (lateral aspect) and posterior paracentral lobule (medial aspect), is concerned with somatosensory sensations –touch, pain, temperature, and limb position (proprioception).The posterior parietal lobe consisting of BA 7, BA 39, and BA 40 (Mesulam, 1998), integrates somatosensory signals with signals from the visual, auditory, and vestibular systems (sensorimotor integration).

The parietal lobe is important in interacting with the world around us (Table 4.1). It operates on a moment-to-moment basis evaluating and responding to environmental stimuli in a bottom-up manner. Movements are scripted here and may be executed in cooperation with the motor cortex with the permission of the prefrontal cortex. The parietal lobe contains and/or has access to one or more maps. It has its own

Table 4.1. Simplified summary of some functions of the parietal lobe and lesions seen following formation of lesions to either the dominant or nondominant side.

Side of lesion	
Dominant	Nondominant
Superior parietal lobule	
Function	
Spatial-motor	Spatial orientation
Lesion	
Aphasia	Spatial agnosia
Agnosia	Sensory neglect
Astereoagnosia	Astereoagnosia
Agraphesthesia	Agraphesthesia
	Dressing apraxia
Inferior parietal lobule	
Ideomotor/ideational apraxia	Aprosodia
Gerstmann syndrome	
Bilateral	
Balint syndrome	
Movement agnosia	

somatotopic map on the postcentral gyrus and has access to the retinotopic map of the occipital cortex. In order to navigate through space we use maps and landmarks. An allocentric map uses an external frame of reference and as with a road map, we identify direction in terms of north, east, south, and west. An egocentric map is one defined by our current location as seen on an automobile global-positioning (GPS) display. We define directions in the case of an egocentric map as ahead, behind, left and right. The allocentric map belongs to the hippocampus (page 177). The egocentric map appears to be located in the lateral parietal area, more strongly on the right side.

The parietal lobe attends to attractive (salient) environmental targets and locates these targets in terms of map coordinates. Input from the temporal lobe gives it information about a target's identity and from past experience, its anticipated weight, texture, and possible value. The parietal lobe formulates motor plans in cooperation with the frontal lobe and subcortical structures to generate eye, head, arm, and hand movements (and presumably leg movements) to intercept these targets. The motor plans are submitted to the frontal lobes including those areas that act as a repository for socially acceptable behavior. The motor plans will be executed unless deemed socially inappropriate or inhibited by voluntary movements generated independently in the motor areas of the frontal lobe. The motor plan formulated by the parietal lobe may range from eye movements used to read text when sitting quietly, to catching a ball in flight while running. In response to visual and auditory cues, the parietal lobe selects and generates speech appropriate to the current social situation, thus contributing to personality.

The parietal lobe responds in an almost automatic mode to sensory signals and attends to the most salient target (e.g., a red balloon in a sea of blue balloons). This is described as bottom-up processing. In contrast, it can be governed by the frontal lobe to search out for a particular target (e.g., trying to spot your mother-in-law as passengers disembark a plane). This is top-down processing, is not as automatic as bottom-up processing, and can require considerable mental effort (Buschman and Miller, 2007; Womelsdorf et al., 2007).

Primary somatosensory cortex (SI)

The primary somatosensory cortex (SI) occupies the postcentral gyrus (BA 3, BA 1, and BA 2). Projections to the postcentral gyrus include thalamocortical fibers from the ventral posteromedial (VPM) and ventral posterolateral (VPL) nuclei of the thalamus (Table 9.1). These nuclei relay somatosensory signals from both sides of the face and from the contralateral body, respectively. Touch and proprioceptive signals project predominantly to BA 1. Pain signals project to BA 3. A somatotopic map of the contralateral body called a sensory homunculus exists along the postcentral gyrus laterally and extends onto the paracentral lobule medially. The leg and genitalia are represented on the medial aspect of the cortex, with the remainder of the body and head on the lateral aspect. Corticothalamic projections from the primary somatosensory cortex project back to the VPM and VPL thalamic nuclei. Sereno and Huang (2006) showed that the superior part of the postcentral gyrus was activated in response to puffs of air directed to various parts of the face. This appears to be an area that codes for the location of objects near to, or in contact with, the face that might be used in feeding.

A lesion of the primary somatosensory cortex produces a temporary loss of sensation over the contralateral body. Recovery may be almost complete with time. Some loss in muscle control may remain. The parietal lobe supplies fibers to the corticospinal tract that project to the ventral region of the dorsal horn of the spinal cord. Here they are believed to regulate incoming sensory signals. They may also be involved in the level and timing of small groups of synergistic muscles during adjustments to sensory input (Drew et al., 2008).

Association fibers from the primary somatosensory cortex pass through the white matter of the parietal lobe and connect the postcentral gyrus with the somatosensory association areas behind it. These higher-order association areas, including the superior and inferior parietal lobules, integrate touch and conscious proprioception with other sensory modalities.

Rauch et al. (1995) reported that cerebral blood flow increased in the somatosensory cortex, as well as in the frontal, cingulate, insular, and temporal cortices, in subjects with simple phobia when they were provoked (snake, rodent, spider, bees). Subjects reported that tactile imagery was the most prominent sensory aspect of the phobic experience.

Secondary somatosensory cortex (SII) and the parietal operculum

The portion of the parietal lobe that makes up the upper bank of the lateral fissure is the parietal operculum. The parietal operculum immediately inferior to SI contains a secondary somatosensory cortex (SII). SII receives input from SI as well as from VPL and VPM of the thalamus. It occupies much of the parietal operculum and extends deep into the lateral fissure. It may overlap and include part of the insula. SII is somatotopically organized but receives input from both sides of the body.

Four areas of the parietal operculum have been described: OP (OPercular) 1–4. OP 1 and OP 2 lie posteriorly and occupy the inferior part of BA 40. OP 3 and OP 4 correspond roughly with BA 43, which lies at the base of BA 1, BA 2, and BA 3 (SI), and extend anteriorly to border on the insular cortex. Areas OP 1, OP 3, and OP 4 appear to be a part of SII (Eickhoff et al., 2006a). OP 2 lies deep inside the lateral fissure just posterior to the insula. OP 2 is recognized as the primary vestibular area (Eickhoff et al., 2006b).

The anatomy of the parietal lobe varies from individual to individual, including that of the parietal operculum. One variation describes an accessory postcentral gyrus accompanied by a parietal operculum of reduced length (Steinmetz et al., 1990). This variation is suggested to be related to impaired receptive language processing and dyslexia (Kibby et al., 2004). Another variation (Steinmetz type IV) in which the lateral fissure transitions into the postcentral sulcus appears to correlate with dyslexia and superior nonverbal processing (Steinmetz et al., 1990; Chiarello et al., 2006; Craggs et al., 2006).

Superior parietal lobule

Brodmann's areas 5 and 7 on the lateral aspect make up the superior parietal lobule (Figures 4.1 and 4.2). BA 7 on the medial aspect is more commonly referred to as the precuneus and is discussed separately below (Figure 2.2).

The SPL receives heavy input from the primary somatosensory cortex. Cortical association fibers connect it with adjacent cortex, including the occipital lobe, temporal lobe, and insular lobe, thus providing direct access to touch, vision, audition and vestibular signals. Reciprocal fibers connect the SPL with the pulvinar, the anterior cingulate gyrus, and the lateral thalamic nuclei (Chapter 9). Pyramidal cells found in the SPL contribute heavily to fibers that project to the brainstem and to the spinal cord. Efferent fibers from the SPL also project to motor control centers such as the red nucleus, basal ganglia, superior colliculus, and pontine tegmentum. Long association bundles connect the SPL with the frontal lobe (Figure 4.5). Commissural connections through the corpus callosum interconnect the left and right SPLs.

The right (nondominant) SPL is part of the posterior attention system. It is critical in selecting one stimulus location among many. It also disengages and shifts attention to a new target when appropriate (Posner and Dahaene, 1994; Chapter 12). The right side attends to stimuli in both visual fields and accounts for the fact that neglect is more severe following right parietal damage (Posner and Petersen, 1990). Norepinephrine input to the right parietal region is greater than to the left, and norepinephrine primes the cortical neurons during times of heightened arousal to react to novel stimuli (Tucker and Williamson, 1984).

The SPL integrates the sensation of touch and proprioception with vision as well as with audition, marking it as a multimodal integrative area. It is especially important in planning and executing visually guided reaching. It is activated during tactile exploration of objects and body part localization (Binkofski et al., 1999, 2001; Felician et al., 2004), and visuomotor tracking (Grafton et al., 1992), as well as when imagining rotary hand movements (Wolbers et al., 2003). It is also activated during attentional switching, i.e., when visual attention is switched between targets (Rees et al., 2002). The parietal lobe is concerned with selecting and attending to a specific target located on the skin or in the nearby extrapersonal space. Anterior superior parietal association area (BA 5) provides the ability to appreciate the weight and texture of an object held in the hand. The anterior SPL (BA 5 and anterior BA 7) is involved in evaluating the shape and size of objects based on touch (Naito et al., 2008).

The SPL is concerned with "where" a target is located (dorsal visual stream) (Figure 6.10). It provides information about the location of the target including the direction and velocity of movement of that target. It can program a plan designed to intercept the target using saccadic eye movements or hand and body movements. Long association fiber bundles from the SPL to the frontal cortex allow for the accurate execution of the developed plan. The anterior SPL is important in the perception of object shape based on feedback of fine finger movements. The right anterior SPL attends to the object being explored while the left anterior SPL maintains information about object shape in working memory (Stoeckel et al., 2004).

The SPL is part of a dorsal network that functions in spatial attention and includes the frontal lobe. The right SPL appears to be an especially important component of this network (Abdullaev and Posner, 2005; Corbetta et al., 2005). Neurons representing various objects compete for representation and it appears that a top-down mechanism exists to bias the final selection (Bisley and Goldberg, 2003). That is, other areas such as the prefrontal cortex, can alert the SPL to narrow its search to attend to a particular target. Both sides play a role in shifts in attention during this process (Behrmann et al., 2004).

Lesions in the left (dominant) SPL can produce dysphasia and agnosias. The dysphasic patient speaks slowly, makes many grammatical errors, and may be mistakenly labeled uncooperative or confused. A lesion bordering the postcentral gyrus can produce tactile agnosia, in which the patient cannot recall the name of an object by touch alone. With eyes closed a patient with astereoagnosia is unable to name a familiar object held in his or her hand based on the weight and three-dimensional characteristics of the object. A number or letter written on the patient's skin will not be recognized by touch following a lesion in the superior parietal lobule (agraphesthesia).

Precuneus

The precuneus is the medial aspect of the SPL represented by BA 7. It is rarely damaged due to strokes or trauma and its function has been revealed only recently by imaging studies. The neurons are not uniform in shape throughout the precuneus. The anterior portion is characterized by larger neurons and the smaller

A 65-year-old right-handed man had progressive difficulty locating items in space or orienting himself in familiar surrounding. He behaved as if blind, unable to either look at or reach for objects in his environment, such as the buttons on his clothes or utensils for eating. When presented with complex scenes, he could not recognize more than one item at a time (simultanagnosia). He could not identify two adjacent but unlinked drawings, large letters made up of smaller ones, or fragmented pictures. When commanded to move his eyes to specific visual objects in his peripheral fields, he could not do so (oculomotor apraxia). When attempting to reach out and touch objects in his peripheral fields with either arm, he would entirely miss them (optic ataxia). In addition to the visuospatial deficits of Balint syndrome, the patient had other impairments. Despite the absence of motor weakness, he was unable to brush his teeth or wave goodbye with his left upper extremity on verbal command (ideomotor apraxia). His attempts at performing these praxis tasks resulted in grotesque motor movements of his left upper extremity. He also had a slow, rigid gait (parkinsonism), abnormal posturing of his right hand and neck (dystonia), and spontaneous jerking of his extremities (myoclonus). Single photon emission tomography imaging showed decreased perfusion in both parietal regions (Figure 4.7). This patient's illness was consistent with corticobasal degeneration, a disorder that includes cortical deficits such as Balint syndrome and ideomotor apraxia, and basal ganglia deficits, such as parkinsonism and dystonia.

posterior portion is populated with smaller neurons, suggesting a regional difference in the function of the precuneus (Zilles *et al.*, 2003). The precuneus receives multimodal sensory input from the lateral parietal cortex including the superior and inferior lobules as well as from the cortex within the intraparietal sulcus (IPS). It has strong reciprocal connections with the frontal lobe, including the premotor and supplementary motor areas, as well as the dorsolateral and ventromedial prefrontal areas. Intermediate between the precuneus and prefrontal lobe in terms of signal processing is the posterior cingulate and the retrosplenial cortices (BA 30) (Figure 12.1). The retrosplenial cortex has reciprocal connections with the precuneus as well as with the medial temporal lobe including the hippocampus. The precuneus has connections with the dorsal thalamus including the pulvinar. Brainstem connections with structures such as the pretectal area, superior colliculus, and reticular formation as well as the frontal eye fields suggest a role in eye movement control (Leichnetz, 2001; Parvizi *et al.*, 2006). The precuneus is recognized as being involved in four general functions: consciousness, body movements in space, self-awareness, episodic memory retrieval, and visuospatial imagery.

Consciousness

Along with the IPL and the ventromedial, dorsomedial prefrontal, and retrosplenial cortices, the precuneus is highly metabolically active during the resting state (Alkire *et al.*, 2008). The precuneus and the retrosplenial cortex and posterior cingulate gyrus make up the "posteromedial cortex." The precuneus is the most active of these areas consuming about 35% more glucose (Gusnard and Raichle, 2001). The precuneus is believed to be tonically active during the resting, waking state. It continuously gathers and processes information about the world within and around us. It receives visual input from the dorsal visual stream so is constantly monitoring the peripheral visual field. It can choose at any time to shift attention to a novel attractive target unless inhibited by the frontal lobe. Joint activation of the precuneus and prefrontal cortex may underlie a state of reflective self-awareness, and activity correlates with mind-wandering (Kjaer and

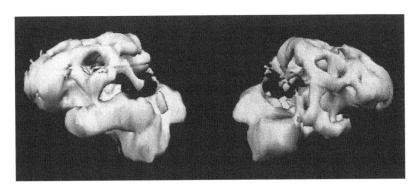

Figure 4.7. This scan is a three-dimensional computerized reconstruction of the patient's single photon emission tomography images. The left hemisphere is on the left side. There are prominent bilateral areas of decreased perfusion in both parietal lobes consistent with his Balint syndrome and ideomotor apraxia. (Reprinted with permission from Mendez, 2000.)

Lou, 2000; Kjaer, et al., 2002). Both these areas show significant deactivation during states of altered consciousness including sleep, hypnosis, dreaming, and persistent vegetative state (Maquet et al., 1997, 1999; Laureys et al., 1999; Rainville et al., 1999; Hobson et al., 2000; Maquet, 2000). Along with the posterior cingulate gyrus, the precuneus becomes progressively deactivated as anesthetic-induced sedation progresses (Alkire et al., 1999; Fiset et al., 1999). It is also one of the first areas to resume activity when consciousness is regained (Laureys et al., 2004, 2006). The precuneus becomes less active during goal-directed cognitive or perceptual tasks, suggesting it is selectively reducing awareness of potentially distracting environmental factors (Gusnard and Raichle, 2001). Its activity is reduced in normal aging but more so in patients with dementia (Lustig et al., 2003).

Body movements in space

The precuneus is activated when preparing to make a movement or when executing a movement in space, especially movements involving pointing, reaching, and saccades. It is activated when an individual just imagines making a movement (Hanakawa, et al., 2003). It also appears to play a key role in attending to a target and shifting attention from one target to another, even if no movement is made (Beauchamp et al., 2001; Simon et al., 2002).

The precuneus is part of a network that elaborates information about maps to help locate one's self on these maps. It can operate using retinotopic coordinates or head-centered coordinates. When imagining moving through an environment with obstacles the precuneus is activated bilaterally along with the right lateral parietal cortex and left supplementary motor cortex (Malouin et al., 2003). It has been suggested that the precuneus acts as the "mind's eye" in these situations, assessing the environment and choosing a navigable route through it (Burgess et al., 2001). In this role it may activate visual images associated with remembered words, objects, and specific autobiographical events as part of episodic memory recall of the meaning of specific environmental landmarks. The anterior precuneus appears to be associated with attention and active recall (visual imagery) whereas the posterior precuneus is more selectively activated during the successful recall of specific events (Cavanna and Trimble, 2006).

Episodic memory retrieval

Evidence suggests that memories of personally experienced events (episodic memory) are retrieved to the precuneus where they are relived and elaborated. It is believed to gather and integrate past information regarding the self and external world especially in the realm of spatial tasks (Gündel et al., 2001; Lou et al., 2004). It provides self-representation, alertness, and "the internal mentation processes of self-consciousness" (Cavanna, 2007).

Self-awareness

Self-awareness includes the recognition of self-ownership and that "I am the initiator of the action and thus that I am causally involved in production of that action" (Gallagher, 2000). Self-awareness allows one to realize that someone else may be the initiator of action in appropriate situations. Action attributed to another produced activity in the right IPL suggesting that it monitors multimodal sensory signals representing movements of both the self and others in an allocentric frame of reference (Farrer and Frith, 2002). The precuneus appears to play a role in self-related tasks whether involving spatial orientation, episodic memory, or social judgments. Along with the posterior cingulate, the precuneus is activated when processing intentions related to the self (Vogeley and Fink, 2003; den Ouden et al. 2005).

The precuneus is believed to be part of a network involved in theory-of-mind processing. Activation of the precuneus and posterior cingulate (BA 31) occurs in situations involving deception and cooperation. It appears to function in a broad sense related to perspective taking as well as attribution, and the processing of emotions and intentions in this situation (Lissek et al., 2008). It shows strong activation when making judgments that require empathy in social situations (Farrow, et al., 2001; Ruby and Decety, 2001). In studies, the left precuneus was preferentially activated when attributing emotions and intentions to the actions of others (Ochsner et al., 2004; Abraham et al., 2008).

Intraparietal sulcus

The IPS (or intraparietal fissure) lies on the lateral aspect, separates the superior from the inferior parietal lobule, and contains the intraparietal cortex. The shape and course of the sulcus are variable but in general it extends from the postcentral sulcus to the occipital lobe. The IPS becomes deeper and its cortex more extensive as it approaches the occipital lobe (Figure 4.8). The more anterior parts in the human are very similar in location to those of the monkey whereas

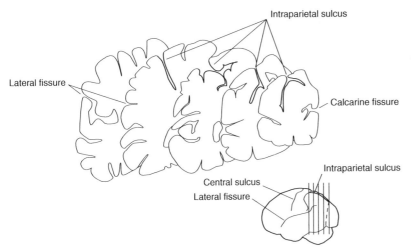

Intraparietal sulcus

Lateral fissure

Calcarine fissure

Intraparietal sulcus

Central sulcus
Lateral fissure

Figure 4.8. The intraparietal sulcus extends from the postcentral sulcus to the occipital lobe. It is the border between the superior and inferior parietal lobules. The sectional views show the depth and complexity of the sulcus as well as the extent of the medial and lateral banks.

those closer to the occipital lobe are more variable. The cortex that makes up the medial and lateral banks within the sulcus has been described as the intraparietal area. It has been subdivided into 17 subregions in the monkey (Lewis and Van Essen, 2000a). The lateral, medial, anterior, ventral, and posterior intraparietal subregions are recognized in the human. The anterior IPS is more concerned with somatosensory processing whereas the posterior IPS processes visual signals. Neurons in the medial bank are more responsive to arm movements, and lateral bank neurons are more responsive to eye movements.

Each area of the IPS functions in response to more than one sensory modality making the cortex of the IPS a multimodal integrative area. The IPS acts to focus attention in space to salient stimuli and especially threat-related stimuli. Fearful faces bias attention toward the threat-related location and increase the gain of face-related signals in the occipital cortex. The timing of these events suggests that negative emotional stimuli can focus attention on a specific location through mechanisms in the IPS (Pourtois and Vuilleumier, 2006).

Information carried by the dorsal visual stream defines target location. Information carried by the ventral visual stream defines target identification. Top-down signals from the frontal lobe can act to preselect targets. An individual in a grocery aisle records the location of all items on the nearby shelf using the dorsal visual stream. The frontal lobe maintains in working memory the specific brand from the shopping list. The ventral visual stream matches the shopping list brand with the package label on the shelf. The ventral visual

stream alerts the dorsal visual stream to create a motor program in the IPS and surrounding region to look at and grasp the desired package ("see and seize").

Lateral intraparietal area (parietal saccade region)

The lateral intraparietal area is one of the most studied subregions in the monkey, in which it makes up the lateral bank of the sulcus near the occipital lobe. In the human the lateral intraparietal area lies close to the occipital lobe but appears to be more medially located in the IPS (Koyama et al., 2004). The lateral intraparietal area receives information regarding objects in the contralateral hemifield. Object location, direction, and velocity are registered, using signals from the visual, auditory, and somatosensory systems (Andersen, 1997; Andersen and Buneo, 2003). It also monitors current eye position with respect to the head and head position and with respect to the body as well as the head's orientation to gravity (i.e., vestibular sense). The lateral intraparietal area determines the relative importance of the object (salience) and then programs and executes a saccade to that object (Ipata et al., 2006). This is a bottom-up control of attention as the attention is determined by the attractiveness of the target (Buschman and Miller, 2007).

Medial intraparietal area (parietal reach region)

A region of the medial bank of the IPS near the occipital lobe and extending laterally onto the surface of the superior parietal lobule is described as the "parietal reach region" (Connolly et al., 2003). It operates in a manner similar to saccade programming but is responsible for planning and executing

45

visually guided reaching movements of the upper limb. Success of the movement is greater if the target is located on the fovea. If the target is in the periphery (e.g., reaching for a cup of coffee while reading the paper) a larger region of parieto-occipital cortex is activated including the precuneus. Continual adjustments are made while reaching for an object in the periphery, suggesting an "automatic pilot" since the individual is unaware of the adjustments (Himmelbach *et al.*, 2006).

Anterior intraparietal area (parietal reach and grasp region)

The anterior intraparietal area is described as the grasp region and occupies the anterior lateral bank of the sulcus (Grol *et al.*, 2007). Neurons of the anterior area are active during fixation and manipulation of objects (Buxbaum *et al.*, 2003). It contains neurons that are sensitive to size, shape, and orientation of objects to be grasped. The objects may be viewed or remembered and the area also monitors hand position and movement (Tunik *et al.*, 2005). The anterior intraparietal area projects to the ventral premotor cortex to provide signals for finger and arm movements involved in reaching and grasping. Pa and Hickok (2007) showed that a region of the anterior intraparietal area was activated by pianists making covert (imagined) playing movements while listening to music, suggesting this is also a region of auditory-manual integration.

Ventral intraparietal area (navigation in space)

The ventral intraparietal area lies deep within the IPS and is believed to contain a crude somatotopic map with most of the map devoted to the head. It receives input from higher order visual processing areas including the middle temporal area (MT) and the middle superior temporal area (MST). It also receives input from motor, somatosensory, auditory, and vestibular areas (Lewis and Van Essen, 2000b). It appears to code for self and object motion and coordinates eye and head movements. Neurons in the ventral intraparietal area are sensitive to the direction and velocity of moving visual targets as well as current head position, velocity, and acceleration. Other neurons in the same area are active during pursuit eye movements (Schlack *et al.*, 2003). Signals from visual, vestibular, and auditory cortices also contribute to the ventral intraparietal area, emphasizing its importance as a multimodal integrative region (Schlack *et al.*, 2002). It plans motor responses to navigate through nearby space while avoiding obstacles (Bremmer, 2005). It may function

to monitor a personal zone of safety surrounding the body (Graziano and Cooke, 2005).

Posterior intraparietal area (three-dimensional analysis)

The posterior intraparietal area in the monkey occupies the lateral bank of the IPS close to the occipital lobe and posterior to the lateral intraparietal area. It receives input from visual areas V3 and V4 and is involved in the analysis of the features of three-dimensional (3D) objects including texture features (Tsutsui *et al.*, 2002). Results indicate that this area is responsible for the short-term memory of object surface features that allows the changing view of an object to be remembered long enough to compare current with past views. Binocular and monocular depth cues and other information from both the dorsal and ventral visual streams are integrated in this region. Signals from the posterior intraparietal region are forwarded to the anterior intraparietal region to code for finger shaping and grasping movements (Grefkes and Fink, 2005).

Lesions involving the IPS may cause neglect or extinction affecting more than one modality. Since the area is head-centered, lesions in this area may account for symptoms seen in visuospatial neglect (Vallar *et al.*, 2003).

In comparison with normally developing controls, IPS depth in children with Asperger syndrome has been reported to be greater. The depth of the IPS correlates with age and IQ (Nordahl *et al.*, 2007). The gray matter density is less in the left IPS in children with dyscalculia (Isaacs *et al.*, 2001). Molko *et al.* (2004) showed that the right IPS was shallower and tended to be shorter in girls with Turner syndrome. This correlated with difficulty during calculation tasks and visuospatial processing.

Inferior parietal lobule

The inferior parietal lobule (IPL) corresponds with the supramarginal gyrus (BA 40) and the angular gyrus (BA 39; Figure 4.2). Further subdivisions have been suggested. Based on its histological and magnetic resonance imaging features, the supramarginal gyrus (BA 40) can be divided into five areas and the angular gyrus (BA 39) into two (Zilles *et al.*, 2003; Caspers *et al.*, 2006). Considerable variability has been found between specimens, as well as left-right differences (asymmetry). The individual variability is believed to be related to the fact that this is one of the last regions of the cortex to mature. The final configuration may be influenced by experience (Caspers *et al.*, 2006). Like the SPL, the IPL has reciprocal connections with the pulvinar and the lateral thalamic nuclei. Short association fibers connect it with nearby occipital and temporal lobes, as well as the SPL and precuneus. Long association fibers link the IPL with the frontal cortex, including the frontal eye fields.

The IPL receives signals representing the sensation of touch, proprioception, and vision and integrates these signals in order to determine the identity of a target (Aguirre and D'Esposito, 1997). The strategic location of the angular gyrus between the occipital lobe and Wernicke's speech area results in it being "the region which turns written language into spoken language and vice versa …" (Geschwind, 1965).

The IPL has been described as where "all the facts can be stored and retrieved" (Bear, 1983). It has also been described as "an association area of association areas" (Geschwind, 1965). Remembering (retrieval of specific content) and knowing (perception that processed information is from the past) activates the IPL as well as portions of the intraparietal sulcus. Remembering also activates the anterior fusiform gyrus bilaterally, which processes visual information related to objects (Wheeler and Buckner, 2004). In one study, the left IPL, extrastriate body area, premotor cortex, and supplementary motor were activated when the viewer saw body movements that were within the range of motor capability of the viewer (i.e., capable of imitation) (Blakemore and Decety, 2001). The IPL plays an important role when the self takes the perspective of others (Ruby and Decety, 2001) and may be part of a "concern mechanism" (Decety and Chaminade, 2003). The IPL functions to encode and retrieve a motor sequence. It is proposed that different areas within the IPL encode different types of sequences. The angular gyrus is particularly involved in evaluating visual messages and selecting an appropriate motor sequence in response (Ruby et al., 2002).

The IPL and the supramarginal gyrus in particular are activated in skill learning (right side) and tool use (left side). It is hypothesized that the supramarginal gyrus stores information about limb and hand positions based on previous experience. Retrieval of a previously formed motor memory may be important in elaborating the skill and adapting it to a new situation (Seidler and Noll, 2008; Vingerhoets, 2008).

Although the left and right IPL are not significantly different in size, asymmetries have been found when sex is included in the analysis. Total IPL volume is greater in males than females and the left IPL is larger in men than women (i.e., leftward asymmetry). The asymmetry is less marked in women in whom

the right IPL is larger than the left (Frederikse et al., 1999; Chen et al., 2007). One subdivision of the supramarginal gyrus (area PFcm) which makes up part of its inferior aspect, accounts for most of the gender difference (Caspers et al., 2008). Weaker leftward asymmetry has been reported for patients with borderline personality disorder. Psychotic symptoms and schizoid personality traits of these patients were correlated with larger right IPL size suggesting a right-sided neurodevelopmental deficit (Irle et al., 2005, 2007). In another study, an increase over controls was observed in the gray matter of the right supramarginal gyrus, which was specific for deficits in social communication and interaction, and repetitive, stereotyped behavior in children with autism spectrum disorder (Brieber et al., 2007).

The supramarginal gyrus of the left IPL works in cooperation with the left dorsolateral prefrontal cortex in support of working memory. Collette et al. (2007) found that these two areas became activated during working memory in control subjects but failed to show activation in patients with posttraumatic stress disorder. This failure in activation appears to reflect a reduction in working memory updating rather than in working memory maintenance operations. The reduction in working memory updating is suggested to relate to the difficulty in concentrating and remembering reported by patients with posttraumatic stress disorder (Moores et al., 2008).

Behavioral considerations

Schizophrenia

Attention deficits are recognized in patients with schizophrenia (Laurens et al., 2005). Since the dorsal visual stream serves areas of the parietal lobe important in attention it has been hypothesized that a defect in this system may underlie attention deficits in this population (Laycock et al., 2007). However, there appears to be limited evidence to support this hypothesis (Skottun and Skoyles, 2008).

Volume reductions were reported for the IPL in patients with schizophrenia (Schlaepfer et al., 1994; Goldstein et al., 1999) and in all parietal subregions in a group of 53 patients with schizophrenia and schizotypal personality disorder (Zhou, et al., 2007). Delusions of passivity in individuals with schizophrenia are associated with hyperactivity coupled with reductions in gray matter volume of the inferior parietal lobe (Dankert et al., 2004; Maruff et al.,

2005). Male but not female patients with schizophrenia have been found to show a reversal of the normal left greater than right angular gyrus (Frederikse *et al.*, 2000; Niznikiewicz *et al.*, 2000). These regions support language and may help explain the language and thought disorders found in schizophrenia (Shenton *et al.*, 2001). Whalley *et al.* (2004) found that during a verbal task subjects at high risk for schizophrenia showed increased activation in the left IPL compared with controls. It was suggested that the overactivation of the IPL is a compensatory action related to attention to task and preparation of a suitable response. Subjects at risk for schizophrenia who showed isolated symptoms, reported difficulties in focusing attention and exhibited a state-related overactivation of the intraparietal sulcus. In another study, gray matter volume was observed to be reduced in the precuneus in men with schizophrenia accompanied by small regions of increased gray matter in the right IPL (Shapleske *et al.*, 2002). The posterior parietal lobe and precuneus have been implicated in distinguishing between self and others (Meltzoff and Decety, 2003).

The IPL is part of frontal-limbic-temporal-parietal network involved in schizophrenia (Torrey, 2007). Reduced asymmetry has been reported for individuals with schizophrenia, with smaller left and larger right IPLs than controls (Frederikse *et al.*, 2000; Niznikiewicz *et al.*, 2000; Nierenberg *et al.*, 2005). The smaller size of the left temporoparietal cortex including the left supramarginal gyrus correlates with the severity of auditory hallucinations in patients with schizophrenia (Gaser *et al.*, 2004).

A group of men with schizophrenia and antisocial personality disorder were compared based on a history of violent behavior with healthy controls, using fMRI. Men with schizophrenia and a history of violent behavior showed reduced activation in the precuneus, right IPL, left frontal gyrus, and anterior cingulate gyrus. Men with antisocial personality disorder also showed reduced activation in the precuneus, left frontal gyrus, and anterior cingulate gyrus. The reduced activation of the right IPL in the subjects with schizophrenia was most strongly associated with ratings of violence. It was hypothesized that the combined involvement of the right IPL and frontal cortex reflected impaired executive control (Kumari *et al.*, 2006). Episodic memory, associated with the precuneus, is reported to be one of the most severely impaired neuropsychological elements in schizophrenia (Reichenberg and Harvey, 2007).

Attention

Three attention networks have been described, all of which involve the parietal cortex. The default network described above is active during resting states (see page 43). It is believed that the default network supports internally directed, mind-wandering processing that includes spontaneous and introspective thoughts, remembering one's role in past events, or planning one's future (Raichle *et al.*, 2001; Fransson and Marrelec, 2008). When either of the other two attention networks (dorsal and ventral) is activated, the default network is suppressed.

Corbetta *et al.* (2000) reported that the dorsal attention network is activated when presented with important external stimuli in a bottom-up manner or when the subject is asked to voluntarily direct attention to a specific cue in a top-down manner. The structures of the dorsal attention network become activated bilaterally and include the cortex of the intraparietal sulcus and the junction of the precentral and superior frontal sulcus (frontal eye field).

The ventral attention network consists of the right temporoparietal junction and the right ventral frontal cortex. When attention is focused, the dorsal network is suppressed to prevent attention to distracting stimuli (Todd *et al.*, 2005). The ventral attention network is thought to act in concert with signals from the dorsal attention network to provide an interrupt or reset signal coincident with shifting attention to a new external target ("Is that my phone ringing?") or to a new thought ("Did I remember to turn off the stove?"). It may be active in reorienting when the individual has no ongoing task; however in most situations it reacts and supports reorientation in response to important novel stimuli selected by the dorsal system (Corbetta *et al.*, 2008).

Spatial neglect

Spatial neglect is considered a visual attention disorder. Patients do not recognize the opposite side of their body and will not dress it (dressing apraxia). Patients are often unaware of the deficit (anosognosia). Inability to correctly copy a simple drawn symmetrical figure (constructional apraxia) is common. The right IPL at the temporoparietal junction traditionally has been implicated (Mort *et al.*, 2003). It has been suggested that there is a map of the contralateral body and peripersonal space in the left IPL, but both an ipsilateral and contralateral map in the right IPL. Loss of the map found in the left hemisphere has little or no effect because of a redundant right hemifield map in the right hemisphere. A lesion in the right hemisphere results in a loss of the map of the left side. It is theorized that since the brain cannot locate objects on the opposite side following a nondominant parietal lobe lesion, the objects cannot be attended to and therefore are ignored.

Spatial neglect can occur following damage to several areas including subcortical sites (caudate nucleus, putamen, and pulvinar), the frontal lobe, and the superior temporal gyrus. Most frequently, however, the IPL and temporoparietal junction in particular, are involved, including the white matter deep to this cortex (Mort *et al.*, 2003; Thiebaut de Schotten *et al.*, 2005). Neglect of personal space correlates with lesions of the supramarginal and postcentral gyri with some involvement of the posterior superior temporal gyrus (Committeri *et al.*, 2007). A lesion restricted to the posterior superior temporal gyrus may also result in spatial neglect (Karnath *et al.*, 2001). Lesions involving white matter pathways between the temporoparietal region and the frontal cortex have been implicated in hemineglect but do not necessarily cause neglect. However, damage to these pathways or to the connections between the dorsal and ventral attention networks may impair shifting from one environment target to another (Doricchi *et al.*, 2008). Since the ventral attention network is localized to the right hemisphere, its loss may inhibit an attempt to direct attention to the contralesional side (He *et al.*, 2007).

Damage to the ventral (temporal) visual stream, concerned with detailed object information, leads to allocentric impairment. Damage to the dorsal (parietofrontal) visual stream results in egocentric deficits (Grimsen *et al.*, 2008). Interestingly, caloric vestibular stimulation has been reported to temporarily improve a number of elements of sensory neglect including anosognosia for left hemiplegia (Vallar *et al.*, 2005; Rode *et al.*, 1998; Bottini *et al.*, 2005). It is proposed that anosognosia of hemiplegia is due to a loss of motor planning ability (Vallar *et al.*, 2003).

Optic ataxia

Optic ataxia can be seen following a lesion on either side involving the dorsal visual processing stream in the posterior superior parietal lobule. It has been seen following lesions in or near the medial IPS (Pisella *et al.*, 2000; Roy *et al.*, 2004). Patients are impaired in the ability to reach for and grasp objects in the contralesional visual field with either hand. Their efforts are inaccurate when using peripheral vision (dorsal visual stream), but accuracy is normal when using foveal vision (ventral visual stream). Pointing errors improve with time in a way that suggests that recovery involves potential interaction between the damaged dorsal visual stream and intact ventral visual stream (Himmelbach and Karnath, 2005; Karnath and Perenin, 2005). The dorsal and ventral streams do not work independently since patients with parietal lesions are usually not successful in completing all visuospatial tasks using intact ventral streams alone (Ellison and Cowey, 2007).

Apraxia

Apraxia is the inability to executed skilled, learned motor acts despite preservation of motor and sensory systems, comprehension, cooperation, and coordination. Ideomotor apraxia is impaired performance in spite of preservation of sensory, motor, and language function (Heilman and Rothi, 2003). The patient cannot perform a meaningful movement of a limb when requested. Many authors include the inability to imitate gestures as part of ideomotor apraxia.

Ideational apraxia is seen as the impaired ability to carry out the appropriate sequential actions of a multistep, complex task. It is a disruption of the space–time movement plan or of its proper activation. The patient cannot form a plan to carry out movements in a proper sequence. Ideational apraxia is associated with lesions of the left parietal lobe alone or in combination with temporal and frontal lesions.

The left parietal lobe is activated when carrying out meaningful limb movements and ideomotor apraxia is seen following a lesion of the left parietal lobe. Since many meaningful movements involve the use of tools, knowledge of the location of tool use is helpful in understanding apraxia and patient rehabilitation (Wheaton, 2007). Specific areas associated with apraxia include the cortex of and around the left IPS and the left middle frontal gyrus (Haaland *et al.*, 2000). Right side lesions can also result in apraxia as well as a lesion of the anterior corpus callosum (Leiguarda and Marsden, 2000; Petreska *et al.*, 2007). A model of praxis proposes that the left inferior parietal lobe is an integrative area that brings together information from the dorsal and ventral visual streams. It is an area that processes representations of body part positions and generates plans for limb movements (Buxbaum *et al.*, 2007). The frontal lobe is responsible for gesture production.

Gerstmann syndrome

Pantomime recognition (recognition of common gestures) may be lost following damage to the dominant IPL. A lesion involving the angular gyrus (BA 39) may produce part or all of Gerstmann syndrome:

- Left–right confusion. (Left–right confusion among neurologically intact adults is seen in 9% of men and 18% of women.)
- Finger agnosia –difficulty in naming fingers.
- Dysgraphia –difficulty with writing.
- Dyscalculia –difficulty with numbers.

Balint syndrome

The patient with Balint syndrome is unable to view the visual field as a whole and is fixed on only one part; a form of tunnel vision (simultanagnosia). Bilateral damage to the posterior IPL, often including adjacent occipital cortex, may produce Balint syndrome:

- Optic apraxia –eyes tend to remain fixed (stuck) on a visual target, although spontaneous eye movements are unaffected.
- Optic ataxia –a deficit in using visual guidance to grasp an object.
- Simultanagnosia –seeing only the components of a visual object; unable to see the object as a whole.

Bilateral damage to the occipitoparietal area, often extending deep enough to involve the precuneus is the most common cause of this disorder (Raichle *et al.*, 2001).

Other considerations

A lesion involving the nondominant IPL may produce a deficit in processing the nonsyntactic component of language (aprosodia). In this situation, patients fail to appreciate aspects of a verbal message that are conveyed by the tone, loudness, and timing of the words (i.e., emotional tone).

Van Essen *et al.* (2006) found that subjects with William syndrome showed reduced asymmetry of the lateral fissure and no asymmetry in the superior temporal sulcus compared with controls. The authors suggested that in light of the relatively intact language skills and heightened emotional responses to music in William syndrome subjects, the abnormalities in cortical folding might reflect altered cortical circuitry rather than a simple size reduction.

Individuals with borderline personality disorder have been shown to have reduced size of the parietal lobes. The right precuneus has been shown to exhibit reduced resting glucose metabolism and reduced size in individuals with borderline personality disorder (Lange *et al.*, 2005; Irle *et al.*, 2007). The right postcentral gyrus was shown to be larger in individuals with a comorbid diagnosis of dissociative amnesia or dissociative identity disorder. Individuals with borderline personality disorder have also been reported to have elevated pain thresholds coupled with reduced activity in the precuneus in response to pain (Schmahl *et al.*, 2006). Irle *et al.* (2007) suggested that the smaller precuneus may relate to symptoms of depersonalization. The increased postcentral gyrus has been speculated to relate to the dissociative amnesia or dissociative identity disorder reflecting severe childhood abuse (Lange *et al.*, 2005; Irle *et al.*, 2007).

Parietal lobe seizures can produce bizarre and transient symptoms that can be confusing to both patients and clinicians. Feelings of paresthesia, numbness, heat, or cold have been described. These feelings can begin locally and spread to other contiguous body parts. Seizures beginning more posteriorly can cause pronounced distortion of body image. Limbs may feel heavier or feel as if they disappear. Even more bizarre, patients have reported feeling that someone is standing close by or the appearance of a phantom third limb. Patients with newly diagnosed schizophrenia are reported to show greater sulcal enlargement in the parietal lobe (Rubin *et al.*, 1993).

The similarities between hysteria and parietal lobe disease should again be stressed. Patients with parietal lobe lesions may show marked inconsistency in task performances, such that he or she may succeed in a task that moments before appeared to be impossible.

Select bibliography

Critchley, M. *The Parietal Lobes.* (London: Edward Arnold, 1953.)

Hecaen, H., and Albert, M.L. *Human Neuropsychology.* (New York: Wiley, 1978.)

Hyvarinen, J. *The Parietal Cortex of Monkey and Man.* (New York: Springer-Verlag, 1982.)

Lishman, W.A. *Organic Psychiatry* (2nd ed.). (Boston: Blackwell Scientific, 1987.)

Milner, A.D., and Goodale, M.A. *The Visual Brain in Action* (2nd ed.). Oxford Psychology Series. (New York: Oxford University Press, 2006.)

Siegel, A.M., Andersen, R.A., Freund, H-J., and Spencer, D.D. *The Parietal Lobes*. Advances in Neurology, Volume 93. (Baltimore: Lippincott Williams & Wilkins, 2003.)

Tilney, F., and Riley, H.A. *The Form and Functions of the Central Nervous System: An Introduction to the Study of Nervous Diseases* (3rd ed.). (New York: Hoeber, 1938.)

Zeki, S. *A Vision of the Brain.* (Boston: Blackwell Scientific Publications, 1993.)

References

Abdullaev, Y., and Posner, M.I. 2005. How the brain recovers following damage. *Nat. Neurosci.* **8**:1424–1425.

Abraham, A., Werning, M., Rakoczy, H., Yves von Cramon, D., and Schubotz, R.I. 2008. Minds, persons, and space: An fMRI investigation into the relational complexity of higher-order intentionality. *Conscious Cogn.* **17**:438–450.

Aguirre, G.K., and D'Esposito, M. 1997. Environmental knowledge is subserved by separable dorsal/ventral neural areas. *J. Neurosci.* **17**:2512–2518.

Alkire, M.T., Pomfrett, C.J.D., Haier, R.J., Gianzero, M.V., Chan, C.M., Jacobsen, B.P., and Fallon, J.H. 1999. Functional brain imaging during anesthesia in humans: Effects of halothane on global and regional cerebral glucose metabolism. *Anesthesiology* **90**:701–709.

Alkire, M.T., Hudetz, A.G., and Tononi, G. 2008. Consciousness and anesthesia. *Science* **322**:876–880.

Andersen, R.A. 1997. Multimodal integration for the representation of space in the posterior parietal cortex. *Phil. Trans. R. Soc. Lond. B* **352**:1421–1428.

Andersen, R.A., and Buneo, C.A. 2003. Senorimotor integration in posterior parietal cortex. *Adv. Neurol.* **93**:159–177.

Anderson, S.W., and Rizzo, M. 1994. Hallucinations following occipital lobe damage: The pathological activation of visual representations. *J. Clin. Exp. Neuropsychol.* **16**:651–653.

Astafiev, S.V., Stanley, C.M., Shulman, G.L., and Corbetta, M. 2005. Extrastriate body area in human occipital cortex responds to the performance of motor actions. *Nat. Neurosci.* **7**:542–548.

Bear, D.M. 1983. Hemispheric specialization and the neurology of emotion. *Arch. Neurol.* **40**:95–202.

Beauchamp, M.S., Petit, L., Ellmore, T.M., Ingeholm, J., and Haxby, J.V. 2001. A parametric fMRI study of overt and covert shifts of visuo-spatial attention. *Neuroimage* **14**:310–321.

Becker, H.G.T., Erb, M., and Haarmeier, T. 2009. Differential dependency on motion coherence in subregions of the human MT+ complex. *Eur. J. Neurosci.* **28**:1674–1685.

Behrens, T.E.J., Johansen-Berg, H., Woolrich, M.W., Smith, S.M., Wheeler-Kingshott, C.A.M., Boulby, P.A.,

Barker, G.J., Sillery, E.L., Sheehan, K., Ciccarelli, O., Thompson, A.J., Brady, J.M., and Matthews, P.M. 2003. Non-invasive mapping of connections between human thalamus and cortex using diffusion imaging. *Nat. Neurosci.* **6**:750–757.

Behrmann, M., Geng, J.J., and Shomstein, S. 2004. Parietal cortex and attention. *Curr. Opin. Neurobiol.* **14**:212–217.

Binkofski, F., Buccino, G., Stephan, K.M., Rizzolatti, G., Seitz, R.J., and Freund, H-J. 1999. A parieto-premotor network for object manipulation: evidence from neuroimaging. *Exp. Brain Res.* **128**:210–213.

Binkofski, F., Kunesch, E., Classen, J., Seitz, R.J., and Freund, H-J. 2001. Tactile apraxia: unimodal apractic disorder of tactile object exploration associated with parietal lobe lesions. *Brain* **124**:132–144.

Bisley, J.W., and Goldberg, M.E. 2003. Neuronal activity in the lateral intraparietal area and spatial attention. *Science* **299**:81–86.

Blakemore, S-J., and Decety, J. 2001. From the perception of action to the understanding of intention. *Nat. Rev. Neurosci.* **2**:561–567.

Bottini, G., Paulesu, E., Gandola, M., Loffredo, S., Scarpa, P., Sterzi, R., Santilli, I., Defanti, C.A., Scialfa, G., Fazio, F., and Vallar, G. 2005. Left caloric vestibular stimulation ameliorates right hemianesthesia. *Neurology* **65**:1278–1283.

Bremmer, F. 2005. Navigation in space –the role of the macaque ventral intraparietal area. *J. Physiol.* **566**:29–35.

Bridge, H., Thomas, O., Jbabdi, S., and Cowey, A. 2008. Changes in connectivity after visual cortical brain damage underlie altered visual function. *Brain* **131**:1433–1444.

Brieber, S., Neufang, S., Burning, N., Kamp-Becker, I., Remschmidt, H., Herpertz-Dahlmann, B., Fink, G.R., and Konrad, K. 2007. Structural brain abhnormalities in adolescents with autism spectrum disorder and patients with attention deficit/hyperactivity disorder. *J. Child Psychol. Psychiatry* **48**:1251–1258.

Britten, K.H. 2008. Mechanisms of self-motion perception. *Annu. Rev. Neurosci.* **31**:389–410.

Buchsbaum, M.S., Wu, J., Haier, R., Hazlett, E., Ball, R., Katz, M., Sokolski, K., Lagunas-Solar, M., and Langer, D. 1987. Positron emission tomography assessment of effects of benzodiazepines on regional glucose metabolic rate in patients with anxiety disorder. *Life Sci.* **40**:2393–2400.

Burgess, N., Becker, S., King, J.A., and O'Keefe, J. 2001. Memory for events and their spatial context: models and experiments. *Phil. Trans. R. Soc. Lond. B* **356**:1493–1503.

Buschman, T.J., and Miller, E.K. 2007. Top-down versus bottom-up control of attention in the prefrontal and posterior parietal cortices. *Science* **315**:1860–1862.

Buxbaum, L.J., Sirigu, A., Schwartz, M.F., and Klatzky, R.L. 2003. Cognitive representations of hand posture in ideomotor apraxia. *Neuropsychologia* **41**: 1091–1113.

Buxbaum, L.J., Kyle, K., Grossman, M., and Coslett, H.B. 2007. Left inferior parietal representations for skilled hand-object interactions: evidence from stroke and corticobasal degeneration. *Cortex* **43**:411–423.

Caspers, S., Geyer, S., Schleicher, A., Mohlberg, H., Amunts, K., and Zilles, K. 2006. The human inferior parietal cortex: cytoarchitectonic parcellation in interindividual variability. *Neuroimage* **33**:430–448.

Caspers, S., Eickhoff, S.B., Geyer, S., Scheperjans, F., Mohlberg, H., Zilles, K., and Amunts, K. 2008. The human inferior parietal lobule in Stereotaxic space. *Brain Struct. Funct.* **212**:481–495.

Cavanna, A.E. 2007. The precuneus and consciousness. *CNS Spectrums* **12**:545–552.

Cavanna, A.E., and Trimble, M.R. 2006. The precuneus: a review of its functional anatomy and behavioural correlates. *Brain* **129**:564–583.

Chen, X., Sachdev, P.S., Wen, W., and Anstey, K.J. 2007. Sex differences in regional gray matter in healthy individuals aged 44–48 years: A voxel-based morphometric study. *Neuroimage* **36**:691–699.

Chiarello, C., Lomvardino, L.J., Kacinik, N.A., Otto, R., and Leonard, C.M. 2006. Neuroanatomical and behavioral asymmetry in an adult compensated dyslexic. *Brain Lang.* **98**:169–181.

Collette, F., Van der Linden, M., Laureys, S., Arigoni, F., Delfiore, G., Degueldre, C.L.A., and Salmon, E. 2007. Mapping the updating process: common and specific brain activations across different versions of the running span task. *Cortex* **43**:146–158.

Committeri, G., Pitzalis, S., Galati, G., Patria, F., Pelle, G., Sabatini, U., Castriota-Scanderbeg, A., Piccardi, L., Guariglia, C., and Pizzamiglio, L. 2007. Neural bases of personal and extrapersonal neglect in humans. *Brain* **130**:431–441.

Connolly, J.D., Andersen, R.A., and Goodale, M.A. 2003. FMRI evidence for a 'parietal reach region' in the human brain. *Exp. Brain Res.* **153**:140–145.

Corbetta, M., Kincade, J.M., Ollinger, J.M., McAvoy, M.P., and Shulman, G.L. 2000. Voluntary orienting is dissociated from target detection in human posterior parietal cortex. *Nat. Neurosci.* **3**:292–297.

Corbetta, M., Tansy, A.P., Stanley, C.M., Astafiev, S.V., Snyder, A.Z., and Shulman, G.L. 2005. A functional MRI study of preparatory signals for spatial location and objects. *Neuropsychologia* **43**:2041–2056.

Corbetta, M., Patel, G., and Shulman, G. 2008. The reorienting system of the human brain: From environment to theory of mind. *Neuron* **58**: 306–324.

Craggs, J.G., Sanchez, J., Kibby, M.Y., Gilger, J.W., and Hynd, G.W. 2006. Brain morphology and neuropsychological profiles in a family displaying dyslexia and superior nonverbal intelligence. *Cortex* **42**:1107–1118.

Critchley, M. 1964. The problem of visual agnosia. *J. Neurol. Sci.* **1**:274–290.

Dankert, K., Saoud, M., and Maruff, P. 2004. Attention, motor control and motor imagery in schizophrenia: implications for the role of the parietal cortex. *Schizophr. Res.* **70**:241–261.

David, N., Cohen, M.X., Newen, A., Bewernick, B.H., Shah, N.J., Fink, G.R., and Vogeley, K. 2007. The extrastriate cortex distinguishes between the consequences of one's own and others' behavior. *Neuroimage* **36**:1004–1014.

Davis, S.W., Dennis, N.A., Daselaar, S.M., Fleck, M.S., and Cabeza, R. 2008. Qué PASA? The posterior-anterior shift in aging. *Cereb. Cortex* **18**:1201–1209.

d'Avossa, G., Tosetti, M., Crespi, S., Biagi, L, Burr, D.C., and Morrone, M.C. 2006. Spatiotopic selectivity of BOLD responses to visual motion in human area MT. *Nat. Neurosci.***10**:249–255.

Decety, J., and Chaminade, T. 2003. Neural correlates of feeling sympathy. *Neuropsychologia* **41**:127–138.

den Ouden, H.E.M., Frith, U., Frith, C., and Blakemore, S-J. 2005. Thinking about intentions. *Neuroimage* **28**:787–796.

DeRenzi, E., and Spinnler, H. 1967. Impaired performance on color tasks in patients with hemispheric damage. *Cortex* **3**:194–216.

Devinsky, O., Bear, D., and Volpe, B.T. 1988. Confusional states following posterior cerebral artery infarction. *Arch. Neurol.* **45**:160–163.

Doricchi, F., Thiebaut de Schotten, M., Tomaiuolo, F., and Bartolomeo, P. 2008. White matter (dis)connections and gray matter (dys)functions in visual neglect: Gaining insights into the brain networks of spatial awareness. *Cortex* **44**:983–995.

Downing, P.E., Jiang, Y., Shuman, M., and Kanwisher, N. 2001. A cortical area selective for visual processing of the human body. *Science* **293**:2470–2473.

Drew, T., Anjujar, J-E., Lajoie, K., and Yakovenko, S. 2008. Cortical mechanisms involved in visuomotor coordination during precision walking. *Brain Res. Rev.* **57**:199–211.

Eickhoff, S.B., Schleicher, A., Zilles, K., and Amunts, K. 2006a. The human parietal operculum. II. Stereotaxic maps and correlation with functional imaging results. *Cereb. Cortex* **16**:268–279.

Eickhoff, S.B., Weiss, P.H., Amunts, K., Fink, G.R., and Zilles, K. 2006b. Identifying human parieto-insular vestibular cortex using fMRI and cytoarchitectonic mapping. *Hum. Brain Mapp.* **27**:611–621.

Ellison, A., and Cowey, A. 2007. Time course of the involvement of the ventral and dorsal visual processing streams in a visuospatial task. *Neuropsychologia* **45**:3335–3339.

Farrer, C., and Frith, C.D. 2002. Experiencing oneself vs another person as being the cause of an action: the neural correlates of the experience of agency. *Neuroimage* **15**:596–603.

Farrow, T.F., Zheng, Y., Wilkinson, I.D., Spence, S.A., Deakin, J.F., Tarrier, N., Griffiths, P.D., and Woodruff, P.W. 2001. Investigating the functional anatomy of empathy and forgiveness. *Neuroreport* **12**:2433–2438.

Felician, O., Romaiguere, P., Anton, J-L., Nazarian, B., Roth, M., Poncet, M., and Roll, J-P. 2004. The role of the human left superior parietal lobule in body part localization. *Ann. Neurol.* **55**:749–751.

ffytche, D.H., Howard, R.J., Brammer, M.J., David, A., Woodruff, P., and Williams, S. 1998. The anatomy of conscious vision: an fMRI study of visual hallucinations. *Nat. Neurosci.* **1**:1247–1260.

Fiset, P., Paus, T., Daloze, T., Plourde, G., Meuret, P., Bonhomme, V., Hajj-Ali, N., Backman, S., and Evans, A.C. 1999. Brain mechanisms of propofol-induced loss of consciousness in humans: a positron emission tomographic study. *J. Neurosci.* **19**:5506–5513.

Fransson, P., and Marrelec, G. 2008. The precuneus/ posterior cingulate cortex plays a pivotal role in the default mode network: Evidence from a partial correlation network analysis. *Neuroimage* **42**:1178– 1184.

Fredrikson, M., Fischer, H., and Wik, G. 1997. Cerebral blood flow during anxiety provocation. *J. Clin. Psychiatry* **58**(Suppl. 16):16–21.

Frederikse, M., Lu, A., Aylward, E., Barta, P., Sharma, T., and Pearlson, G. 2000. Sex differences in inferior parietal lobule volume in schizophrenia. *Am. J. Psychiatry* **157**:422–427.

Frederikse, M.E., Lu, A., Aylward, E.H., Barta, P.E., and Pearlson, G.D. 1999. Sex differences in the inferior parietal lobule. *Cereb. Cortex* **9**:896–901.

Frederikse, M.E., Lu, A., Aylward, E., Barta, P., Sharma, T., and Pearlson, G. 2000. Sex differences in inferior parietal lobule volume in schizophrenia. *Am. J. Psychiatry* **157**:422–427.

Gallagher, S. 2000. Philosophical conceptions of the self: Implications for cognitive science. *Trends Cogn. Sci.* **4**:14–21.

Gaser, C., Nenadic, I., Volz, H.P., Büchel, C., and Sauer, H. 2004. Neuroanatomy of 'hearing voices': a frontotemporal brain structural abnormality associated with auditory hallucinations in schizophrenia. *Cereb. Cortex* **14**:91–96.

Geschwind, N. 1965. Disconnection syndromes in animals and man. Part I and II. *Brain* **88**:237–294, 585–644.

Goldstein, J.M., Goodman, J.M., Seidman, L.J., Kennedy, D.N., Makris, N., Lee, H., Tourville, J., Caviness, V.S. Jr., Faraone, S.V., and Tsuang, M.T. 1999. Cortical abnormalities in schizophrenia identified by structural magnetic resonance imaging. *Arch. Gen. Psychiatry* **56**:537–547.

Grafton, S.T., Mazziotta, J.C., Woods, R.P., and Phelps, M.E. 1992. Human functional anatomy of visually guided finger movements. *Brain* **115**:565–587.

Graziano, M.S.A., and Cooke, D.F. 2005. Parieto-frontal interactions, personal space, and defensive behavior. *Neuropsychologia* **44**:845–859.

Grefkes, C., and Fink, G.R. 2005. The functional organization of the intraparietal sulcus in humans and monkeys. *J. Anat.* **207**:3–17.

Grimsen, C., Hildebrandt, H., and Fahle, M. 2008. Dissociation of egocentric and allocentric coding of space in visual search after right middle cerebral artery stroke. *Neuropsychologia* **46**:902–914.

Grol, M.J., Majdandžic, J., Stephan, K.E., Verhagen, L., Kijkerman, H.C., Bekkering, H., Verstraten, F.A.J., and Toni, I. 2007. Parieto-frontal connectivity during visually guided grasping. *J. Neurosci.* **27**:11877– 118887.

Gündel, H., O'Connor, M-F., Littrell, L., Fort, C., and Lane, R.D. 2001. Functional neuroanatomy of Grief: An fMRI study. *Am. J. Psychiatry* **160**:1946–1953.

Gusnard, D.A., and Raichle, M.E. 2001. Searching for a baseline: functional imaging and the resting human brain. *Nat. Rev. Neurosci.* **2**:685–694.

Haaland, K.Y., Harrington, D.L., and Knight, R.T. 2000. Neural representations of skilled movement. *Brain* **123**:2306–2313.

Hadjikhani, N., Sanchez del Rio, M., Wu, O., Schwartz, E., Bakker, D., Fischl, B., Kwong, K.K., Cutrer, F.M., Rosen, B.R., Tootel, R.H., Sorensen, A.G., and Moskowitz, M.A. 2001. Mechanisms of migraine aura revealed by functional MRI in human visual cortex. *Proc. Natl. Acad. Sci. USA.* **98**:4687–4692.

Hanakawa, T., Immisch, I., Toma, K, Dimyan, M.A., Van Gelderen, P., and Hallett, M. 2003. Functional properties of brain areas associated with motor execution and imagery. *J. Neurophysiol.* **89**:989–1002.

He, B.J., Snyder, A.Z., Vincent, J.L., Epstein, A., Shulman, G.L., and Corbetta, M. 2007. Breakdown of functional connectivity in frontoparietal networks underlies behavioral deficits in spatial neglect. *Neuron* **53**: 905–918.

Hecaen, H., and Albert, M.L. 1978. *Human Neuropsychology.* (New York: Wiley.)

Heilman, K.M., and Rothi, L.J.G. 2003. Apraxia. In: K.M.Heilman and E.Valenstein (eds.) *Clinical Neuropsychology.* (New York: Oxford University Press, pp. 215–235.)

Hendry, S.H.C., and Reid, R.C. 2000. The koniocellular pathway in primate vision. *Annu. Rev. Neurosci.* **23**: 127–153.

Hermann, D., Smolka, M.N., Klein, S., Heinz, A., Mann, K., and Braus, D.F. 2007. Reduced fMRI activation of an occipital area in recently detoxified alcohol-dependent patients in a visual and acoustic paradigm. *Addict. Biol.* **12**:117–121.

Himmelbach, M., and Karnath, H-O. 2005. Dorsal and ventral stream interaction: contributions from optic ataxia. *J. Cogn. Neurosci.* **17**:632–640.

Himmelbach, M., Karnath, H.-O., Perenin, M.-T., Franz, V.H., and Stockmeier, K. 2006. A general deficit of the 'automatic pilot' with posterior parietal cortex lesions? *Neuropsychologia* **44**:2749–2756.

Hobson, J.A., Pace-Schott, E.F., and Stickgold, R. 2000. Dreaming and the brain; Toward a cognitive neuroscience of conscious states. *Behav. Brain Sci.* **23**:793–1121.

Ipata, A.E., Gee, A.L., Goldberg, M.E., and Bisley, J.W. 2006. Activity in the lateral intraparietal area predicts the goal and latency of saccades in a free-viewing visual search task. *J. Neurosci.* **26**:3656–3661.

Irle, E., Lange, E., and Sachsse, U. 2005. Reduced size and abnormal asymmetry of parietal cortex in women with borderline personality disorder. *Biol. Psychiatry* **57**:173–182.

Irle, E., Lange, E., Weniger, G., and Sachsse, U. 2007. Size abnormalities of the superior parietal cortices are related to dissociation in borderline personality disorder. *Psychiatry Res.* **156**:139–149.

Isaacs, E.B., Edmonds, C.J., Lucas, A., and Gadian, D.G. 2001. Calculation difficulties in children of very low birthweight: A neural correlate. *Brain* **124**:1701–1707.

James, T.W., Culham, J., Humphrey, G.K., Milner, A.D., and Goodale, M.A. 2003. Ventral occipital lesions impair object recognition but not object-directed grasping: an fMRI study. *Brain* **126**:2463–2475.

Joseph, R. 1996. *Neuropsychology, Neuropsychiatry, and Behavioral Neurology.* Baltimore: Williams and Wilkins.

Karnath, H-O., and Perenin, M-T. 2005. Cortical control of visually guided reaching: evidence from patients with optic ataxia. *Cereb. Cortex* **15**:1561–1569.

Karnath, H.-O., Ferber, S., and Himmelbach, M. 2001. Spatial awareness is a function of the temporal not the posterior parietal lobe. *Nature* **411**:950–953.

Kastner, A., and Ungerleider, L.G. 2001. The neural basis of biased competition in human visual cortex. *Neuropsychologia* **39**:1263–1276.

Kibby, M.Y., Kroese, J.M., Morgan, A-E., Hiemenz, J.R., Cohen, M.J., and Hynd, G.W. 2004. The relationship between perisylvian morphology and verbal short term functioning in children with neurodevelopmental disorders. *Brain Lang.* **89**:122–135.

Koyama, M., Hasegawa, I., Osada, T., Adachi, Y., Nakahara, K., and Miyashita, Y. 2004. Functional magnetic resonance imaging of macaque monkeys performing visually guided saccade tasks: comparison of cortical eye fields with humans. *Neuron* **41**:795–807.

Kjaer, T.W., and Lou, H.C. 2000. Interaction between precuneus and dorsolateral prefrontal cortex may play a unitary role in consciousness: a principal component of analysis of rCBF. *Conscious Cogn.* **9**:S59.

Kjaer, T.W., Nowak, M., and Lou, H.C. 2002. Reflective self-awareness and conscious states: PET evidence for a common midline parietofrontal core. *Neuroimage* **17**:1080–1086.

Kumari, V., Aasen, I., Taylor, P., Ffytche, D.H., Das, M., Barkataki, I., Goswami, S., O'Connell, P., Howlett, M., Williams, S.C.R., and Sharma, T. 2006. Neural dysfunction and violence in schizophrenia: an fMRI investigation. *Schizophr. Res.* **84**:144–164.

Lange, C., Kracht, L., Herholz, K., Sachsse, U., and Irle, E. 2005. Reduced glucose metabolism in temporo-parietal cortices of women with borderline personality disorder. *Psychiatry Res.* **139**:115–126.

Laurens, K.R., Kiehl, D.A., Bates, A.T., and Liddle, P.F. 2005. Attention orienting dysfunction during salient stimulus processing in schizophrenia. *Schizophr. Res.* **75**:159–171.

Laureys, S., Goldman, S., Phillips, C., Van Bogaert, P., Aerts, J., Luxen, A., Franck, G., and Maquet, P. 1999. Impaired effective cortical connectivity in vegetative state. *Neuroimage* **9**:377–382.

Laureys, S., Owen, A.M., and Schiff, N.D. 2004. Brain function in coma, vegetative state and related disorders. *Lancet Neurol.* **3**:537–546.

Laureys, S., Boly, Mélanie, B., and Maquet, P. 2006. Tracking the recovery of consciousness from coma. *J. Clin. Invest.* **116**:1823–1825.

Laycock, R., Crewther, S.G., and Crewther, D.P. 2007. Attention orienting dysfunction during salient novel stimulus processing in schizophrenia. *Schizophr. Res.* **75**:159–171

Leichnetz, G.R. 2001. Connections of the medial posterior parietal cortex (area 7m) in the monkey. *Anat. Rec.* **263**, 215–236.

Leiguarda, R.C., and Marsden, C.D. 2000. Limb apraxias: higher-order disorders of sensorimotor integration. *Brain* **123**:860–879.

Lewis, J.W., and Van Essen, D.C. 2000a. Mapping of architectonic subdivisions in the macaque monkey, with emphasis on parieto-occipital cortex. *J. Comp. Neurol.* **428**:79–111.

Lewis, J.W., and Van Essen, D.C. 2000b. Corticocortical connections of visual, sensorimotor, and multimodal processing areas in the parital lobe of the macaque monkey. *J. Comp. Neurol.* **428**:112–137.

Lou, H.C., Luber, B., Crupain, M., Keenan, J.P., Nowak, M., Kjaer, T.W., Sackeim, H.A., and Lisanby, S.H. 2004.

Parietal cortex and representation of the mental self. *Proc. Natl. Acad. Sci. USA*. **101**:6827–6832.

Lustig, C., Snyder, A.Z., Bhakta, M., O'Brien, K.C., McAvoy, M., Raichle, M.E., Morris, J.C., and Buckner, R.L. 2003. Functional deactivations: change with age and dementia of the Alzheimer type. *Proc. Natl. Acad. Sci. USA*. **100**:14504–14509.

Malouin, F., Richards, C.L., Jackson, P.L., Dumans, F., and Doyon, J. 2003. Brain activations during motor imagery of locomotor-related tasks: a PET study. *Hum. Brain Mapp*. **19**:47–62.

Maquet, P. 2000. Functional neuroimaging of normal human sleep by positron emission tomography. *J. Sleep Res*. **9**:207–231.

Maquet, P., Degueldre, C., Delfiore, G., Aerts, J., Péters, J-M., Luxen, A., and Georges Franck, G. 1997. Functional neuroanatomy of human slow wave sleep *J. Neurosci*. **17**:2807–2812.

Maquet, P., Faymonville, M.E., Degueldre, C., Delfiore, G., Franck, G., Luxen, A., and Lamy, M. 1999. Functional neuroanatomy of hypnotic state. *Biol. Psychiatry* **45**:327–333.

Maruff, P., Wood, S.J., Velakoulis, D., Smith, D.J., Soulsby, B., Suckling, J., Bullmore, E.T., and Pantelis, C. 2005. Reduced volume of parietal and frontal association areas in patients with schizophrenia characterized by passivity delusions. *Psychol. Med*. **35**:783–789.

Mendez, M.F. 2000. Corticobasal ganglionic degeneration with Balint's syndrome. *J. Neuropsychiatry Clin. Neurosci*. **12**:273–275.

Mendez, M.F. 2001. Visuospatial deficits and preserved reading ability in a patient with posterior cortical atrophy. *Cortex* **37**:535–543.

Meltzoff, A.N., and Decety, J. 2003. What imitation tells us about social cognition: a rapprochement between developmental psychology and cognitive neuroscience. *Phil. Trans. R. Soc. Lond. B* **358**:491–500.

Mesulam, M.M. 1998. From sensation to cognition. *Brain* **121**:1013–1052.

Mitelman, S.A., and Buchsbaum, M.S. 2007. Very poor outcome schizophrenia: Clinical and neuroimaging aspects. *Int. Rev. Psychiatry* **19**:347–359.

Molko, N., Cachia, A., Riviere, D., Mangin, J.R., Bruander, M., LeBihan, D., Cohen, L., and Dehaene, S. 2004. Brain anatomy in Turner Syndrome: Evidence for impaired social and spatial-numerical networks. *Cereb. Cortex* **14**:840–850.

Moores, K.A., Clark, C.R., McFarlane, A.C., Brown, G.C., Puce, A., and Taylor, D.J. 2008. Abnormal recruitment of working memory updating networks during maintenance of trauma-neutral information in post-traumatic stress disorder. *Psychiatry Res* **163**:156–170.

Morland, A.B., Le, S., Carroll, E., Hoffmann, M.B., and Pambakian, A. 2004. The role of spared calcarine cortex and lateral occipital cortex in the responses of human hemianopes to visual motion. *J. Cogn. Neurosci*. **16**:204–218.

Moro, V., Urgesi, C., Pernigo, S., Lanteri, P., Pazzaglia, M., and Aglioti, S.M. 2008. The neural basis of body form and body action agnosia. *Neuron* **60**:235–246.

Mort, D.J., Malhotra, P., Mannan, S.K., Rorden, C., Pambakian, A., Kennard, C., and Husain, M. 2003. The anatomy of visual neglect. *Brain* **126**:1986–1997.

Nagaratnam, N., Virk, S., and Brdarevic, O. 1996. Musical hallucinations associated with recurrence of a right occipital meningioma. *Br. J. Clin. Pract*. **50**:56–57.

Naito, E., Scheperjans, F., Eickhoff, S.B., Amuns, K., Roland, P.E., Zilles, K., and Ehrsson, H.H. 2008. Human superior parietal lobule is involved in somatic perception of bimanual interaction with an external object. *J. Neurophysiol*. **99**:695–703.

Nierenberg, J., Salisbury, D.F., Levitt, J.J., David, E.A., McCarley, R.W., and Shenton, M.E. 2005. Reduced left angular gyrus volume in first-episode schizophrenia. *Am. J. Psychiatry* **162**:1539–1541.

Niznikiewicz, M., Donnino, R., McCarley, R.W., Nestor, P.G., Iosifescu, D.V., O'Donnell, B., Levitt, J., and Shenton M.E. 2000. Abnormal angular gyrus asymmetry in schizophrenia. *Am. J. Psychiatry* **157**:428–437.

Nordahl, C.W., Dierker, D., Mostafavi, I., Schumann, C.M., Rivera, S.M., Amaral, D.G., and Van Essen, D.C. 2007. Cortical folding abnormalities in autism revealed by surface-based morphometry. *J. Neurosci*. **27**:11725–11735.

Nuding, U., Ono, S., Mustari, M.J., Buttner, U., and Glasauer, S. 2008. Neural activity in cortical areas MST and FEF in relation to smooth pursuit gain control. *Prog. Brain Res*. **171**:261–264.

Ochsner, K.N., Knierim, K., Ludlow, D.H., Hanelin, J., Ramachandran, T., Glover, G., and Mackey, S. 2004. Reflecting upon feelings: An fMRI study of neural systems supporting the attribution of emotion to self and other. *J. Cogn. Neurosci*. **16**:1746–1772.

O'Donnell, B.R., Bismark, A., Hetrick, W.P., Bodkins, M., Vohs, J.L., and Anatha, S. 2006. Early stage vision in schizophrenia and schizotypal personality disorder. *Schizophr. Res*. **86**:89–98.

Ono, S., and Mustari, M.J. 2006. Extraretinal signals in MSTd neurons related to volitional smooth pursuit. *J. Neurophysiol*. **96**:2819–2825.

Orban, G.A. 2008. Higher order visual processing in macaque extrastriate cortex. *Physiolog. Rev*. **88**:59–89.

Pa, J., and Hickok, G. 2007. A parietal-temporal sensory-motor integration area for the human vocal tract: Evidence from an fMRI study of skilled musicians. *Neuropsychologia* **46**:362–368.

Panayiotopoulos, C.P. 1999. Visual phenomena and headache in occipital epilepsy: a review, a systematic study and differentiation from migraine. *Epileptic Disord.* **1**:205–216.

Parekh, P.I., Spencer, J.W., George, M.S., Gill, D.S., Ketter, T.A., Andreason, P., Herscovitch, P., and Post, R.M. 1995. Procaine-induced increases in limbic rCBF correlate positively with increases in occipital and temporal EEG fast activity. *Brain Topogr.* **7**:209–216.

Parvizi, J., Van Hoesen, G.W., Buckwalter, J., and Damasio, A. 2006. Neural connections of the posteromedial cortex in the macaque. *Proc. Natl. Acad. Sci. USA.* **103**:1563–1568.

Pelphrey, K.A., Viola, R.J., and McCarthy, G. 2004. When strangers pass: processing of mutual and averted social gaze in the superior temporal sulcus. *Psychol. Sci.* **15**:598–603.

Pessoa, L., Kastner, S., and Ungerleider, L. 2002. Attentional control of the processing of neural and emotional stimuli. *Brain Res.* **15**:31–45.

Petreska, B., Adriani, M., Blanke, O., and Billard, A.G. 2007. Apraxia: A review. *Prog. Brain Res.* **164**:61–83.

Pisella, L., Grea, H. Tilikete, C., Vighetto, A., Desmurget, M., Rode, G., Boisson, D., and Rossetti, Y. 2000. An "automatic pilot" for the hand in human posterior parietal cortex, toward reinterpreting optic ataxia. *Nat. Neurosci.* **3**:729–736.

Posner, M., and Petersen, S.E. 1990. The attention system of the brain. *Annu. Rev. Neurosci.* **13**:25–42.

Posner, M.I., and Dahaene, S. 1994. Attentional networks. *Trends Neurosci.* **17**: 75–79.

Pourtois, G., and Vuilleumier, P. 2006. Dynamics of emotional effects on spatial attention in the human visual cortex. *Prog. Brain Res.* **156**:67–91.

Pourtois, G., Grandjean, D., Sander, D., and Vuilleumier, P. 2004. Electrophysiological correlates of rapid spatial orienting towards fearful faces. *Cereb. Cortex* **14**:619–633.

Raichle, M.E., MacLeod, A.M., Snyder, A.Z., Powers, W.J., Gusnard, D.A., and Shulman, G.L. 2001. A default mode of brain function. *Proc. Natl. Acad. Sci. USA.* **98**:676–682.

Rainville, P., Hofbauer, R.K., Paus, T., Duncan, G.H., Bushnell, M.C., and Price, D.D. 1999. Cerebral mechanisms of hypnotic induction and suggestion. *J. Cogn. Neurosci.* **11**:110–125.

Rauch, S.L., Savage, C.R., Alpert, N.M., Miguel, E.C., Baer, L., Breiter, H.C., Fischman, A.J., Manzo, P.A., Moretti, C., and Jenike, M.A. 1995. A positron emission tomographic study of simple phobic symptom provocation. *Arch. Gen. Psychiatry* **52**:20–28.

Redlich, F.C., and Dorsey, J.E. 1945. Denial of blindness by patients with cerebral disease. *Arch. Neurol. Psychiatry* **53**:407–417.

Rees, G. 2007. Neural correlates of the contents of visual awareness in humans. *Philos. Trans. R. Soc. Lond.* **362**:877–886.

Rees, G. 2008. The anatomy of blindsight. *Brain* **131**:1414–1415.

Rees, G., Kreiman, G., and Koch, C. 2002. Neural correlates of consciousness in humans. *Nat. Rev. Neurosci.* **3**: 261–270.

Reichenberg, A., and Harvey, P.D. 2007. Neuropsychological impairments in schizophrenia: Integration of performance-based and brain imaging findings. *Psycholog. Bull.* **133**:833–858.

Rode, G., Perenin, M.T., Honoré, J., and Boisson, D. 1998. Improvement of the motor deficit of neglect patients through vestibular stimulation: evidence for a motor neglect component. *Cortex* **34**:253–261.

Roy, A.C., Stefanini, S., Pavesi, G., and Gentilucci, M. 2004. Early movement impairments in a patient recovering from optic ataxia. *Neuropsychologia* **42**:847–854.

Rubin, P., Karle, A., Moller-Madsen, S., Hertel, C., Povlsen, U.J., Noring, U., and Hemmingsen, R. 1993. Computerised tomography in newly diagnosed schizophrenia and schizophreniform disorder. A controlled blind study. *Br. J. Psychiatry* **163**:604–612.

Ruby, P., and Decety, J. 2001. Effect of subjective perspective taking during simulation of action: a PET investigation of agency. *Nat. Neurosci.* **4**:546–550.

Ruby, P., Sirigu, A ., and Decety, J. 2002. Distinct areas in parietal cortex involved in long-term and short term action planning: a PET investigation. *Cortex* **38**: 321–339.

Santhouse, A.M., Howard, R.J., and ffytche, D.H. 2000. Visual hallucinatory syndromes and the anatomy of the visual brain. *Brain* **123**:2055–2064.

Saxe, R. 2006. Uniquely human social cognition. *Curr. Opin. Neurobiol.* **16**:235–239.

Saxe, R., Jamal, N., and Powell, L. 2005. My body or yours? The effect of visual perspective on cortical body representation. *Cereb. Cortex* **16**:178–182.

Schlaepfer, T.E., Harris, G.J., Tien, A.Y., Peng, L.W., Lee, S., Federman, E.B., Chase, G.A., Barta, P.E., and Pearlson, G.D. 1994. Decreased regional cortical gray matter volume in schizophrenia. *Am. J. Psychiatry* **151**:842–848.

Schlack, A., Hoffmann, K.P., and Bremmer, F. 2002. Interaction of linear vestibular and visual stimulation in the macaque ventral intraparietal area (VIP). *Eur. J. Neurosci.* **16**:1877–1886.

Schlack, A., Hoffmann, K-P., and Bremmer, F. 2003. Selectivity of macaque ventral intraparietal area (area VIP) for smooth pursuit eye movements. *J. Physiol.* **2**:551–561.

Schmahl, C., Bohus, M., Esposito, F., Treede, R.D., Di Salle, F., Greffrath, W., Ludaescher, P., Jochims, A., Lieb, K., Scheffler, K., Hennig, J., and Seifritz, E. 2006. Neural correlates of antinociception in borderline personality disorder. *Arch. Gen. Psychiatry* **63**:659–667.

Seidler, R.D., and Noll, D.C. 2008. Neuroanatomical correlates of motor acquisition and motor transfer. *J. Neurophysiol.* **99**:1836–1845.

Selemon, L.D., Rajkowska, G., and Goldman-Rakic, P.S. 1995. Abnormally high neuronal density in two widespread areas of the schizophrenic cortex. A morphometric analysis of prefrontal area 9 and occipital area 17. *Arch. Gen. Psychiatry* **52**:808–818.

Sereno, M.I., and Huang, R-S. 2006. A human parietal face area contains aligned head-centered visual and tactile maps. *Nat. Neurosci.* **9**:1337–1343.

Shapleske, J., Rossell, S.L., Chitnis, X.A., Suckling, J., Simmons, A., Bullmore, E.T., Woodruff, P.W., and David, A.S. 2002. A computational morphometric MRI study of schizophrenia: effects of hallucinations. *Cereb. Cortex* **12**:1331–1341.

Shenton, M.E., Dickey, C.C., Frumin, M., and McCarley, R.W. 2001. A review of MRI findings in schizophrenia. *Schizophr. Res.* **49**:1–52.

Silvanto, J. 2008. A re-evaluation of blindsight and the role of striate cortex (V1) in visual awareness. *Neuropsychologia* **46**:2869–2871.

Simon, O., Mangin, J.F., Cohen, L., Le Bihan, D., and Dehaene, S. 2002. Topographical layout of hand, eye, calculation, and language-related areas in the human parietal lobe. *Neuron* **33**:475–487.

Sincich, L.C., Park, K.F., Wohlgemuth, M.J., and Horton, J.C. 2004. Bypassing V1: a direct geniculate input to area MT. *Nat. Neurosci.* **7**:1123–1128.

Skottun, B.C., and Skoyles, J.R. 2008. A few remarks on attention and magnocellular deficits in schizophrenia. *Neurosci. Biobehav. Rev.* **32**:118–122.

Steinmetz, H., Ebeling, D.U., Huang, Y., and Kohn, T. 1990. Sulcus topography in the parietal opercular region: An anatomic and MR study. *Brain Lang.* **38**:515–533.

Stoeckel, M.C., Weder, B., Binkofski, F., Choi, H-J., Amunts, K., Pieperhoff, P., Shah, N.J., and Seitz, R.J. 2004. Left and right superior parietal lobule in tactile object discrimination. *Eur. J. Neurosci.* **19**:1067–1072.

Tamietto, M., and de Gelder, B. 2007. Affective blindsight in the intact brain; Neural interhemispheric summation for unseen fearful expressions. *Neuropsychologia* **46**:820–828.

Thiebaut de Schotten, M., Urbanski, M., Daffau, H., Volle, E, Lévy, R., Dubois, B., and Bartolomeo, P. 2005. Direct evidence for a parietal-frontal pathway subserving spatial awareness in humans. *Science* **309**:2226–2228.

Todd, J.J., Fougnie, D., and Marois, R. 2005. Visual short-term memory load suppresses temporo-parietal junction activity and induces inattentional blindness. *Psychol. Sci.* **16**:965–972.

Torrey, E.F. 2007. Schizophrenia and the inferior parietal lobule. *Schizophr. Res.* **97**:215–225.

Tsutsui, K., Jiang, M., Sakata, H., and Taira, M. 2003. Short-term memory and perceptual decision for three-dimensional visual features in the caudal intraparietal sulcus (Area CIP). *J. Neurosci.* **23**:5486–5495.

Tsutsui, K.I., Sakata, H., Naganuma, T., and Taira, M. 2002. Neural correlates for perception of 3D surface orientation from texture gradient. *Science* **298**: 409–412.

Tucker, D.M., and Williamson, P.A. 1984. Asymmetric neural control systems in human self regulation. *Psychol. Rev.* **91**:185–215.

Tunik, E., Frey, S.H., and Grafton, S.T. 2005. Virtual lesions of the anterior intraparietal area disrupt goal-dependent on-line adjustments of grasp. *Nat. Neurosci.* **2005**:505–511.

Vallar, G., Guariglia, C., and Rusconi, M.L. 1997. Modulation of the neglect syndrome by sensory stimulation. In: P.Thier and H.-O.Karnath (eds.) *Parietal Lobe Contributions to Orientation in 3D space.* New York: Springer, pp. 555–578.

Vallar, G., Bottini, G., and Sterzi, R. 2003. Anosognosia for left-sided motor and sensory deficits, motor neglect, and sensory hemiinattention: is there a relationship? *Prog. Brain Res.* **142**:289–301.

Van Essen, D.C., Dierker, D., Snyder, A.Z., Raichle, M.E., Reiss, A.L., and Korenberg, J. 2006. Symmetry of cortical folding abnormalities in Williams syndrome revealed by surface-based analyses. *J. Neurosci.* **26**:5470–5483.

Vingerhoets, G. 2008. Knowing about tools: Neural correlates of too familiarity and experience. *Neuroimage* **40**:1380–1391.

Vogeley, K., and Fink, G.R. 2003. Neural correlates of the first-person-perspective. *Trends Cogn. Sci.* **7**:38–42.

Weiskrantz, L. 2004. Roots of blindsight. *Prog. Brain Res.* **144**:229–241.

Whalley, H.C., Simonotto, E., Flett, S., Marshall, L., Ebmeier, K.P., Owens, D.G.C., Goddard, N.H., Johnstone, E.C., and Lawrie, S.M. 2004. fMRI correlates of state and trait effects in subjects at genetically enhanced risk of schizophrenia. *Brain* **127**:478–490.

Wheaton, L.A. 2007. Parietal representations for hand-object interactions. *J. Neurosci.* **27**:969–970.

Wheeler, M.E., and Buckner, R.L. 2004. Functional–anatomic correlates of remembering and knowing. *Neuroimage* **21**:1337–1349.

Wilkinson, F. 2004. Auras and other hallucinations: Windows on the visual brain. *Prog. Brain Res.* **144**: 305–320.

Williams, L. M., Das, P., Liddell, B. J., Kemp, A. H., Rennie, C. J., and Gordon, E. 2006. Mode of functional connectivity in amygdala pathways dissociates level of awareness for signals of fear. *J. Neurosci.* **26**:9264–9271.

Wik, G., Fredrikson, M., Ericson, K., Eriksson, L., Stone-Elander, S., and Grieitz, T. 1992. A functional cerebral response to frightening visual stimulation. *Psychiatry Res.* **50**:15–24.

Wolbers, T., Weiller, C., and Büchel, C. 2003. Contralateral coding of imagined body parts in the superior parietal lobe. *Cereb. Cortex* **13**:392–399.

Womelsdorf, T., Schoffelen, J-M., Oostenveld, R., Singer, W., Desimone, R., Engel, Andreas K., and Fries, P. 2007. Modulation of neuronal interactions through neuronal synchronization. *Science* **316**:1609–1612.

Zhou, S-Y., Suzuki, M., Takahashi, T., Hagion, H., Kawasaki, Y., Matsui, M., Seto, H., and Kurachi, M. 2007. Parietal lobe volume deficits in schizophrenia spectrum disorders. *Schizophr. Res.* **89**:35–48.

Zilles, K., Eickhoff, S., and Palomero-Gallagher, N. 2003. The human parietal cortex: a novel approach to its architectonic mapping. *Adv. Neurol.* **93**:1–21.

Zohar, J., Insel, Berman, K.F., Foa, E.B., Hill, J.L., and Weinberger, D.R. 1989. Anxiety and cerebral blood flow during behavioral challenge: Dissociation of central from peripheral and subjective measures. *Arch. Gen. Psychiatry* **46**:505–510.

Chapter 5

Temporal lobe: Neocortical structures

Functional anatomy

Emil Kraepelin (1919) suggested that abnormalities in the frontal lobe were responsible for problems in reasoning and that damage to the temporal lobe resulted in delusions and hallucinations in patients with dementia praecox (schizophrenia). The classical findings of Klüver and Bucy in the 1930s clearly and strongly linked the temporal lobes to behavior (Klüver and Bucy, 1939). Their work provided the basis from which the concept of the limbic system has developed.

The temporal lobe can be divided into two regions: dorsolateral and ventromedial. The dorsolateral region supports cognitive functions associated with several sensory systems, especially language. It is now accepted that dysfunction of the dorsolateral region of the temporal lobe may be associated with several psychopathological states. Temporal lobe lesions due to a variety of neurological insults can lead a patient to present with signs and symptoms that are more consistent with a psychiatric diagnosis than with a traditional neurological one. The dorsolateral temporal cortex is recognized as neocortex and is the focus of this chapter. The ventromedial region of the temporal lobe contains major portions of the limbic system and thus contributes significantly to emotional tone. The ventromedial, limbic temporal lobe is discussed in Chapter 11.

The temporal lobe lies ventral to the lateral fissure (of Sylvius) and anterior to the parietal lobe. It also forms part of the anterior border of the occipital lobe (Figure 5.1). The superior temporal gyrus is bordered by the lateral fissure above and the superior temporal sulcus below. Both sulci are particularly deep. The middle and inferior temporal gyri make up the lateral surface below the superior temporal sulcus.

The dorsolateral temporal lobe is recognized as important in auditory processing and speech analysis. Language is an important means of social communication. Other methods of communication such as gestures have been found to be analyzed by the temporal lobe as well.

Auditory areas

The transverse gyrus of Heschl [Brodmann's area (BA) 41] is located on the superior surface of the superior temporal gyrus (Figure 2.3). Heschl's gyrus is recognized as the primary auditory area and corresponds

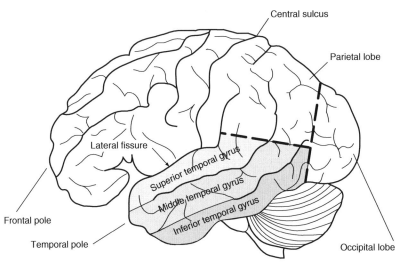

Figure 5.1. The dashed lines indicate the imaginary boundaries between the parietal, occipital, and temporal lobes. The temporal lobe lies below the lateral fissure and below the parietal lobe, and to the front of the occipital lobe. The dashed line demarcating the occipital from the parietal and temporal lobes is an imaginary line that runs from the parieto-occipital sulcus above to the preoccipital notch below.

Central sulcus

Parietal lobe

Lateral fissure

Superior temporal gyrus

Middle temporal gyrus

Inferior temporal gyrus

Frontal pole

Temporal pole

Occipital lobe

Clinical vignette

A 68-year-old left-handed man had difficulty under-standing speech after a stroke sustained during cor-onary artery bypass surgery. When he awoke from anesthesia, he could not understand what people were saying, as if they were "speaking too fast or in Chinese." His own speech was not affected, and he could read and write perfectly. In addition, envir-onmental sounds became indistinct and difficult to understand. On examination, he was very talkative, but, when spoken to, he appeared confused and per-plexed. His audiometry testing was adequate, and he could discriminate pure tones based on frequency, intensity, or duration. In contrast, he had difficulty understanding spoken commands, and he could not understand simple sounds, such as a birdcall or a train whistle. This patient had auditory agnosia for spoken words (word deafness) and environmental sounds. These problems were consequent to a stroke involv-ing the right temporal auditory cortex (Figure 5.2). Whereas right temporal lesions can produce auditory agnosia for environmental sounds, the presence of the additional word deafness was probably due to a greater right hemisphere role in auditory-language pathways in this left-handed person.

Clinical vignette

A 71-year-old language teacher complained of a progressive loss of the ability to use and understand Spanish and German. The patient had difficulty under-standing even common nouns in Spanish, and he was no longer able to understand any German words. His English was impaired as well. The patient had lost the meaning of many words such as cuff, lapel, and eyelashes and, on an aphasia battery, his word com-prehension was moderately impaired. Moreover, the patient was losing the ability to identify many of the objects that he could not name. This patient's presen-tation was compatible with the syndrome of seman-tic dementia characterized by early loss of word comprehension followed by more pervasive inability in the identification of objects. His magnetic reson-ance imaging (MRI) studies showed anterior inferior temporal atrophy in the left hemisphere (Figure 5.3) (Mendez *et al.*, 2004).

with the core area described in the monkey. BA 42 is the secondary auditory cortex and surrounds Heschl's gyrus on all but the medial side. It corresponds with the belt and parabelt areas described in the monkey (Saleem *et al.*, 2008; Shapleske *et al.*, 1999).

The superior, middle, and inferior temporal gyri cor-respond roughly with BA 22, 21, and 20, respectively. The cortex of the temporal pole is BA 38. The posterior

portion of the middle and inferior temporal gyri which lie inferior to the parietal lobe constitutes BA 37. These areas may be described as the auditory association cor-tex. If the lips of the lateral fissure are pulled apart, the insular cortex is seen to lie deep within the lateral fissure.

Gyri and sulci are more variable on the inferior sur-face of the temporal lobe (Figure 5.4). Three parallel gyri can be recognized. The most lateral is the infer-ior temporal gyrus. The fusiform (lateral occipitotem-poral) gyrus lies next to it and is separated from it by the occipitotemporal sulcus. The lingual gyrus (medial occipitotemporal gyrus) is separated from the fusiform gyrus by the collateral sulcus. The lingual gyrus is con-tinuous anteriorly with the parahippocampal gyrus.

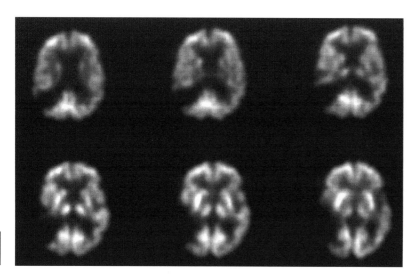

Figure 5.2. The patient's 18-fluorode-oxyglucose positron emission tomog-raphy showed focal right temporal lobe hypometabolism affecting his auditory cortex. (Reprinted with permission from Mendez, 2001.)

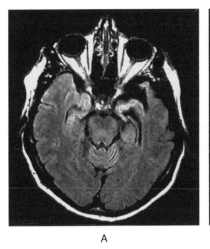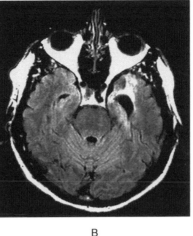

A   B

Figure 5.3. A, B. T2-weighted magnetic resonance image showed bilateral anterior inferior temporal atrophy disproportionately affecting the left temporal lobe. (Reprinted with permission from Mendez and Cummings, 2003.)

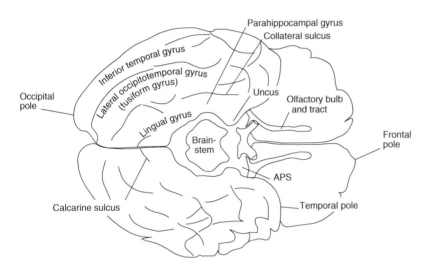

Figure 5.4. The boundary between the temporal lobes and the occipital lobe is indistinct on the ventral surface of the brain. The isthmus of the cingulate gyrus is continuous with the parahippocampal gyrus. APS, anterior perforated substance.

The collateral sulcus and its anterior extension, the rhinal fissure, mark the lateral extent of the parahippocampal (hippocampal) gyrus. The parahippocampal gyrus expands at its anterior pole to form the uncus (Chapter 11).

Heschl's gyrus (primary auditory area; BA 41)

Heschl's gyrus receives projections from the medial geniculate body of the thalamus. There are often two Heschl's gyri on the right but only one on the left (Leonard *et al.*, 1998). The size of Heschl's gyrus is variable between individuals and may be asymmetrical in the same individual. It is generally larger on the left (Dorsaint-Pierre, *et al.*, 2006), and it is consistently larger bilaterally in females than in males (Rademacher *et al.*, 2001). Heschl's gyrus contains a tonotopic map

that reflects the distribution of frequency-dependent cells along the organ of Corti. The auditory cortex consists of cell columns in an arrangement similar to that of other sensory cortical areas.

All incoming sound signals are first processed bilaterally in BA 41. Neurons in Heschl's gyrus of the monkey respond maximally to pure tones. It is not until signals reach the auditory association area that individual neurons respond maximally to complex sounds including species-specific vocalizations (Rauschecker *et al.*, 1995; Kosaki *et al.*, 1997).

The gray matter volume of BA 41 has been reported to be significantly greater and to show greater activity in professional musicians than in nonmusicians. The size of the gyrus correlates with the degree of musical aptitude (Schneider *et al.*, 2002; Pa and Hickok, 2008).

Electrical stimulation of the primary auditory region produces elementary hallucinations, including ringing, buzzing, or whispering. On the rare occasion when tumors involve this area, there is often a repetitive quality that makes the experience more disagreeable. Word deafness may result if the pathway from the primary auditory cortex to the auditory association cortex is interrupted. Occasionally, in patients with complex partial seizures, more meaningful sounds such as footsteps or music can be experienced.

Auditory association area (BA 42)

The auditory association area (BA 42) extends anterior and posterior to BA 41 along the superior temporal gyrus (Figure 2.3). Sounds received by BA 41 are next handled by the auditory association cortex. Sound processing in the human appears to proceed from BA 41 in two directions resulting in two auditory streams. The two auditory streams are believed to be analogous to the "what" and "where" visual streams. The auditory stream proceeding anteriorly from BA 41 is designated the anterior/ventral stream and is believed to be more involved in identification of an object or person based on sounds or speech. For example, voice gender recognition takes place in an area rostral to the BA 41 on the right (Lattner *et al.*, 2005). The stream proceeding posteriorly is designated the posterior/dorsal stream and is more involved in speech content and identification of location of the source of the sound. Signals proceeding posteriorly move from BA 42 to the posterior planum temporale and then laterally onto the exposed surface of the superior temporal gyrus.

Mummery *et al.* (1999) demonstrated bilateral activation in the superior temporal gyrus anterior to Heschl's gyrus in response to speech and complex nonspeech sounds. At the same time, a similar response was observed from the posterior superior temporal gyrus/superior temporal sulcus on the left. In another study, the anterior/ventral stream was activated only by intelligible sounds whereas the posterior left superior temporal gyrus/superior temporal sulcus responded to phonic cues whether or not they were intelligible (Scott *et al.*, 2000). Fibers from the anterior superior temporal gyrus/superior temporal sulcus project to anterior and lateral prefrontal cortex (BA 9, BA 10, BA 46). The posterior superior temporal gyrus/superior temporal sulcus has reciprocal connections via the arcuate fasciculus with the dorsolateral prefrontal cortex (Jones and Powell, 1970; Gloor, 1997). The posterior/dorsal stream provides auditory spatial information to aid in directing attention. It is speculated that the posterior/dorsal "where" stream is important in verbal working memory and acts to keep auditory-based representations available. It directs motor responses that are useful in repeating back vocalizations or mimicking words and phrases, and nonspeech sounds (Wise *et al.*, 2001). The posterior/dorsal auditory stream projects dorsoposteriorly to the parietal lobe and then to frontal regions (Hickok and Poeppel, 2004).

Planum temporale

The planum temporale makes up the superior surface of the superior temporal gyrus from BA 41 to the parietal lobe. The planum temporale includes portions of BA 42 and BA 22. The posterior extent of the planum temporale is variably defined (Zetzsche *et al.*, 2001). This has led to variability in estimates of the size and degree of asymmetry of the planum temporale (Westbury *et al.*, 1999). The planum temporale is reported to exhibit asymmetry in many individuals with the left side larger than the right. The leftward asymmetry, however, does not directly relate to asymmetry of language processing in all individuals (Dorsaint-Pierre *et al.*, 2006). More detailed analysis of planum temporale asymmetry has indicated that the anterior planum temporale is responsible for the greater part of the asymmetry (Zetzsche *et al.*, 2001).

The anterior planum temporale (BA 42) is auditory unimodal association cortex. The posterior planum temporale (BA 22) is a multimodal auditory association area and the heart of Wernicke's receptive language area. The exact borders of Wernicke's area are vague although the area is usually described as the posterior portion of BA 22. Inferior parts of the parietal lobe are sometimes included. Reciprocal transcortical projections interconnect BA 41 and the anterior planum temporale. A second set of fibers interconnects the anterior with the posterior planum temporale in a stepwise fashion (Galuske *et al.*, 2000; Brugge *et al.*, 2003). There are strong connections via the corpus callosum with homologous areas in the contralateral hemisphere (Hackett *et al.*, 1999).

The planum temporale is concerned with analysis of complex sounds including sounds that change frequency over time such as found in language. The left planum temporale is related to speech perception (Griffiths and Warren, 2002; Jäncke *et al.*, 2002). The right planum temporale plays a role in spatial attention (Karnath *et al.*, 2001). The planum temporale on the left responds to moving sounds presented to the right ear. However, the planum temporale on the right responds to moving sounds from both sides (Krumbholz *et al.*,

2005). The size of the right planum temporale has been found to correlate inversely with the degree of absolute pitch discrimination (Keenan *et al.*, 2001).

Auditory processing beyond Heschl's gyrus exhibits some degree of asymmetry. Tonal pitch perception and melody are processed in the right superior temporal gyrus (Peretz and Zatorre, 2005; Limb, 2006). Activation patterns indicate that voice pitch is processed close to the right Heschl's gyrus and a "pitch center" is proposed lateral to Heschl's gyrus (Schonwiesner and Zatorre, 2008). Voice spectral information is processed in posterior parts of the right superior temporal gyrus and areas surrounding the planum temporale bilaterally. BA 22, in addition to contributing to the planum temporale, forms part of the lateral surface of the superior temporal gyrus and even curves anteriorly to make up part of the superior temporal gyrus anterior to Heschl's gyrus. BA 22 anterior to Heschl's gyrus is part of the anterior/ventral auditory system. Imaging studies have shown that speech processing also activates the cortex within the superior temporal sulcus.

Superior temporal gyrus and superior temporal sulcus

The superior temporal gyrus includes all of BA 41 and BA 42 as well as parts of BA 22 posteriorly and BA 38 of the temporal pole anteriorly. It extends beyond the planum temporale to include cortex on the lateral aspect. Much of the cortex of the superior temporal gyrus lies within the lateral fissure where it forms the floor. It extends inferiorly on the lateral aspect to the superior temporal sulcus. The superior temporal sulcus refers to the cortex that forms the roof, floor, and fundus (depth) of the sulcus. The cortex of the superior temporal sulcus also includes cortex of the superior and middle temporal gyri located on the lateral surface immediately above and below the superior temporal sulcus.

Speech sounds including cadence and word meaning are processed in the left hemisphere involving the superior temporal gyrus/superior temporal sulcus and planum temporale, even in infants (Dehaene-Lambertz *et al.*, 2002). Simple auditory tasks such as passive listening to tones, white noise, or constant vowel sounds result in activation of restricted areas of the surface of the superior temporal gyrus (Rimol *et al.*, 2005). Activity can spread anteriorly and posteriorly from the area of Heschl's gyrus but the degree of spread varies from individual to individual. Pure tones and simple vowel sounds cause activation to spread more than white noise (Binder *et al.*, 2000). Meaningful and nonmeaningful sounds activate the superior temporal sulcus bilaterally (Lewis *et al.*, 2005). The rhythm of music is processed on the left involving temporal lobe language areas as well as Broca's speech area of the frontal lobe (Limb, 2006). Some other sounds including those involved in spatial location are processed on the left (Zatorre *et al.*, 2002). Meaningful sounds (speech, laughter, sounds from animals, tools, running water, etc.) are left lateralized (Belin *et al.*, 2000, 2004; Engelien *et al.*, 2006). Exposure to rapidly changing sounds such as those in speech result in activation of the left superior and middle temporal gyri (Zaehle *et al.*, 2008). More complex sounds such as single words, tone and patterns result in the spread of activity to involve the entire superior surface as well as the lateral aspect of the superior temporal gyrus. Intelligible speech (easy sentences) produced significantly more activation than pseudo-word sentences in the anterior left superior temporal gyrus/superior temporal sulcus (Roder *et al.*, 2002). Activation is greater in response to stories than to individual sentences (Xu *et al.*, 2005). It is hypothesized that voice-selective regions of the superior temporal sulcus are the counterpart of the face-selective regions of the visual cortex (Belin *et al.*, 2000).

The superior temporal gyrus/superior temporal sulcus is activated during exposure to auditory stimuli and when imagining tone when no acoustical stimulus is present (Halpern *et al.*, 2004). The response may be modified as a function of learning or early environmental exposure. Signals from other sensory areas converge on the posterior superior temporal gyrus and act to modify the interpretation of language. For example, the image of a dog opening its mouth anticipates the sound of a bark, not a meow (Zatorre, 2007). The McGurk effect demonstrates that speech analysis uses input from more than one sensory modality (McGurk and MacDonald, 1976). The McGurk effect occurs when a subject hears a syllable (or word) and simultaneously sees a print version that differs slightly. The subject's interpretation, processed in the superior temporal gyrus/superior temporal sulcus, is modified by the visual input.

Speech analysis extends beyond the temporal lobe. It is proposed that a sequence of areas is activated during speech analysis. The first area activated is the superior temporal area, followed by the inferior parietal area and finally inferior frontal areas (Campbell, 2008). Wise *et al.*, (2001) showed that sound processing may be further specialized. Two regions of the posterior superior temporal sulcus process single words. One area in the posterior superior temporal sulcus is involved in response to the sound of single words and retrieval of words from memory, but not our own utterances. The second is at the junction of the posterior superior temporal gyrus with the posterior inferior temporal cortex. This second area is activated by the motor act of speech, independent of the speaker's own utterances. Wise *et al.* also showed that the left planum temporale was activated by the speaker's own voice and complex nonspeech sounds. The authors proposed that the left posterior superior temporal sulcus acts as an interface between hearing words (perception) and matching them with words held in long-term memory (Wise *et al.*, 2001).

Sign language and communicative gestures also result in activation of the superior temporal sulcus (MacSweeney *et al.*, 2004). Activation is greater for sign language than gestures and the degree of activation appears to be proportional to the meaningfulness of the information signed (Gallagher and Frith, 2004). Pauses used in word retrieval and speech planning that relate to speech cadence are associated with activation of the left superior temporal sulcus (BA 22 and BA 39) (Kircher *et al.*, 2004).

The posterior superior temporal gyrus/superior temporal sulcus is involved in more than just auditory processing since it becomes activated when individuals view biological movements including gaze shifts and mouth movements. Auditory language, visualized gestures and gaze are all used in combination as social communication signals and can affect social attention (Puce *et al.*, 1998; Allison *et al.*, 2000; Hoffman and Haxby, 2000; Puce and Perrett, 2003; Redcay, 2008). Biologically important social signals (head, arm, and hand gestures) result in stronger activation of the posterior superior temporal gyrus/superior temporal sulcus on the right (Blakemore and Decety, 2001). Body movements, gestures, and gaze that are clearly goal directed have a greater influence than those that are not goal directed. The source of the sound can also modify interpretation. Integration of face and voice, helpful in the identification of a person in social situations, results in activation of the posterior superior temporal sulcus (Campanella and Belin, 2007; Redcay 2008). Young adults of both genders listening to voices exhibit a stronger response in this region to the sound of a female voice (Lattner *et al.*, 2005).

A bilateral lesion of the temporal lobe including the auditory radiations can result in central deafness. Many patients show initial profound hearing loss followed by some degree of recovery. A smaller lesion that includes the superior temporal gyrus bilaterally

can result in auditory agnosia. Three forms have been described: for words (word deafness), music (amusia), and environmental sounds (environmental-sound agnosia) (Griffiths, 2002). The patient can hear sounds and can locate them in the environment apparently using lower level structures, but the meaning of the sounds is lost.

Temporal association areas

The cortex in the ascending limb of the superior temporal sulcus close to the occipital lobe is recognized as visual area V5/MT. This area is associated with the dorsal visual stream and is important in eye movement control. See Chapter 4 for a detailed description.

Posterior portions of the middle and inferior temporal gyri adjacent to the occipital lobe are heavily involved with visual processing. Visual signals that enter the posterior temporal lobe are matched with embedded constructs for object recognition (e.g., box, sphere, face; Figure 5.6). Lesions in this area in rhesus monkeys render them unable to distinguish one complex visual image from another (as a human would distinguish one object from another) (Ungerleider and Mishkin, 1982). Reciprocal connections with the anterior inferior temporal gyrus and temporal pole provide recognition of the object (e.g., edible, predator). These same posterior gyri also have extensive reciprocal connections with the ventromedial temporal cortex. It is through these connections that emotional values are assigned to visual objects (Figure 5.6).

The superior temporal sulcus and inferior temporal gyrus function to detect meaningful movement patterns. The areas did not show the same response when only portions of the walker were shown in motion (Thompson *et al.*, 2005). The left posterior inferior temporal area (BA 37) functions to process letters and words and is an association area that integrates input from several areas (Scott *et al.*, 2006). This area is activated in blind as well as in sighted individuals processing a variety of word forms (Büchel *et al.*, 1998). Stevens and Weaver (2009) found that subjects blind since early life showed similar areas of activation compared with sighted subjects but were more sensitive to low signal volume. There is reduced activation of the same area in individuals with dyslexia (Brunswick *et al.*, 1999).

Fusiform gyrus and fusiform face area

The posterior fusiform gyrus (BA 37), described as the fusiform face area (Figure 5.4), is an extrastriate visual area that becomes activated when viewing faces

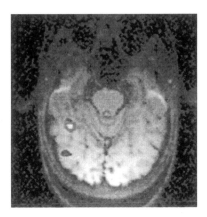

Figure 5.5. This functional magnetic resonance image shows activation of the "fusiform face area" responsive to human faces. The right hemisphere appears on the left. The brain images at the left show (in color in the color plate) the voxels that produced a significantly higher magnetic resonance signal intensity during the epochs containing faces than during those containing objects. These significance images are overlaid on a T1-weighted anatomical image of the same slice. In each image, the region of interest is shown outlined in green. (Reproduced with permission from Kanwisher et al., 1997.) See also color plate.

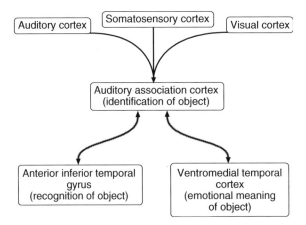

Figure 5.6. The predominant flow of information is from the auditory association cortex to the anteroinferior temporal gyrus (recognition of object) and to the ventromedial temporal cortex (emotional meaning of object).

(Figure 5.5) (Narumoto et al., 2001), even in 2-month-old infants (Tzourio-Mazoyer et al., 2002; Gathers et al., 2004). It is hypothesized to detect motion related to facial expression (Cipolotti et al., 1999; Blair et al., 2002). The fusiform face area is activated whether the face is clearly defined or is implied by surrounding, contextual cues (Cox et al., 2004). The right side is more sensitive to emotional than to neutral expressions and face recognition is better if the image is presented in the left visual

field (Vuilleumier et al., 2001). The fusiform face area also distinguishes between consciously remembered and forgotten faces (Lehmann et al., 2004). It responds to objects other than faces and appears to be sensitive to complex attributes common to both faces and familiar objects (Haxby et al., 2001; Hasson et al., 2004). For example, it is sensitive to image classes with which an individual may have particular experience, e.g., birds to an ornithologist or old cars to an antique automobile enthusiast (Gauthier et al., 2000).

Visual signals from the fusiform face area are relayed to the amygdala to evaluate emotional content. Activation of the amygdala can potentiate responses of the fusiform gyrus in a top-down fashion. The amygdala in turn, feeds back to the occipital cortex probably through the parietal cortex to attend to and amplify signals from emotionally salient faces (Tabert et al., 2001).

Temporal pole and theory-of-mind

The temporal pole corresponds with BA 38 and covers the anterior aspect of the temporal lobe (Figure 5.4). It is sometimes included as part of the perirhinal cortex, which is usually defined as medial temporal lobe (BA 35 and BA 36). The temporal pole has strong connections with the amygdala and orbital prefrontal cortex and is sometimes recognized as a component of the paralimbic region. It also has connections with the basal forebrain and hypothalamus. It receives input from auditory association cortex, extrastriate visual cortex of the inferior temporal lobe, insula, and piriform olfactory cortex. The temporal pole is recognized as association cortex involved with multimodal analysis, and is believed to be particularly important in social and emotional processing. It is hypothesized to act to match sensory stimuli from sensory or multimodal association areas with emotional sensations (Olson et al., 2007). For example, in one study the right temporal pole, along with the left frontal lobe, was activated during the correct identification of a familiar voice (Nakamura et al., 2001).

The left temporal pole is associated with semantic memory, i.e., memory for meanings, names, and general impersonal facts. Damage to the left temporal pole often results in semantic memory impairments (Snowden et al., 2004). The right temporal pole is believed to store personal, episodic memories and is more closely associated with emotion and socially relevant memory (Nakamura et al., 2000).

Patients with damage to the right temporal pole may present with apathy, irritability, depression, emotional blunting, and an expression of being ill at ease with social company (Thompson et al., 2003). These individuals exhibit a reduced ability to recognize or recall information about famous or family faces and memories related to these faces (Tsukiura et al., 2003).

There is some evidence to indicate there are specialized regions within the temporal pole. The dorsal portion of the temporal pole receives input from auditory association areas and is believed to link auditory stimuli with emotional reactions. Activation of this area was reported in response to emotionally evocative sounds including a baby crying (Lorberbaum et al., 2002) and a woman screaming (Royet et al., 2000).

The ventral portion of the temporal pole is activated in response to complex visual stimuli including faces, cartoons, and photographs of houses that evoke both positive (humor) and negative (sadness, anger, disgust, and anxiety) emotions (Damasio et al., 2000,

2004; Levesque et al., 2003; Mobbs et al., 2003). For example, in one study, young men exposed to sexually arousing, erotic film excerpts showed activation of the right anterior temporal pole along with activation of the hypothalamus and right amygdala (Beauregard et al., 2001).

Frontal temporal dementia results from a degeneration of the frontal and anterior temporal lobes. Patients with right, but not left, temporal pole atrophy exhibit changes in personality and socially appropriate behavior. The patient with primarily temporal pole involvement (temporal variant) often becomes introverted, cold, and lacks empathy (Mycack et al., 2001; Rankin et al., 2006). Personal hygiene may decline and indiscriminate eating behavior can result in weight gain (Gorno-Tempini et al., 2004).

The temporal pole is believed to be a critical component of the theory-of-mind network. Theory of mind is the ability to understand and predict the mental state of another, to infer their emotions, desires, intentions, and to recognize that the view point of another may be different from our own. It is believed that the areas in our brain that become active when viewing another person experiencing and expressing an emotion are the same as those that are activated in that other person. The process by which we read the mental state of another person is called mentalizing. (For more detail on theory-of-mind see Premack and Woodruff, 1978; Frith and Frith, 2003, 2007; Frith, 2007; George and Conty, 2008; Hein and Knight, 2008.) The temporal pole acts as a convergence zone where features of situations, persons, and objects are brought together. The identity and/or disposition of the situation, person, or object may be determined by the context in which it appears (Ganis and Kutas, 2003). Based on the evaluation of the situation, specific thoughts and/or feelings are appreciated. In studies, the temporal pole was activated when subjects were asked to think about other's thoughts and emotions, and to make moral decisions (Moll et al., 2002; Heekeren et al., 2003; Vollm et al., 2006).

Temporoparietal junction and the social brain

Portions of the temporal lobe, prefrontal cortex, cingulate cortex, and amygdala make up the social brain (Frith and Frith, 2007). More specifically the neuroanatomical components include the orbital prefrontal cortex, medial prefrontal cortex and adjacent cingulate cortex, temporal pole, anterior insula, posterior superior temporal sulcus, and temporoparietal junction

(Brothers, 1990; Amodio and Frith, 2006). The social brain is involved with social cognition (Adolphs, 2009). (See also social brain in Chapter 6.)

Signals are routed into the social brain by way of the intraparietal sulcus, superior temporal sulcus, fusiform face area as well as associative sensory regions of the parietal and occipital cortex (Nelson *et al.*, 2005). This network functions to decipher the social properties of incoming sensory stimuli (Blakemore, 2008).

The temporoparietal junction is a major player in the social brain. It consists of the posterior superior temporal sulcus, parts of the supramarginal gyrus, and dorsal anterior parts of the occipital gyri. It represents a posterior multimodal sensory convergence area and integrates information that arrives from the thalamus, visual, auditory, and somatosensory areas, as well as limbic system (Figure 5.7). The temporoparietal junction has reciprocal connections with the prefrontal and temporal cortices.

The temporoparietal junction is involved in multisensory, body-related processing including self-awareness and theory-of-mind (Saxe and Wexler, 2005; Lawrence *et al.*, 2006). Functions associated with the temporoparietal junction include attention to salient, socially important environmental stimuli (Astafiev *et al.*, 2006). The temporoparietal junction compares ongoing events based on previous experience to predict the outcome of a social situation (Decety and Lamm, 2007). During social processing it can direct attention to specific salient sensory signals in order to focus on critical events and suppress distracting stimuli (Astafiev *et al.*, 2006; Shulman *et al.*, 2007). It provides the ability to adopt the perspective of another and to empathize (Ruby and Decety, 2003). It also functions to adopt a sense of agency, i.e., recognizing that I am the source of my own actions, desires, and thoughts (Farrer *et al.*, 2003), and allows us to distinguish self from nonself (Uddin *et al.*, 2006). Multisensory body-related processing, along with processing vestibular input in the temporoparietal junction, supports the sensation of self and embodiment (Lenggenhager *et al.*, 2006). The right temporoparietal junction is activated when the person must distinguish between self and other (i.e., agency) indicating the right temporoparietal junction is more involved with higher level social processing than the left temporoparietal junction (Farrer *et al.*, 2003).

The right temporal/parietal region plays a role in comprehending nonliteral language, understanding jokes, and many aspects of general discourse (Bartolo *et al.*, 2006; Van Lancker Sidtis, 2006; Virtue *et al.*, 2006). Patients with lesions involving the right (nondominant) temporal/parietal region may lose their capacity to discern the emotional content of speech (receptive aprosodia). These patients misperceive paralinguistic social-emotional messages. After the onset of the lesion they may notice that the voices of friends and relatives sound different. Patients then may become progressively paranoid and delusional.

Damage to the temporoparietal junction has resulted in anosognosia (denial of illness), asomatognosia (lack of awareness of all or parts of one's own body), and somatoparaphrenia (delusional beliefs about the body) (Decety and Lamm, 2007).

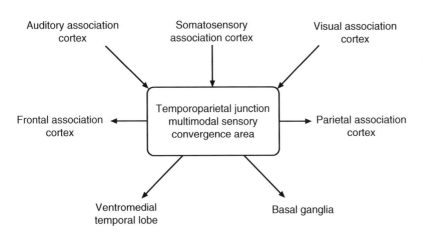

Figure 5.7. The temporoparietal junction is a multimodal sensory convergence area that receives input from all sensory association areas and projects to the frontal and parietal association areas as well as to the basal ganglia and ventromedial temporal cortex.

Insula

The insular cortex lies deep within the lateral fissure, centrally located between the posterior sensory cortex and anterior motor cortex (Figure 9.1). It consists of several long gyri located more posteriorly that parallel the lateral fissure, and five short gyri located more anteriorly. The anterior and posterior regions are divided by the middle cerebral artery, which passes across the surface of the insular cortex. The insular cortex consists of a core area surrounded by several belt areas. The insula receives input from the somatosensory cortex, auditory cortex, and sensory relay nuclei of the thalamus. Efferent projections go to the motor cortex and temporal lobe including the temporal pole. The insula has reciprocal connections with the parietal operculum, basal ganglia, and many limbic structures, including the cingulate gyrus, and the orbital and medial prefrontal cortices.

Anterior insula

The anterior insula is particularly involved with monitoring signals generated in the viscera (Critchley *et al.*, 2004). It is important in the detection and interpretation of certain internal bodily states, "interoceptive awareness," and has been described as an "alarm center" for internal, visceral sensations (Critchley *et al.*, 2004). Many of the sensory signals conveyed by the vagus nerve terminate here. It is thought that emotional responses to visceral signals are processed in the anterior insula. Connections between the anterior insula and amygdala are particularly strong (Augustine, 1996).

The insula along with the amygdala plays a role in anxiety (Etkin and Wager, 2007). Increased activity in the anterior insula (more so on the right) was seen in response to images of emotional faces in a group of anxiety-prone compared with anxiety-normative undergraduate students. Bilateral increased amygdala activity was also reported (Stein *et al.*, 2007). In other studies, both the anterior insula and amygdala showed increased activation over controls in subjects with posttraumatic stress disorder, social anxiety disorder, and generalized and specific phobia (Lorberbaum, *et al.*, 2004; Etkin and Wager, 2007; Lindauer *et al.*, 2007). The right insula was reported to be more highly activated in subjects with posttraumatic stress disorder than controls when viewing images of faces expressing fear (Felmingham *et al.*, 2008). The anterior/middle insula is activated in control subjects in anticipation of negative compared with positive stimuli (Schunck

et al., 2008). The same areas of the insula were hyperactivated in subjects with posttraumatic stress disorder (Simmons *et al.*, 2008a). The insula and amygdala were activated in young anxiety-prone individuals during an emotion-processing task. The degree of activation corresponded with measures of anxiety sensitivity (Stein *et al.*, 2007).

The anterior insula is considered part of the social brain (Frith and Frith, 2007). Game theory has revealed that the anterior insula plays an important role in sustaining and/or repairing cooperation during social exchange, especially when shared expectations about fairness are violated. It is activated when the individual is faced with a choice that has both positive and negative social outcomes. Activation precedes the rejection of low-risk gambles (Knutson and Greer, 2008). Control subjects showed activation levels of the anterior insula proportional to monetary rewards received and repaid to their partner. Subjects with borderline personality disorder showed activation only proportional to the amount of money repaid to their partner, not to the amount offered to the subject. The diminished response to the amount offered reflects atypical social norms and correlates with low levels of trust (King-Casas *et al.*, 2008).

The anterior insula has been called cardiac control cortex. It provides the basis of conscious awareness of visceral activity (e.g., heart beat) and subjective feelings of visceral awareness (Critchley *et al.*, 2004; Kringelbach *et al.*, 2004). It, along with its close ties with the amygdala, may be responsible for the unexplained anxiety that is reported to sometimes accompany coronary thrombosis.

The anterior insula is involved with appetite. Taste signals from the ipsilateral solitary nucleus that relay in the ventral posteromedial nucleus of the thalamus terminate in the anterior insula. The anterior insula along with the adjoining frontal operculum is recognized as the primary taste cortex (Rolls, 2006). The left anterior insula is activated in response to all odors whereas the right insula is activated specifically by disgusting odors (Heining *et al.*, 2003). The anterior insula is one of several areas that are activated during sexual arousal in both men and women (Stoléru *et al.*, 1999; Yang *et al.*, 2008).

The insula is involved with pain. Visceral afferent signals conveying pain information including that relayed from the vagus nerve terminate in the insula bilaterally (Brooks *et al.*, 2005). Bladder filling sensations produce activation in the insula. The area of activation shifts anteriorly as the sensation becomes stronger and more unpleasant (Griffiths and Tadic, 2008). Pain sensitivity is reportedly reduced following strokes involving the insula (Schön *et al.*, 2008). A decrease in gray matter of the insula is common to many pain syndromes (May, 2008), and patients with migraine headaches and chronic head pain showed decreased insula gray matter (Rocca *et al.*, 2006). The decrease correlates positively with headache duration in years (Schmidt-Wilcke *et al.*, 2007). In contrast, an increase in insular gray matter volume has been reported in patients with panic disorder (Graeff and Del-Ben, 2008).

The right anterior insula is involved in sympathetic arousal to pain. The insula in cooperation with the basal ganglia may function to match pain signals with the appropriate autonomic response (Leone *et al.*, 2006). Two regions are described as key regions of the "shared circuit" for self and other pain (Danziger *et al.*, 2009). Both the anterior insula and anterior cingulate are activated during the experience of pain in self and perception of pain in others (Singer *et al.*, 2004, 2006). It is suggested that both areas function to recruit systems that determine the emotional and/or affective level of pain experienced by the self or by another person (Saarela *et al.*, 2007; Zaki *et al.*, 2007). In contrast to negative aspects, the anterior insula is activated during feelings of maternal attachment and reward (Elliott *et al.*, 2003; Bartels and Zeki, 2004).

Posterior insula

The posterior insula processes information related to somatic and auditory sensation and control of somatic musculature. The posterior insula on the left is identified as part of neural circuit that is involved in affective processing, particularly in anxious individuals (Simmons *et al.*, 2006). Other structures in this circuit are the bilateral middle temporal and superior frontal gyri, and the right inferior frontal gyrus. The left posterior insula along with the other structures in this circuit showed significantly greater activation in anxiety-prone over normative subjects when performing an affective appraisal task (Simmons *et al.*, 2008b).

Behavioral considerations

Schizophrenia

The insula is part of the articulatory loop that is important in processing verbal material (Paulesu *et al.*, 1993). It is activated during inner-speech generation (Shergill

et al., 2000). When an individual speaks the brain is aware that it is the self that is speaking by way of connections between the temporal and frontal lobes (efference copy and forward model) (Miall and Wolpert, 1996). Activity in the auditory cortex is reduced in response to the sound of one's own voice when one is speaking. This suppression is not seen in patients with schizophrenia, especially those with auditory hallucinations (Ford *et al.*, 2001). The connectivity (coherence) between the frontal and temporal areas as measured by electroencephalography is increased in control subjects when they are speaking. The increase in connectivity is not seen in patients with schizophrenia (Ford *et al.*, 2002). It is hypothesized that a dysfunction in the neuroanatomical basis of the forward model plays a role in hallucinations and delusions in schizophrenia (Frith, 2005).

Abnormalities of temporal cortex are well documented in patients with schizophrenia (Wright *et al.*, 2000; Shenton *et al.*, 2001). The left lateral fissure is larger in this population, evidently the result of reduction in gray mater volume of the underlying left superior temporal gyrus (Meisenzahl *et al.*, 2008). A reduction in volume of the superior temporal gyrus in schizophrenia has been suspected for some time and has been confirmed more recently (Southard, 1910; Barta *et al.*, 1990; Hirayasu *et al.*, 2000). The effect appears to be lateralized to the dominant cortex, especially in males (Reite *et al.*, 1997; O'Donnell *et al.*, 2005). Subregions such as the left Heschl's gyrus and left planum temporale show consistent abnormalities in schizophrenia (Honea *et al.*, 2005). Kasai *et al.* (2003) found that gray matter volume of the left planum temporale and Heschl's gyrus bilaterally was reduced in patients with schizophrenia.

Relative metabolism in the posterior superior temporal region is decreased in patients with schizophrenia as they hallucinate (Cleghorn *et al.*, 1992). Blood flow to the left superior temporal cortex increases in patients with schizophrenia as they experience auditory hallucinations. The activity decreases as the hallucinations resolve (Suzuki *et al.*, 1993). A lower glucose metabolic rate has been reported in patients with schizophrenia with predominantly negative symptoms in the ventral stream including the right inferotemporal area and fusiform gyrus (Potkin *et al.*, 2002). This is consistent with difficulties seen in this group in correctly identifying and expressing the emotional content of both faces and scenes (Borod *et al.*, 1993; Bryson *et al.*, 1998).

There is a strong correlation between the increase of thought disorder and volume reduction in the left posterior superior temporal gyrus (McCarley *et al.*, 1993). By comparison, there is a close association between auditory hallucinations and volume reduction in more anterior regions of the superior temporal gyrus especially on the left (Barta *et al.*, 1990; Shapleske *et al.*, 2002). The severity of hallucinations has been reported to correlate with volume loss in the left Heschl's gyrus as well as the left supramarginal gyrus (parietal lobe) and the right middle and inferior frontal gyri (Gaser *et al.*, 2004). These findings are consistent with the findings that there is greater impairment in auditory processing than in visual processing in schizophrenia and suggest that auditory hallucinations originate from the left hemisphere (Hugdahl *et al.*, 2008).

Abnormalities are also seen in the middle and inferior temporal gyri. Volume reductions of 13% have been reported in both the left superior and left middle temporal gyri, accompanied by a 10% reduction in the inferior temporal gyrus and fusiform gyrus bilaterally. The severity of hallucinations correlated with the reduced volume of involved left hemisphere structures (Onitsuka *et al.*, 2004). Smaller left superior temporal gyrus and reduced gray matter volume of the middle temporal gyrus bilaterally have been reported in patients with first-episode schizophrenia but not in patients with affective psychosis. In the same study, smaller posterior inferior temporal gyri were common to both groups. These results indicate that smaller volumes in the superior and middle temporal gyri may be specific to schizophrenia and related to auditory hallucinations (Kuroki *et al.*, 2006; Aguilar *et al.*, 2008; Galderisi *et al.*, 2008).

The planum temporale is also reduced in volume in schizophrenia (Kwon *et al.*, 1999). Schizophrenia is associated with a decrease in the normal left–right asymmetry of the planum temporale (McCarley *et al.*, 1993). Some patients exhibit a reversal of normal left–right asymmetry (Petty *et al.*, 1995; Kwon *et al.*, 1999). In addition, gray matter reductions in the temporal pole, middle and lateral superior temporal gyri (BA 21, 22), and in the temporal-occipital junction (BA 37) have been reported in patients with particularly poor outcome schizophrenia (Metelman and Buchsbaum, 2007). Using functional MRI (fMRI), Lawrie *et al.* (2002) showed reduced coupling between the left dorsolateral prefrontal cortex and the left superior temporal gyrus (frontotemporal connectivity) in patients with schizophrenia compared with controls. The coupling was reduced further in patients experiencing auditory hallucinations. It was hypothesized that reduced frontotemporal connectivity is responsible for the failure of normal constraint of inner speech.

Meisenzahl *et al.* (2008) reported gray matter volume reductions in the left superior temporal gyrus and left insula in a group of 40 untreated subjects at risk for schizophrenia. Fifteen of the group developed a psychotic disorder within two and half years of the date of the initiation of the study. Morgan *et al.* (2007) observed gray matter reductions in the left insula and left fusiform gyrus in patients with affective psychosis when compared with controls. The gray matter volume and surface area of the insula were reduced in patients with schizophrenia. Abnormal activation of the insula can result in auditory or visual hallucinations. It has been suggested that hallucinations in the absence of external stimuli common to schizophrenia result from activation of the posterior insula (Nagai *et al.*, 2007). A group of 22 patients with first-episode schizophrenia showed significant reduction in fusiform gyrus volume (Lee *et al.*, 2002). Differences are less in first-episode patients, suggesting that tissue loss progresses over time (McIntosh and Lawrie, 2004).

A key feature of schizotypal personality disorder is language abnormalities. Greater activation is reported in the superior temporal gyrus bilaterally in tasks involving pure tones differing in pitch and duration. Heschl's gyrus volume did not differ from controls (Kiang and Kutas, 2006; Dickey *et al.*, 2008).

Depression

The insula is one of the most consistently identified regions in a network that is associated with depression. Depression symptoms have been reported to correlate with increased metabolism in the right insula (Harrison *et al.*, 2003). In contrast, activation is decreased in the insula of patients with depression (Fitzgerald *et al.*, 2009). Other areas showing decreased activation include the left middle frontal, anterior cingulate, inferior frontal, and right cingulate cortices (Li *et al.*, 2005).

Vagus nerve stimulation in patients has been effective when used in patients with drug-resistant depression. Vagus nerve stimulation was monitored in a population of patients with depression. Decreased activation of ventral medial prefrontal cortex and other limbic areas has been reported, coupled with increased activity in the right insula (Kraus *et al.*, 2007; Nahas *et al.*, 2007).

Recalled sadness in normal individuals produces activation of the anterior insula (Lane *et al.*, 1997). Studies suggest that the anterior insular cortex participates in the emotional response to particularly distressing cognitive or interoceptive sensory stimuli (Reiman *et al.*, 1997). Activation of the insular cortex during emotional situations may reflect its role in cardiac control by altering heart rate (Oppenheimer, 1993).

Disgust is believed to play a role in obsessive-compulsive disorder (Berle and Phillips, 2006). Shapira *et al.* (2003) found that patients with obsessive-compulsive disorder compared with controls showed significantly greater activation in the right insula in response to disgust-inducing photos.

The observation that patients in complex partial seizure status (continuous complex partial seizures) can be awake and even responsive can be explained (at least partially) by the existence of anatomical connections between the two temporal lobes that do not involve most of the other brain regions (noncallosal connections). If a seizure is generalized through the corpus callosum, it is very likely that consciousness will be totally lost (e.g., generalized seizures). One patient, while undergoing electrical stimulation of the left superior temporal gyrus as she counted out loud, reported that she heard her speech as an "echo" and at the same time felt "frightened" (Fried, 1997).

Reduplicative paramnesia

Reduplicative paramnesia is a delusional belief that a place has been duplicated. It is postulated that a combination of right posterior parietal lesion and frontal pathology leads to the development of this syndrome. The posterior right hemisphere lesion causes visuoperceptual dysfunction involving identification of person or place, and the frontal pathology makes it impossible to resolve the conflicting information, resulting in delusional ideas. The related syndromes described below may involve the temporal lobe more directly.

As many as 40% of patients with schizophrenia exhibit symptoms of delusional misidentification syndrome (Cutting, 1994). These syndromes include Capgras delusion. The patient with Capgras syndrome believes that well-known persons, including family members, are impostors or may be identical doubles, or both. Two lesions may be needed to produce this syndrome. Right temporal lobe lesions may cause distortion in the sense of familiarity of a person. Frontal damage (usually bilateral) results in the inability to resolve the conflict and hence the feeling

of unfamiliarity that results in the belief that the loved one is an impostor (Malloy *et al.*, 1992). Cotard delusion is an extreme example of depersonalization in a misidentification syndrome (Sno, 1994; see clinical vignette, page 67).

Seizures

Temporal lobe seizures involving the posterolateral cortex are characterized by aphasia if the seizure is localized to the dominant lobe, as well as auditory, visual, and vestibular disturbances. In contrast, mesial temporal seizures are characterized by the presence of an aura, followed by staring and behavioral arrest. Oroalimentary automatism is common (Fried, 1997).

One patient, while being stimulated in the left inferotemporal cortex, reported familiar music and vivid visual images of personal importance, but was aware that they were unreal (Fried, 1997). Epileptic discharges in the middle and inferior temporal gyri can result in complex hallucinations or confusional episodes, or may cause an abnormal attribution of emotional significance to otherwise neutral thoughts and external stimuli. Hallucinations become increasingly complex as the disturbance expands from primary to more complex association areas. A variety of emotional reactions can occur during the course of a temporal lobe seizure. Fear is the most frequently reported emotion during a seizure. Other reported emotions include anxiety, pleasure, displeasure, depersonalization, depression, familiarity, and unfamiliarity.

Receptive aphasia

Lesions of the posterior parts of the left temporal lobe with extension into the ventral parietal lobe can cause a receptive aphasia (Wernicke's aphasia) in which a severe comprehension deficit to spoken language develops. Extension of the lesion up into the parietal lobe can produce a similar deficit in the appreciation of written language. Expressive speech may become hyperfluent, with the patient using nonsense words. Such patients can be mistaken for being acutely psychotic, particularly if they have a past psychiatric history. The arcuate fasciculus connects Wernicke's area with Broca's area in the frontal lobe. Lesions limited to the arcuate fasciculus cause a form of aphasia characterized by difficulty with repetition (conduction aphasia).

Autoscopic phenomena

Vestibular signals reach the thalamus bilaterally and relay in the ventral posterolateral nucleus before terminating in the posterior insular cortex. The posterior insular cortex adjacent to the parietal lobe is a vestibular sensory area and may be involved in autoscopic phenomena (Duque-Parra, 2004).

Autoscopic phenomena are illusions involving the entire body in terms of embodiment and body ownership. Four autoscopic phenomena are: autoscopic hallucination, heautoscopy, out-of-body experience, and feeling-of-a-presence. A fifth related phenomenon is the room-tilt illusion. They have been reported following damage to the temporoparietal, frontoparietal, or parieto-occipital cortex. More recently focus has been on the temporoparietal junction (Blanke and Arzy, 2005). During an out-of-body experience the patient is often supine. They localize themselves outside the body and see their body from the disembodied location. Lesions related to out-of-body experience involve the right temporoparietal junction (Blanke et al., 2004; De Ridder et al., 2007).

A patient experiencing heautoscopy reports seeing a second own (illusory) body in their extrapersonal space and localizes himself in the second body. Heautoscopy may follow damage to the left temporoparietal junction. Autoscopy is similar to heautoscopy in that there is a second, illusory body. However, in autoscopy the patient does not localize themselves in the second body. Autoscopy is associated with a lesion of the right parieto-occipital junction (Blanke and Mohr, 2005; Blanke and Castillo, 2007; Lopez et al., 2008).

The lesion associated with feeling-of-a-presence is lateralized to the right and usually involves the frontoparietal cortex. It often accompanies hemineglect. The patient feels (senses but does not see) the presence of another body in the extrapersonal space. The body may be attributed to a person familiar to the patient (Brugger et al., 1996).

The room-tilt illusion is a sudden upside-down reversal that lasts from seconds to hours. The patient does not mislocalize their own body (Brandt and Dieterich, 1999). The room-tilt illusion may be due to a lesion of the brainstem and/or vestibulocerebellar system but also may be due to lesions of the parieto-occipital and frontal cortices (Solms et al., 1988). The room-tilt illusion often has in common with autoscopic phenomena feelings of elevation and floating, along with a disturbance of personal and extrapersonal space (Blanke et al., 2004). It is suggested that the room-tilt illusion is the result of a transient mismatch between visual and vestibular information at the cortical level (Brandt, 1997). The inversion illusion is similar to the room-tilt illusion in which there is a feeling of misalignment with gravity. The inversion illusion is a feeling of being upside-down and is commonly experienced in outer space (Lackner, 1992; Kornilova, 1997).

Vestibular sensations are often reported during autoscopic experiences. Several regions of the cortex receive vestibular information. The vestibular area is defined as the temporoparietal junction and posterior insula, and has been referred to as the parieto-insular vestibular cortex (Grüsser et al., 1994). Projections from the parieto-insular vestibular cortex to the frontal eye fields and the premotor and primary motor areas are believed to be in support of eye movement control. The vestibular cortex appears to be more strongly represented on the right, and the integration of proprioceptive and vestibular signals seems to focus on the right temporoparietal junction (Bottini et al., 2001).

Autism

The temporal lobe appears to be involved in autism. Tasks requiring emotional processing in a social setting have been shown to be associated with decreased activation of the insula in autism (Di Martino et al., 2009). Individuals with autism exhibit abnormal folding of the cortex of the insula (Nordahl et al., 2007).

The fusiform face area has been reported to show significantly little or no activity when viewing facial images. Activation and volume of the amygdala was also significantly reduced when compared with control subjects (Schultz et al., 2000; Pierce et al., 2001). In contrast, the left dorsolateral superior temporal area that includes Wernicke's receptive speech area has been found to show increased activity in high-functioning children with autism and/or Asperger syndrome during sentence comprehension tasks coupled with decreased activity in the left inferior frontal area (Broca's area) (Just et al., 2004). In addition, heightened activity has been reported in the superior temporal gyrus, peristriate cortex and inferior temporal gyrus when viewing images of faces (Critchley et al., 2000; Schultz et al., 1997). These latter areas are usually activated when confronted with face versus nonface images. The combination of reduced activity in higher order face processing areas with increased activity in lower order face processing areas have led to the suggestion that individuals with autism rely on low-level processing. As a result they rely on details for facial recognition and fail to completely integrate information regarding the person (Belmonte et al., 2004). This reduces their ability to form a model of the mental state of another person (theory of mind) (Levy, 2007).

Dyslexia

A number of brain areas are identified as associated with dyslexia including the left inferior frontal cortex, occipital cortex, thalamus, cerebellum, precuneus, and superior temporal gyrus (Maisog et al., 2008). The area most frequently reported is the left middle and inferior temporal gyri (BA 21) and the fusiform gyrus (BA 37). These areas are described as underactivated and show reduced gray matter density (Silani et al., 2005). A more anterior section of the fusiform gyrus of the right side (BA 20) is also reported to be underactivated with accompanying atrophy (Eden et al., 2004).

It is hypothesized that neurons in the left fusiform gyrus develop the ability to recognize the visual forms of familiar words. Injury or insufficient/atypical activation of this area may result in a specific reading deficit such as dyslexia (Proverbio et al., 2008). It is suggested that during reading, dyslexic readers have a deficiency in recruiting left hemisphere language areas in the region of the temporoparietal junction (Maisog et al., 2008).

Increased activity compared with controls has been reported in dyslexic adults in the primary auditory, posterior superior temporal and inferior parietal cortices when comparing pseudo-words and pure tones in auditory working memory (Conway et al., 2008). The left inferior temporal-occipital area has been reported to show increased activity in children with dyslexia following remedial training (Simos et al., 2002).

Prosopagnosia

Prosopagnosia (face blindness) is a disorder in which the ability to recognize faces is impaired while the ability to recognize other objects remains intact. One form is congenital although most cases follow damage to the fusiform face area. Prosopagnosia is usually associated with bilateral occipitotemporal damage and the fusiform face area in particular (Moro et al., 2008). In some instances damage to only the right fusiform face area can produce this deficit (Yovel et al., 2008).

Individuals with developmental prosopagnosia have good object recognition but are unable to recognize faces including those of family members. It may have a familial basis. Imaging studies indicate the fusiform face area is functional in these individuals (Duchaine and Nakayama, 2006). Neutral faces trigger lower activation level compared to controls but

facial expressions produce the same level of activation (Van den Stock et al., 2008). Body recognition is also affected. It is hypothesized that the network used in the initial process of face and body recognition is faulty (Righart and de Gelder, 2007).

Stuttering

Individuals who stutter are reported to be slower in phonological encoding, a task associated with the planum temporale (Sasiekaran et al., 2006). Increases but no decreases in gray matter density have been reported in individuals who stutter. The region exhibiting the greatest increase is the right superior temporal gyrus including Heschl's gyrus (BA 41), the planum temporale and adjacent lateral BA 22 extending into the middle temporal gyrus (BA 21) (Jäncke et al., 2004). A small increase has been reported in the same area on the left (Beal et al., 2007).

Brown et al. (2005) reported that people who stutter showed an increase in activity in the cerebellar vermis and right anterior insula accompanied by a decrease in activity in the auditory areas. They exhibited overactivity compared with control subjects in the anterior insula, cerebellum, and midbrain bilaterally and reduced activity in the ventral premotor cortex, inferior frontal gyrus, and Heschl's gyrus on the left. Reduced white matter was also seen in the area underlying the premotor and inferior frontal gyrus. It is hypothesized that stuttering is due to a disruption of the function of the involved gray matter areas along with the underlying subcortical neural systems represented by the white matter connections (Watkins et al., 2008).

Other behavioral considerations

Insular tumors have been reported to elicit partial seizures that begin with sensations of butterflies in the throat or tingling in the arm followed by a warm flush (Roper et al., 1993). Patients who develop panic symptoms with lactate infusion exhibit blood flow increase bilaterally in the temporal lobes, insular cortex, brainstem superior colliculus, and putamen (Reiman et al., 1989).

A stroke involving the insula has been reported to lead to the loss of the urge to smoke in patients who smoked prior to the stroke. It is proposed that the insula anticipates the pleasure that accompanies use of the drug (Naquvi et al., 2007). An infarct involving the parietal lobe has a high association with a subsequent heart attack. The authors proposed that the parietal lobe has a buffering effect on the insular cortex that is removed following loss of parietal lobe input (Rincon *et al.*, 2008).

Select bibliography

Ellis, H.D., Luaute, J.-P., and Retterstol, N. 1994. Delusional misidentification syndromes. *Psychopathology* **27**:117–120 (1 of 25 articles on this topic in this issue of Psychopathology).

Gloor, P. *The Temporal Lobe and Limbic System.* (New York: Oxford University Press, 1997.)

Lishman, W.A. *Organic Psychiatry.* (Oxford: Blackwell Scientific, 1987.)

Rhawn, J. *Neuropsychology, Neuropsychiatry, and Behavioral Neurology.* (New York: Plenum Press, 1989.)

Willis, W. Jr., and Grossman, R. *Medical Neurobiology.* (St. Louis: Mosby, 1977.)

References

Adolphs, R. 2009. The social brain: neural basis of social knowledge. *Annu. Rev. Psychol.* **60**:693–716.

Aguilar, E.J., Sanjuan, J., Garcia-Marti, G., Lull, J.J., and Robles, M. 2008. MR and genetics in schizophrenia: focus on auditory hallucinations. *Eur. J. Radiol.* **67**:434–439.

Allison, T., Puce, A., and McCarthy, G. 2000. Social perception from visual cues: role of the STS region. *Trends Cogn. Sci.* **4**:267–278.

Amodio, D.M., and Frith, C.D. 2006. Meeting of the minds: the medial frontal cortex and social cognition. *Nat. Rev. Neurosci.* **7**:268–277.

Astafiev, S.V., Shulman, G.L., and Corbetta, M. 2006. Visuospatial reorienting signals in the human temporo-parietal junction are independent of response selection. *Eur. J. Neurosci.* **23**:591–596.

Augustine, J.R. 1996. Circuitry and functional aspects of the insular lobe in primates including humans: A full-length review. *Brain Res. Rev.* **22**:229–244.

Barta, P.E., Pearlson, G.D., Powers, R.E., Richards, S.S., and Tune, L.E. 1990. Auditory hallucinations and smaller superior temporal gyral volume in schizophrenia. *Am. J. Psychiatry* **147**:1457–1462.

Bartels, A., and Zeki, S. 2004. The neural correlates of maternal and romantic love. *Neuroimage* **21**:1155–1166.

Bartolo, A., Benuzzi, F., Nocetti, L., Baraldi, P., and Nichelli, P. 2006. Humor comprehension and appreciation: An fMRI study. *J. Cogn. Neurosci.* **18**:1789–1798.

Beal, D.S., Gracco, V.L., Lafaille, S.J., and De Nil, L.F. 2007. Voxel-based morphometry of auditory and speech-related cortex of stutters. *Neuroreport* **18**:1257–1260.

Beauregard, M., Levesque, J., and Bourgouin, P. 2001. Neural correlates of the conscious self-regulation of emotion. *J. Neurosci.* **21**:RC165.

Belin, P., Zatorre, R.J., Lafaille, P., Ahad, P., and Pike, B. 2000. Voice-selective areas in human auditory cortex. *Nature* **403**:309–312.

Belin, P., Fecteau, S., and Bedard, C. 2004. Thinking the voice: neural correlates of voice perception. *Trends Cogn. Sci.* **8**:129–135.

Belmonte, M.K., Cook Jr, E.H., Anderson, G.M., Rubenstein, J.L.R., Greenough, W.T., Beckel-Mitchener, A., Courchesne, E., Boulanger, L.M., Powell, S.B., Levitt, P.R., Perry, E.K., Jiang, Y.H., DeLorey, T.M., and Tierney, E. 2004. Autism as a disorder of neural information processing: Directions for research and targets for therapy. *Mol. Psychiatry* **9**:646–663.

Berle, D., and Phillips, E.S. 2006. Disgust and obsessive-compulsive disorder: An update. *Psychiatry* **69**:228–238.

Binder, J.R., Frost, J.A., Hammeke, T.A., Bellgowan, P.S.F., Springer, J.S., Kaufman, J.N, and Possing, E.T. 2000. Human temporal lobe activation by speech and nonspeech sounds. *Cereb. Cortex* **10**:512–528.

Blair, R.J., Frith, U., Smith, N., Abell, F., and Cipolotti, L. 2002. Fractionation of visual memory: agency detection and its impairment in autism. *Neuropsychologia* **40**:108–118.

Blakemore, S-J. 2008. The social brain in adolescence. *Nat. Rev. Neurosci.* **9**:267–276.

Blakemore, S-J., and Decety, J. 2001. From the perception of action to the understanding of intention. *Nat. Rev. Neurosci.* **2**:561–567.

Blanke, O., and Arzy, S. 2005. The out-of-body experience: disturbed self-processing at the temporo-parietal junction. *Neuroscientist* **11**:16–24.

Blanke, O., and Mohr, C., 2005. Out-of-body experience, heautoscopy, and autoscopic hallucination of neurological origin. Implications for neurocognitive mechanisms of corporeal awareness and self-consciousness. *Brain Res. Brain Res. Rev.* **50**:184–199.

Blanke, O., and Castillo, V. 2007. Clinical neuroimaging in epileptic patients with autoscopic hallucinations and out-of-body experiences. *Epileptologie* **24**:90–96.

Blanke, O., Landis, T., Spinelli, L., and Seeck, M. 2004. Out-of-body experience and autoscopy of neurological origin. *Brain* **127**:243–258.

Borod, J.C., Martin., C.C., Alpert, M., Brozgold, A., and Welkowitz, J. 1993. Perception of facial emotion in schizophrenic and right brain-damaged patients. *J. Nerv. Ment. Dis.* **181**:494–502.

Bottini, G., Karnath, H.O., Vallar, G., Sterzi, R., Frith, C.D., Frackowiak, R.S., and Paulesu, E. 2001. Cerebral representations for egocentric space: functional-anatomical evidence from caloric vestibular stimulation and neck vibration. *Brain* **134**:1182–1196.

Brandt, T. 1997. Cortical matching of visual and vestibular 3D coordinate maps. *Ann. Neurol.* **42**:983–984.

Brandt, T., and Dieterich, M. 1999. The vestibular cortex, its locations, functions, and disorders. *Ann. N. Y. Acad. Sci.* **871**:293–312.

Brooks, J.C.W., Zambreanu, L., Godinez, A., Craig, A.D., and Tracey, I. 2005. Somatotopic organization of the human insula to painful heat studied with high resolution functional imaging. *Neuroimage* **27**:201–209.

Brothers, L. 1990. The social brain: a project for integrating primate behavior and neurophysiology in a new domain. *Concepts Neurosci.* **1**:27–51.

Brown, S., Ingham, R. J., Ingham, J. C., Laird, A. R., and Fox, P. T. 2005. Stuttered and fluent speech production: An ale meta-analysis of functional neuroimaging studies. *Hum. Brain Mapp.* **25**:105–117.

Brugge, J.F., Volkov, I.O., Garell, P.C., Reale, R. A., and Howard, M.A. III 2003. Functional connections between auditory cortex on Heschl's gyrus and on the lateral superior temporal gyrus in humans. *J. Neurophysiol.* **90**:3750–3763.

Brugger, P., Regard, M., and Landis, T., 1996. Unilaterally felt "presences": the neuropsychiatry of one's invisible Doppelgänger. *Neuropsychiatry, Neuropsychol. Behavioral. Neurol.* **9**:114–122.

Brunswick, N., McCrory, E., Price, C., Frith, C.D., and Frith, U. 1999. Explicit and implicit processing of words and pseudowords by adult developmental dyslexics a search for Wernick's Wortschatz? *Brain* **122**:1901–1917.

Bryson, G., Bell, M., Kaplan, E., Greig, T., and Lysaker, P. 1998. Affect recognition in deficit syndrome schizophrenia. *Psychiatry Res.* **77**:113–120.

Büchel, C., Price, C.J., and Friston, K.J. 1998. A multimodal language area in the ventral visual pathway. *Nature* **394**:274–277.

Campbell, R. 2008. The processing of audio-visual speech: empirical and neural bases. *Phil. Trans. R. Soc. Lond. B* **363**:1001–1010.

Campanella, S., and Belin, P. 2007. Integrating face and voice in person perception. *Trends Cogn. Sci.* **11**:535–543.

Cipolotti, L., Robinson, G., Blair, J., and Frith, U. 1999. Fractionation of visual memory: evidence from a case with multiple neurodevelopmental impairments. *Neruropsychologia* **37**:329–332.

Cleghorn, J.M., Franco, S., Szechtman, B., Kaplan, R.D., Szechtman, H., Brown, G.M., Nhmias, C., and Garnett, E.S. 1992. Toward a brain map of auditory hallucinations. *Am. J. Psychiatry* **149**:1062–1069.

Conway, T., Heilman, K.M., Gopinath, K., Peck, K., Bauer, R., Briges, R.W., Torgesen, J.K., and Crosson, B. 2008. Neural substrates related to auditory working memory comparisons in dyslexia: an fMRI study. *J. Int. Neuropsychol. Soc.* **14**:629–639.

Cox, D., Meyers, E., and Sinha, P. 2004. Contextually evoked object-specific responses in human visual cortex. *Science* **304**:115–117.

Critchley, H., Daly, E., Phillips, M., Brammer, M., Bullmore, E., Williams, S., Van Amelsvoort, T., Robertson, D., David, A., and Murphy, D. 2000. The functional neuroanatomy of social behaviour: Changes in cerebral blood flow when people with autistic disorder process facial expressions. *Brain* **123**:2203–2212.

Critchley, H.D., Wiens, S., Rothstein, P., Ohman, A., and Dolan, R.J. 2004. Neural systems supporting interoceptive awareness. *Nat. Neurosci.* **7**:189–195.

Cutting, J. 1994. Evidence for right hemisphere dysfunction in schizophrenia. In: A.S.David and J.C.Cutting (eds.) *The Neuropsychology of Schizophrenia*. Hove, England: Erlbaum, pp. 321–242.

Damasio, A.R., Grabouski, T.J., Bechara, A., Damasio, H., Ponto, L.L., Parvizi, J., and Hichwa, R.D. 2000. Subcortical and cortical brain activity during the feeling self-generated emotions. *Nat. Neurosci.* **3**:1049–1056.

Damasio, H., Tranel, D., Grabowski, T., Adolphs, R., and Damasio, A. 2004. Neural systems behind word and concept retrieval. *Cognition* **92**:179–229.

Danziger, N., Faillenot, I., and Peyron, R. 2009. Can we share a pain we never felt? Neural correlates of empathy in patients with congenital insensitivity to pain. *Neuron* **61**:203–212.

Decety, J., and Lamm, C. 2007. The role of the right temporoparietal junction in social interaction: how low-level computational processes contribute to mega-cognition. *Neuroscientist* **13**:580–593.

Dehaene-Lambertz, G., Dehaene, S., and Hertz-Pannier, L. 2002. Functional neuroimaging of speech perception in infants. *Science* **298**:2013–2015.

De Ridder, D., Van Laere, K., Dupont, P., Menovsky, T., and Van de Heyning, P. 2007. Visualizing out-of-body experience in the brain. *N. Engl. J. Med.* **357**:1829–1833.

Dickey, C.C., Morocz, I.A., Niznikiewicz, M.A., Voglmaier, M., Toner, S., Khan, U., Dreusicke, M., Yoo, S.S., Shenton, M.E., and McCarley, R.W. 2008. Auditory processing abnormalities in schizotypal personality disorder: an fMRI experiment using tones of deviant pitch and duration. *Schizophr. Res.* **103**:26–39.

Di Martino, A., Ross, K., Uddin, L.Q., Sklar, A.B., Castellanos, F.X., and Milham, M.P. 2009. Functional brain correlates of social and nonsocial processes in autism spectrum disorders: An activation likelihood estimation meta-analysis. *Biol. Psychiatry* **65**:63–74.

Dorsaint-Pierre, R., Penhune, V.B., Watkins, K.E., Neelin, F.P., Lerch, J.P., Bouffard, M., and Zatorre, R.J. 2006. Asymmetries of the planum temporale and Heschl's gyrus: relationship to language lateralization. *Brain* **129**:1164–1176.

Drake, M.E. 1987. Postictal Capgras syndrome. *Clin. Neurol. Neurosurg.* **89**:4.

Duchaine, B.C., and Nakayama, K. 2006. Developmental prosopagnosia: a window to content-specific face processing. *Curr. Opin. Neurobiol.* **16**:166–173.

Duque-Parra, J.E., 2004. Perspective on the vestibular cortex throughout history. *Anat. Rec. B New Anat.* **280**:15–19.

Eden, G.F., Jones, K.M., Cappell, K., Gareau, L., Wood, F.B., Zeffiro, T.A., Dietz, N.A.E., Agnew, J.A., and Lynn Flowers, D.L. 2004. Neural changes following remediation in adult developmental dyslexia. *Neuron* **44**:411–422.

Elliott, R., Newman, J.L., Longe, O.A., and Deakin, J.F. 2003. Differential response patterns in the striatum and orbitofrontal cortex to financial reward in humans: A parametric functional magnetic resonance imaging study. *J. Neurosci.* **23**:303–307.

Engelien, A., Tuscher, O., Hermans, W., Isenberg, N., Eidelberg, D., Frith, C., Stern, E., and Silbersweig, D. 2006. Functional neuroanatomy of non-verbal semantic sound processing in humans. *J. Neural. Transm.* **113**:599–608.

Etkin, A., and Wager, T.D. 2007. Functional neuroimaging of anxiety: a meta-analysis of emotional processing in PTSD, social anxiety disorder, and specific phobia. *Am. J. Psychiatry* **164**:1476–1488.

Farrer, C., Franck, N., Frith, C.D., Decety, J., and Jennerod, M. 2003. Modulating the experience of agency: a PET study. *Neuroimage* **18**:324–333.

Felmingham, K., Kemp, A.H., Williams, L., Falconer, E., Olivieri, G., Peduto, A., and Bryant, R. 2008. Dissociative responses to conscious and non-conscious fear impact underlying brain function in post-traumatic stress disorder. *Psychol. Med.* **38**:1771–1780.

Fitzgerald, P.B., Hoy, K., Daskalakis, Z.J., and Kulkarni, J. 2009. A randomized trial of the anti-depressant effects of low- and high-frequency transcranial magnetic stimulation in treatment-resistant depression. *Depress. Anxiety* **26**:229–234.

Ford, J.M., Mathalon, D.H., Kalba, S., Whitfield, S., Faustman, W.O., and Roth, W.T. 2001. Cortical responsiveness during talking and listening in schizophrenia: An event-related brain potential study. *Biol. Psychiatry* **50**:540–549.

Ford, J.M., Mathalon, D.H., Whitefield, S., Faustman, W.O., and Roth, W.T. 2002. Reduced communication between frontal and temporal lobes during talking in schizophrenia. *Biol. Psychiatry* **51**:485–492.

Fried, I. 1997. Auras and experiential responses arising in the temporal lobe. *J. Neuropsychiatry Clin. Neurosci.* **9**:420–428.

Frith, C.D. 2005. The neural basis of hallucinations and delusions. *C.R. Biologies* **328**:169–175.

Frith, C.D. 2007. The social brain? *Phil. Trans. R. Soc. Lond. B* **362**:671–678.

Frith, W., and Frith, C.D. 2003. Development and neurophysiology of mentalizing. *Phil. Trans. R. Soc. Lond. B* **358**:459–473.

Frith, C.D., and Frith, U. 2007. Social cognition in humans. *Curr. Biol.* **17**:724–732.

Galderisi, S., Quarantelli, M., Volpe, U., Mucci, A., Cassano, G.B., Invernizzi, G., Rossi, A., Vita, A., Pini, S., Cassano, F., Daneluzzo, E., De Peri, L., Stratta, P., Brunetti, A., and Maj, M. 2008. Patterns of structural MRI abnormalities in deficit and nondeficit schizophrenia. *Schizophr. Bull.* **34**:393–401.

Gallagher, H.L., and Frith, C.D. 2004. Dissociable neural pathways for the perception and recognition of expressive and instrumental gestures. *Neuropsycholgia* **42**:1725–1736.

Galuske, R.A., Schlote, W., Bratzke, H., and Singer, W. 2000. Interhemispheric asymmetries of the modular structure in human temporal cortex. *Science* **289**:1646–1949.

Ganis, G., and Kutas, M. 2003. An electrophysiological study of scene effects on object identification. *Cogn. Brain Res.* **16**:123–144.

Gaser, C., Nenadie, I., Volz, H-P., Büchel, C., and Sauer, H. 2004. Neuroanatomy of "hearing voices": A frontotemporal brain structural abnormality associated with auditory hallucinations in schizophrenia. *Cereb. Cortex* **14**:91–96.

Gathers, A.D., Bhatt, R., Corbly, C.R., Farley, A.B., and Joseph, J.E. 2004. Developmental shifts in cortical loci for face and object recognition. *Neuroreport* **15**:1549–1553.

Gauthier, I., Skudlarski, P., Gore, J.C., and Anderson, A.W. 2000. Expertise for cars and birds recruits brain areas involved in face recognition. *Nat. Neurosci.* **3**:191–197.

George, N., and Conty, L. 2008. Facing the gaze of others. Le regard de l'autre. *Neurophysiol. Clin.* **38**:197–207.

Gloor, P. 1997. *The Temporal Lobe and Limbic System.* New York: Oxford University Press.

Gorno-Tempini, M.L., Rankin, K.P., Woolley, J.D., Rosen, H.J., Phengrasamy, L, and Miller, B.L. 2004. Cognitive and behavioral profile in a case of right anterior temporal lobe neurodegeneration. *Cortex* **40**:631–644.

Graeff, F.F., and Del-Ben, C.M. 2008. Neurobiology of panic disorder: from animal models to brain neuroimaging. *Neurosci. Biobehav. Rev.* **32**:1326–1335.

Griffiths, D., and Tadic, S.D. 2008. Bladder control, urgency, and urge incontinence: evidence from functional brain imaging. *Neurourol. Urodyn.* **27**:166–474.

Griffiths, T.D. 2002. Central auditory pathologies. *Br. Med. Bull.* **63**:107–120.

Griffiths, T.D., and Warren, J.D. 2002. The planum temporale as a computational hub. *Trends Neurosci.* 25:348–353.

Grüsser, O.J., Guldin, W.O., Mirring, S., and Salah-Eldin, A.1994. Comparative physiological and anatomical studies of the primate vestibular cortex. In: B. Albowitz, K. Albus, U. Kuhnt, H.C. Nothdurf, and P. Wahle (eds.) *Structural and Functional Organization of the Neocortex.* Berlin: Spinger-Verlag, pp. 358–371.

Hackett, T.A., Stepniewska, I., and Kaas, J.H. 1999. Callosal connections of the parabelt auditory cortex in macaque monkeys. *Eur. J. Neurosci.* 11:856–866.

Halpern, A.R., Zatorre, R.J., Bouffard, M., and Johnson, J.A. 2004. Behavioral and neural correlates of perceived and imagined musical timbre. *Neuropsychologia* 42:1281–1292.

Harrison, L., Penny, W.D., and Friston, K. 2003. Multivariate autoregressive modeling of fMRI time series. *Neuroimage* 19:1477–1491.

Hasson, U., Nir, Y., Levy, I., Fuhrmann, G., and Rafael, M. 2004. Intersubject synchronization of cortical activity during natural vision. *Science* 303:1634–1640.

Haxby, J.V., Gobbini, M.I., Furey, M.L., Ishai, A., Schouten, J.L., and Pietrini, P. 2001. Distributed and overlapping representations of faces and objects in ventral temporal cortex. *Science* 293:2425–2430.

Heekeren, H.R., Wartenburger, I., Schmidt, H., Schwintowski, H-P., and Villringer, A. 2003. An fMRI study of simple ethical decision-making. *Neuroreport* 14:1215–1219.

HeinG., and Knight, R.T. 2008. Superior temporal sulcus –It's my area: or is it? *J. Cogn. Neurosci.*20:2125–2136.

Heining, M., Young, A.W., Ioannou, G., Andrew, C.M., Brammer, M.J., Gray, J.A., and Phillips, M.L. 2003. Disgusting smells activate human anterior insula and ventral striatum. *Ann. N. Y. Acad. Sci.* 1000:380–384.

Hickok, G., and Poeppel, D. 2004. Dorsal and ventral streams: a framework for understanding aspects of the functional anatomy of language. *Cognition* 92:67–99.

Hirayasu, Y., McCarley, R.W., Salisbury, D.F., Tanaka, S., Kwon, J.S., Frumin, M., Snyderman, D., Yurgelun-Todd, D., Kikinis, R., Jolesz, F.A., and Shenton, M.E. 2000. Planum temporale and Heschl gyrus volume reduction in schizophrenia: a magnetic resonance imaging study of first-episode patients. *Arch. Gen. Psychiatry* 57:692–699.

Hoffman, E.A., and Haxby, J.V. 2000. Distinct representations of eye gaze and identity in the distributed human neural system for face perception. *Nat. Neurosci.* 3:80–84.

Honea, R., Crow, T.J., Passingham, D., and Mackay, C.E. 2005. Regional deficits in brain volume in schizophrenia: A meta-analysis of voxel-based morphometry studies. *Am. J. Psychiatry* 162:2233–2245.

Hugdahl, K., Løberg, E-M., Jørgensen, H.A., Lundervold, A., Lund, A., Green, M.F., and Rund, B. 2008. Left hemisphere lateralisation of auditory hallucinations in schizophrenia: A dichotic listening study. *Cogn. Neuropsychiatry* 13:166–179.

Jäncke, L., Wustenberg, T., Scheich, H., and Heinz, H.J. 2002. Phonetic perception and the temporal cortex. *Neuroimage* 15:733–746.

Jäncke, L., Hanggi, J., and Steinmetz, H. 2004. Morphological brain differences between adult stutterers and non-stutterers. *BMC Neurol.* 4:1–8.

Jones, E.G., and Powell, T.P. 1970. An anatomical study of converging sensory pathways within the cerebral cortex of the monkey. *Brain* 93:793–820.

Just, M.A., Cherkassky, V.L., Keller, T.A., and Minshew, N.J. 2004. Cortical activation and synchronization during sentence comprehension in high-functioning autism: evidence of underconnectivitiy. *Brain* 127:1811–1821.

Kanwisher, N., McDermott, J., and Chun, M.M. 1997. The fusiform face area: A module in human extrastriate cortex specialized for face perception. *J. Neurosci.* 17:4302–4311.

Karnath, H.O., Ferber, S., and Himmelbach, M. 2001. Spatial awareness is a function of the temporal not the posterior parietal lobe. *Nature* 411:950–953.

Kasai, K., Shenton, M.E., Salisbury, D.F., Hirayasu, Y., Onitsuka, T., Spencer, M.H., Yurgelun-Todd, D.A., Kikinis, R., Jolesz, F.A., and McCarley, R.W. 2003. Progressive decrease of left Heschl gyrus and planum temporale gray matter volume in first-episode schizophrenia. *Arch. Gen. Psychiatry* 60:766–775.

Keenan, J.P. Thangaraj, V., Halpern, A. R., and Schlaug, G. 2001. Absolute pitch and planum temporale. *Neuroimage* 14:1402–1408.

Kiang, M., and Kutas, M. 2006. Abnormal typicality of responses on a category fluency task in schizotypy. *Psychiatry Res.*145:119–126.

King-Casas, B., Sharp, C., Lomax-Bream, L., Lohrenz, T., Fonagy, P., and Montague, P.R. 2008. The rupture and repair of cooperation in borderline personality disorder. *Science* 321:806–810.

Kircher, T.T.J., Brammer, M.J., Levelt, W., Bartels, M., and McGuire, P.K. 2004. Pausing for thought: engagement of the left temporal cortex during pauses in speech. *Neuroimage* 21:84–90.

Klüver, H., and Bucy, P.C. 1939. Preliminary analysis of functions of the temporal lobes in monkeys. *Arch. Neurol. Psychiatry* 42:979–1000.

Knutson, B., and Greer, S.M. 2008. Anticipatory affect: Neural correlates and consequences for choice. *Proc. R. Soc. Lond. B* 363:3771–3786.

Kornilova, L.N. 1997. Orientation illusions in spaceflight. *J. Vestibular Res.* 7:429–439.

Kosaki, H., Hashikawa, T., He, J., and Jones, E.G. 1997. Tonotopic organization of auditory cortical fields delineated by pavalbumin immuno-reactivity in macaque monkeys. *J. Comp. Neurol.* 386:304–316.

Kraepelin, E. 1919/1971. *Dementia Praecox*. Barclay, E., and Barclay, S. (trans.). New York: Churchill Livingstone.

Kraus, T., Host, K., Kiess, O., Schanze, A., Kornhuber, J., and Forster, C. 2007. BOLD fMRI deactivation of limbic temporal brain structures and mood enhancing effect by transcutaneous vagus nerve stimulation. *J. Neural. Transm.* 114:1485–1493.

Kringelbach, M.L., de Araujo, I.E.T., and Rolls, E.T. 2004. Taste-related activity in the human dorsolateral prefrontal cortex. *Neuroimage* 21:781–788.

Krumbholz, K., Schonwiesner, M., von Cramon, D., Yves, R., Shah, N.J., Zilles, K., and Fink, G.R. 2005. Representation of interaural temporal information from left and right auditory space in the human planum temporale and inferior parietal lobe. *Cereb. Cortex* 15:317–324.

Kuroki, N., Shenton, M.E., Salisbury, D.F., Hirayasu, Y., Onitsuka, T., Ersner-Hershfield, H., Yurgelun-Todd, D., Kikinis, R., Jolesz, F.A., and McCarley, R.W. 2006. Middle and inferior temporal gyrus gray matter volume abnormalities in first-episode schizophrenia: An MRI study. *Am. J. Psychiatry* 1463:2103–2110.

Kwon, J.S., McCarley, R.W., Hirayasu, Y., Anderson, J.E., Fischer, I.A., Kikinis, R., Jolesz, F.A., and Shenton, M.E. 1999. Left planum temporale volume reduction in schizophrenia. *Arch. Gen. Psychiatry* 56:142–148.

Lackner, J.R. 1992. Spatial orientation in weightless environments. *Perception* 21:803–812.

Lane, R., Reiman, E.M., Ahern, G.L., Schwartz, G.E., and Davidson, R.J. 1997. Neuroanatomical correlates of happiness, sadness, and disgust. *Am. J. Psychiatry* 154:926–933.

Lattner, S., Meyer, M.E., and Friederici, A.D. 2005. Voice perception: Sex, pitch, and the right hemisphere. *Hum. Brain Mapp.* 24:11–20.

Lawrence, E.J., Shaw, P., Giampietro, V.P., Surguladze, S., Brammer, J.J., and David, A.S. 2006. The role of "shared representations" in social perception and empathy: an fMRi study. *Neuroimage* 29:1173–1184.

Lawrie, S.M., Buechel, C., Whalley, H.C., Frith, C.D., Friston, K.J., and Johnstone, E.C. 2002. Reduced frontotemporal functional connectivitiy in schizophrenia associated with auditory hallucinations. *Biol. Psychiatry* 51:1008–1011.

Lee, C.U., Shenton, M.E., Salisbury, D.F., Kasi, K., Onitsuka, T., Dickey, C.C., Yurgelun-Todd, D., Kikinis, R., Jolesz, F.A., and McCarley, R.W. 2002. Fusiform gyrus volume reduction in first-episode schizophrenia: an MRI study. *Arch. Gen. Psychiatry* 59:775–781.

Lehmann, C., Mueller, T., Federspiel, A., Hubl, D., Schroth, G., Huber, O., Strik, W., and Dierks, T. 2004. Dissociation between overt and unconscious face processing in fusiform face area. *Neuroimage* 21:75–83.

Lenggenhager, B., Smith, S.T., and Blanke, O. 2006. Functional and neural mechanisms of embodiment: importance of the vestibular system and the temporal parietal junction. *Rev. Neurosci.* 17:643–657.

Leonard, C.M., Puranik, C., Kuldau, J.M., and Lombardino, L.J. 1998. Normal variation in the frequency and location of human auditory cortex landmarks. Heschl's gyrus: Where is it? *Cereb. Cortex* 8:397–406.

Leone, M., Proietti Cecchini, A., Mea, E., Tullo, V., Curone, M., and Bussone, G. 2006. Neuroimaging and pain: a window on the autonomic nervous system. *Neurol. Sci.* 27:S134–S137.

Levesque, J., Eugene, F., Joanette, Y., Paquette, V., Mensour, B., Beaudoin, G., Leroux, J-M., Bourgouin, P., and Beauregard, M. 2003. Neural circuitry underlying voluntary suppression of sadness. *Biol. Psychiatry* 53:502–510.

Levy, F. 2007. Theories of autism. *Aust. N. Z. J. Psychiatry* 41:859–868.

Lewis, J.W., Brefczyniski, J.A., Phinney, R.E., Janik, J.J., and DeYoe, E.A. 2005. Distinct cortical pathways for processing tool versus animal sounds. *J. Neurosci.* 25:5148–5158.

Li, C-S.R., Kosten, T.R., and Sinha, R. 2005. Sex differences in brain activation during stress imagery in abstinent cocaine users: a functional magnetic resonance imaging study. *Biol. Psychiatry* 57:487–494.

Limb, C.J. 2006. Structural and functional neural correlates of music perception. *Anat. Rec. A Discov. Mol. Cell Evol. Biol.* 288A:435–446.

Lindauer, R.J.L., Booij, J., Habraken, J.B.A., van Meijel, E.P.M., Uylings, H.B.M., Olff, M., Carlier, I.V.E., den Heeten, G.J., van Eck-Smit, B.L.F., and Gersons, B.P.R. 2007. Effects of psychotherapy on regional cerebral blood flow during trauma imagery in patients with post-traumatic stress disorder: a randomized clinical trial. *Psychol. Med.* 38:543–554.

Lopez, C., Halje, P., and Blanke, O., 2008. Body ownership and embodiment: Vestibular and multisensory mechanisms. *Clin. Neurorphysiol.* 38:149–161.

Lorberbaum, J.P., Newman, J.D., Horwitz, A.R., Dubno, J.R., Lydiard, R.B., Hamner, M.B., Bohning, D.E., and George, M.S. 2002. A potential role for thalamocingulate circuitry in human maternal behavior. *Biol. Psychiatry* 51:431–445.

Lorberbaum, J.P., Kose, S., Johnson, M.R., Arana, G.W., Sullivan, L.K., Hamner, M.B., Ballenger, J.C., Lydiard,

R.B., Brodrick, P.S., Bohning, D.E., and George, M.S. 2004. Neural correlates of speech anticipatory anxiety in generalized social phobia. *Neuroreport* **15**:2701–2705.

MacSweeney, M., Campbell, R., Woll, B., Giampietro, V., David, A.S., McGuire, P.K., Calvert, GA., and Brammer, M.J. 2004. Dissociating linguistic and nonlinguistic gestural communication in the brain. *Neuroimage* **22**:1605–1618.

Maisog, J.M., Einbinder, E.R., Flowers, D.L., Turkeltaub, P.E., and Eden, G.F. 2008. A meta-analysis of functional neuroimaging studies of dyslexia. *Ann. N. Y. Acad. Sci.* **1145**:234–259.

Malloy, P., Cimino, C., and Westlake, R. 1992. Differential diagnosis of primary and secondary Capgras delusions. *Neuropsychiatry Neuropsychol. Behav. Neurol.* **5**:83–96.

May, A. 2008. Chronic pain may change the structure of the brain. *Pain* **137**:7–15.

McCarley, R.W., Shenton, M.E., O'Donnell, B.F., and Nestor, P.G. 1993. Uniting Kraepelin and Bleuler: The psychology of schizophrenia and the biology of temporal lobe abnormalities. *Harvard Rev. Psychiatry* **1**:36–56.

McIntosh, A., and Lawrie, S. 2004. Structural magnetic resonance imaging. In: S.Lawrie, E.Johnstone, and D.Weinberger (eds.) *Schizophrenia from Neuroimaging to Neuroscience.* Oxford: Oxford University Press, pp. 21–57.

McGurk, H., and MacDonald, J. 1976. Hearing lips and seeing voices. *Nature* **264**:746–748.

Mega, M.S., Cummings, J.L., Salloway, S., and Malloy, P. 1997. The limbic system: an anatomic, phylogenetic, and clinical perspective. *J. Neuropsychiatry Clin. Neurosci.* **9**:315–330.

Meisenzahl, E.M., Koutsouleris, N., Gaser, C., Bottlender, R., Schmitt, G.J.E., McGuire, P., DeckerP., Burgermeister, B., Born, C., Reiser, M., and Moller, H-J. 2008. Structural brain alterations in subjects at high-risk of psychosis: a voxel-based morphometric study. *Schizophr. Res.***102**:150–162.

Mendez, M.F. 2001. Generalized auditory agnosia with spared music recognition in a left-hander. Analysis of a case with a right temporal stroke. *Cortex* **37**:139–50.

Mendez, M.F., and Cummings, J.L. 2003. *Dementia: A Clinical Approach,* 3rd ed. New York: Butterworth-Heinemann, p. 206.

Mendez, M.F., Saghafi, S., and Clark, D.G. 2004. Semantic dementia in multilingual patients. *J. Neuropsychiatry Clin. Neurosci.* **16**:381.

Metelman, S.A., and Buchsbaum, M.S. 2007. Very poor outcome schizophrenia: Clinical and neuroimaging aspects. *Int. Rev. Psychiatry* **19**:347–359.

Miall, R.C., and Wolpert, D.M. 1996. Forward models for physiological motor control. *Neural Netw.* **9**:1265–1279.

Mobbs, D., Greicius, M.D., Abdel-Azim, E., Menon, V., and Reiss, A.L. 2003. Humor modulates the mesolimbic reward centers. *Neuron* **40**:1041–1048.

Moll, J., de Oliveira-Souza, R., Eslinger, P.J., Bramati, I.E., Mourao-Miranda, J., Andreiuolo, P.A., and Pessoa, L. 2002. The neural correlates of moral sensitivity: a functional magnetic resonance investigation of basic and moral emotions. *J. Neurosci.* **22**:2730–2736.

Morgan, K.D., Dazzan, P., Orr, K.G., Hutchinson, G., Chitnis, X., Suckling, J., Lythgoe, D., Pollock, S-J. Rossell, S., Shapleske, J., Fearon, P., Morgan, C., David, A., McGuire, P.K., Jones, P.B., Leff, J., and Murray, R.M. 2007. Grey matter abnormalities in first-episode schizophrenia and affective psychosis. *Br. J. Psychiatry* –Supp **51**:S111–116.

Moro, V., Urgesi, C., Pernigo, S., Lanteri, P., Pazzaglia, M., and Aglioti, S.M. 2008. The neural basis of body form and body action agnosia. *Neuron* **60**:235–246.

Mummery, C.J., Ashburner, J., Scott, S.K., and Wise, R.J. 1999. Funtional neuroimaging of speech perception in six normal and two aphasic subjects. *J. Acoust. Soc. Am.* **106**:449–447.

Mycack, P., Kramer, J.H., Boone, K.B., and Biller, B.L. 2001. The influence of right frontotemporal dysfunction on social behavior in frontotemporal dementia. *Neurology* **56**:11–15.

Nagai, M., Kishi, K., and Kato, S. 2007. Insular cortex and neuropsychiatric disorders: A review of recent literature. *Eur. J. Psychiatry.* **22**:387–394.

Nahas, Z., Teneback, C., Chae, J-H., Mu., Q., Molnar, C., Kozel, F.A., Walker, J., Anderson, B., Koola, J., Kose, S., Lomarev, M., Bohning, D.E., and Geroge, M.S. 2007. Serial vagus nerve stimulation functional MRI in treatment-resistant depression. *Neuropsychopharmacology* **32**:1649–1660.

Nakamura, K., Kawashima, R., Sato, N., Nakamura, A., Sugiura, M., Kato, T., Hatano, K, Ito, K., Fukuda, H., Schormann, T., and Zilles, K. 2000. Functional delineation of the human occipito-temporal areas related to face and scene processing: a PET study. *Brain* **123**:1903–1912.

Nakamura, K., Kawashima, R., Sugiura, M., Kato, T., Nakamura, A., Hatano, K., Nagumo, S., Kubota, K., Fukuda, H., Ito, K., and Kojima, S. 2001. Neural substrates for recognition of familiar voices: a PET study. *Neuropsychologia* **39**:1047–1054.

Naqvi, N.H., Rudrauf, D., Damasio, H., and Bechara, A. 2007. Damage to the insular disrupts addiction to cigarette smoking. *Science* **315**:531–534.

Narumoto, J., Ikada, T., Sadato, N., Fukui, K. and Yonekura, Y. 2001. Attention to modulate fMRI activity in human right superior temporal sulcus. *Brain Res. Cogn. Brain Res.* **12**:225–231.

Nelson, E.E., Leibenluft, E., McClure, E.B., and Pine, D.S. 2005. The social re-orientation of adolescence: A neuroscience perspective on the process and its relation to psychopathology. *Psychol. Med.* **35**:163–174.

Nordahl, C.W., Dierker, D., Mostafavi, I., Schumann, C.M., Rivera, S.M., Amaral, D.G., and Van Essen, D.C. 2007. Cortical folding abnormalities in autism revealed by surface-based morphometry. *J. Neurosci.* **27**:11725–11735.

O' Donnell, B.F., Vohs, J.L., Hetrick, W.P., Carroll, C.A., and Shekhar, A. 2005. Auditory event-related potential abnormalities in bipolar disorder and schizophrenia. *Int. J. Psychophysiol.* **53**:45–55.

Olson, I.R., Plotzker, A., and Ezzyat, Y. 2007. The enigmatic temporal pole: a review of findings on social and emotional processing. *Brain* **130**:1718–1731.

Onitsuka, T., Shenton, M.E., Salisbury, D.F., Dickey, C.C., Kasai, K., Toner, S.K., Frumin, M., Kikinis, R., Jolesz, F.A., and McCarley, R.W. 2004. Middle and inferior temporal gyrus gray matter volume abnormalities in chronic schizophrenia: An MRI Study. *Am. J. Psychiatry* **161**:1603–1611.

Oppenheimer, S. 1993. The anatomy and physiology of cortical mechanisms of cardiac control. *Stroke* 24(Suppl. 12): I3–I5.

Pa, J., and Hickok, G. 2008. A parietal-temporal sensory-motor integration area for the human vocal tract: Evidence from an fMRI study of skilled musicians. *Neuropsychologia* **46**:362–368.

Paulesu, E., Frith, C.D., and Frackowiak, R.S.J. 1993. The neural correlates of the verbal component of working memory. *Nature* **362**:342–344.

Peretz, I., and Zatorre, R.J. 2005. Brain organization for music processing. *Annu. Rev. Psychol.* **56**:89–114.

Petty, R.G., Barta, P.E., Pearlson, G.D., McGilchrist, I.K., Lewis, R.W., Tien, A.Y., Pulver, A., Vaughn, D.D., Casanova, M.F., and Powers, R.E. 1995. Reversal of asymmetry of the planum temporale in schizophrenia. *Am. J. Psychiatry* **152**:715–721.

Pierce, K., Müller, R.-A., Ambrose, J., Allen, G., and Courchesne, E. 2001. Face processing occurs outside the fusiform "face area" in autism: Evidence from functional MRI. *Brain* **124**:2059–2073.

Potkin, S.G., Alva, G., Fleming, K., Anand, R., Keator, D., Carreon, D., Doo, M., Jin, Y., Wu, J.C., and Fallon, J.H. 2002. A PET study of the pathophysiology of negative symptoms in schizophrenia. Positron emission tomography. *Am. J. Psychiatry* **159**:227–237.

Premack, D.G., and Woodruff, G. 1978. Does the chimpanzee have a theory of mind? *Behav. Brain Sci.* **1**:515–526.

Proverbio, A.M., Zani, A., and Adorni, R. 2008. The left fusiform area is affected by written frequency of words. *Neuropsychologia* **48**:2292–2299.

Puce, A., Allison, T., Bentin, S., Gore, J.C., and McCarthy, G. 1998. Temporal cortex activation in humans viewing eye and mouth movements. *J. Neurosci.* **18**:2188–2199.

Puce, A., and Perrett, D. 2003. Electrophysiology and brain imaging of biological motion. *Phil. Trans. Roy. Soc. Lond. B* **358**:435–445.

Rademacher, J., Morosan, P., Schleicher, A., Freund, H.J., and Zilles, K. 2001. Human primary auditory cortex in women and men. *Neuroreport* **12**:1561–1566.

Rankin, K.P., Gorno-Tempini, M.L., Allison, S.C., Stanley, C.M., Glenn, S., Weiner, M.W., and Miller, B.L. 2006. Structural anatomy of empathy in neurodegenerative disease. *Brain* **129**:2945–2956.

Rauschecker, J.P., Tian, B., and Hauser, M. 1995. Processing of complex sounds in the macaque nonprimary auditory cortex. *Science* **268**:111–114.

Redcay, E., 2008. The superior temporal sulcus performs a common function for social and speech perception: Implications for the emergence of autism. *Neurosci. Biobehav. Rev.* **32**:123–142.

Reiman, E.M., Raichle, M.E., Robins, E., Mintun, M.A., Fusselman, M.J., Fox, P.T., Price, J.L., and Hackman, K.A. 1989. Neuroanatomical correlates of a lactate-induced anxiety attack. *Arch. Gen. Psychiatry* **46**: 493–500.

Reiman, E.M., Lane, R.D., Ahern, G.L., Schwartz, G.E., Davidson, R.J., Friston, K.J., Yun, L.-S., and Chen, K. 1997. Neuroanatomical correlates of externally and internally generated human emotion. *Am. J. Psychiatry* **154**:918–925.

Reite, M., Sheeder, J., Teale, P., Adams, M., Richardson, D., Simon, J., Jones, R.H., and Rojas, D.C. 1997. Magnetic source imaging evidence of sex differences in cerebral lateralization in schizophrenia. *Arch. Gen. Psychiatry* **54**:433–440.

Righart, R., and de Gelder, B. 2007. Impaired face and body perception in developmental prosopagnosia. *Proc. Natl. Acad. Sci. USA.* **104**:17234–1 7238.

Rimol, L.M., Specht, K., Weis, S., Savoy, R., and Hugdahl, K. 2005. Processing of sub-syllabic speech units in the posterior temporal lobe: an fMRI study. *Neuroimage* **26**:1059–1067.

Rincon, F., Dhamoon, M., Moon, Y., Paik, M.C., Boden-Albala, B., Homma, S., Di Tullio, M.R., Sacco, R.L., and Elkind, M.S.V. 2008. Stroke Location and Association With Fatal Cardiac Outcomes: Northern Manhattan Study (NOMAS). *Stroke* **39**:2425–2431.

Rocca, M.A., Ceccarelli, A., Falini, A., Colombo, B., Tortorella, P., Bernasconi, L, Comi, G., Scotti, G., and Filippi, M. 2006. Brain gray matter changes in migraine patients with T2-visible lesions: a 3-T MRI study. *Stroke* **37**:1765–1770.

Roder, B., Stock, O., Neville, H., Bien, S., and Rosler, F. 2002. Brain activation modulated by the comprehension of normal and pseudo-word sentences of different processing demands: a functional magnetic resonance imaging study. *Neuroimage* **15**:1003–1014.

Rolls, E.T. 2006. Brain mechanisms underlying flavour and appetite. *Phil Trans. Roy. Soc. Lond. Sci.* **361**:1123–1136.

Roper, S.N., Levesque, M.F., Sutherling, W.W., and Engel, J. Jr. 1993. Surgical treatment of partial epilepsy arising from the insular cortex. *J. Neurosurg.* **79**:266–269.

Royet, J-P., Zald, D., Versace, R., Costes, N., Lavenne, F., Koenig, O., and Gervais, R. 2000. Emotional responses to pleasant and unpleasant olfactory, visual, and auditory stimuli: a positron emission tomography study. *J. Neurosci.* **20**:7752–7759.

Ruby, P., and Decety, J. 2003. What you believe versus what you think they believe: A neuroimaging study of conceptual perspective-taking. *Eur. J. Neurosci.* **17**:2475–2480.

Saarela, M.V., Hiushchuk, Y., Willaims, A.C., Schurmann, M., Kalso, E., and Hari, R. 2007. The compassionate brain: Humans detect intensity of pain from another's face. *Cereb. Cortex* **17**:230–237.

Saleem, K.S., Kondo, H., and Price, J.L. 2008. Complementary circuits connecting the orbital and medial prefrontal networks with the temporal, insular, and opercular cortex in the macaque monkey. *J. Comp. Neurol.* **506**:659–693.

Sasiekaran, J., De Nil, L.F., Smyth, R., and Johnson, C. 2006. Phonological encoding in the silent speech of persons who stutter. *J. Fluency Disord.* **31**:1–21.

Saxe, R., and Wexler, A. 2005. Making sense of another mind: the role of the right temporo-parietal junction. *Neuropsychologia* **43**:1391–1399.

Schmidt-Wilcke, T., Leinisch, E., Straube, A., Kampfe, N., Draganski, B., Diener, H.C., Bogdahn, U., and May, A. 2007. Gray matter decrease in patients with chronic tension type headache. *Neurology* **65**:1483–1486.

Schneider, P., Scherg, M., Dosch, H.G., Specht, H.J., Gutschalk, A., and Rupp, A. 2002. Morphology of Heschl's gyrus reflects enhanced activation in the auditory cortex of musicians. *Nat. Neurosci.* **5**:688–694.

Schön, D., Rosenkranz, M,. Regelsberger, J., Dahme1, B., Büchel, C., and von Leupold.A. 2008. Reduced perception of dyspnea and pain after right insular cortex lesions. *Am. J. Respir. Crit. Care Med.* **178**:1173–1179.

Schonwiesner, M., and Zatorre, R.J. 2008. Depth electrode recordings show double dissociation between pitch processing in lateral Heschl's gyrus and sound onset processing in medial Heschl's gyrus. *Exp. Brain Res.* **187**:97–105.

Schultz, R.T., Gauthier, I., Klin, A., Fulbright, R.K., Anderson, A.W., Volkmar, F., Skudlarski, P., Lacadie, C., Cohen, D.J., and Gore, J.C. 2000. Abnormal ventral temporal cortical activity during face discrimination among individuals with autism and Asperger syndrome. *Arch. Gen. Psychiatry* **57**:331–340.

Schunck, T., Erb, G., Mathis, A., Jacob, N., Gilles, C., Namer, I.J., Meier, D., and Luthringer, R. 2008. Test-retest reliability of a functional MRI anticipatory anxiety paradigm in healthy volunteers. *J. Magn. Reson. Imaging* **27**:459–168.

Scott, S.K., Blank, C., Rosen, S., and Wise, R.J.S. 2000. Identification of a pathway for intelligible speech in the left temporal lobe. *Brain* **123**:2400–2406.

Scott, S.K., Rosen, S., Lang, H., and Wise, R.J.S. 2006. Neural correlates of intelligibility in speech investigated with noise vocoded speech –a positron emission tomography study. *J. Acoust. Soc. Am.* **120**:1075–1083.

Shapira, N.A., Liu, Y., He, A.E., Bradley, M.B., Lessig, M.C., James, G.A., Stein, D.J., Lang, P.J., and Goodman, W.K. 2003. Brain activation by disgust-inducing pictures in obsessive-compulsive disorder. *Biol. Psychiatry* **54**:751–756.

Shapleske, J., Rossell, S.L., Woodruff, P.W., and David, A.S. 1999. The planum temporale: a systematic, quantitative review of its structural, functional and clinical significance. *Brain Res. Rev.* **29**:26–49.

Shapleske, J., Rossell, S.L., Chitnis, X.A., Suckling, J., Simmons, A., Bullmore, E.T., Woodruff, P.W., and David, A.S. 2002. A computational morphometric MRI study of schizophrenia: effects of hallucinations. *Cereb. Cortex* **12**:1331–1341.

Shenton, M.E., Dickey, C.C., Frumin, M., and McCarley, R.W. 2001. A review of MRI findings in schizophrenia. *Schizophr. Res.* **49**:1–52.

Shergill, S.S., Bullmore, E., Simmons, A., Murray, R., and McGuire, P. 2000. Functional anatomy of auditory verbal imagery in schizophrenic patients with auditory hallucinations. *Am. J. Psychiatry* **157**:1691–1693.

Shulman, G.I., Astafiev, S.V., McAvoy, M.P., d'Avossa, G., and Corbetta, M. 2007. Right TPJ deactivation during visual search functional significance and support for a filter hypothesis. *Cereb. Cortex* **17**:2625–2633.

Schultz, W., Tremblay, L., and Hollerman, J. 1997. Reward processing in primate orbitofrontal cortex and basal ganglia. *Cereb. Cortex* **10**:272–283.

Silani, G., Frith, U., Demonet, J.F., Fazio, F., Perani, D., Price, C., Frith, C.D., and Paulesu, E. 2005. Brain abnormalities underlying altered activation in dyslexia: a voxel based morphometry study. *Brain* **128**:2453–2461.

Simmons, A., Strigo, I., Matthews, S.C., Paulus, M.P., and Stein, M.B. 2006. Anticipation of aversive visual stimuli is associated with increased insula activation in anxiety-prone subjects. *Biol. Psychiatry* **60**:402–409.

Simmons, A.N., Paulus, M.P., Thorp, S.R., Matthews, S.C., Norman, S.B., and Stein, M.B. 2008a. Functional activation and neural networks in women with posttraumatic stress disorder related to intimate partner violence. *Biol. Psychiatry* **64**:681–690.

Simmons, A., Matthews, S.C., Feinstein, J.S., Hitchcock, C., Paulus, M.P., and Stein, M.B. 2008b. Anxiety vulnerability is associated with altered anterior cingulate response to an affective appraisal task. *Neuroreport* **19**:1033–1037.

Simos, P.G., Fletcher, J.M., Bergman, E., Breier, J.I., Foorman, B.R., Castillo, E.M., Davis, R.N., Fitzgerald, M., and Papanicolaou, A.C. 2002. Dyslexia-specific brain activation profile becomes normal following successful remedial training. *Neurology* **58**:1203–1213.

Singer, T., Seymour, B., O'Doherty, J., Kaube, H., Dolan, R.J., and Frith, C.D. 2004. Empathy for pain involves the affective but not sensory components of pain. *Science* **303**:1157–1162.

Singer, T., Seymour, B., O'Doherty, J., Stephan, K., Dolan, R.J., and Frith, D.D. 2006. Empathic neural responses are modulated by the perceived fairness of others. *Nature* **439**:466–469.

Sno, H.N. 1994. A continuum of misidentification symptoms. *Psychopathology* **27**:144–147.

Snowden, J.S., Thompson, J., C., and Neary, D. 2004. Knowledge of famous faces and names in semantic dementia. *Brain* **127**:860–867.

Solms, M., Kaplan-Solms, K., Saling, M., and Miller, P. 1988. Inverted vision after frontal lobe disease. *Cortex* **24**:499–509.

Southard, E.E. 1910. A study of the dementia praecox group in the light of certain cases showing anomalies or scleroses in particular brain regions. *Am. J. Insanity* **67**:119–176.

Stein, M.B., Simmons, A.N., Feinstein, J.S., and Paulus, M.P. 2007. Increased amygdala and insula activation during emotion processing in anxiety-prone subjects. *Am. J. Psychiatry* **164**:318–327.

Stevens, A.A., and Weaver, K.E. 2009. Functional characteristics of auditory cortex in the blind. *Behav. Brain Res.* **196**:134–138.

Stoléru, S., Grégoire, M-C., Gérard, D., Decety, J., Lafarge, E., Cinotti, L, Lavenne, F., LeBars, D., Vernet-Maury, E., Rada, H., Collet, C., Mazoyer, B., Forest, M.G., Magnin, F., Spira, A., and Comar, D. 1999. Neuroanatomical correlates of visually evoked sexual arousal in human males. *Arch. Sex. Behav.* **28**:1–21.

Suzuki, M., Yuasa, S., Minabe, Y., Murata, M., and Kurachi, M. 1993. Left superior temporal blood flow increases in schizophrenia and schizophreniform patients with auditory hallucination: A longitudinal case study using 123I-IMP SPECT. *Eur. Arch. Psychiatry Clin. Neurosci.* **242**:257–261.

Tabert, M.H., Borod, J.C., Tang, C.Y., Lange, G., Wei, T.C., Johnson, R., Nusbaum, A.O., and Buchsbaum, M.S. 2001. Differential amygdala activation during emotional decision and recognition memory tasks using unpleasant words: an fMRI study. *Neuropsychologia* **39**:556–573.

Thompson, J.C., Clarke, M., Stewart, T., and Puce, A. 2005. Configural processing of biological motion in human superior temporal sulcus. *J. Neurosci.* **25**: 9059–9066.

Thompson, S.A., Patterson, K., and Hodges, J.R. 2003. Left/right asymmetry of atrophy in semantic dementia: behavioral-cognitive implications. *Neurology* **61**:1196–1203.

Tsukiura, T., Namiki, M., Fujii, T., and Iijima, T. 2003. Time-dependent neural activations related to recognition of people's names in emotional and neutral face-name associative learning: an fMRI study. *Neuroimage* **20**:784–794.

Tzourio-Mazoyer, N., Schonen, S.D., Crivello, F, Reutter, B., Aujard, Y. and Mazoyer, B. 2002. Neural correlates of woman face processing by 2-month-old infants. *Neuroimage* **15**:454–461.

Uddin, L.Q., Molnar-Szakacs, I., Zaide, I. E., and Iacoboni, M. 2006. rTMS to the right inferior parietal lobule disrupts self-other discrimination. *Soc. Cogn. Affect. Neurosci.* **1**:65–71.

Ungerleider, L.G., and Mishkin, M. 1982. Two cortical visual systems. In: D.J.Ingle, M.H.Goodale, and R.J.W.Mansfield (eds.) *The Analysis of Visual Behavior.* Cambridge, MA: M.I.T. Press.

Van den Stock, J., van de Rit, W.A.C., Righart, R., and de Gelder, B. 2008. Neural correlates of perceiving emotional faces and bodies in developmental prosopagnosia: an event-related fMRI-study. *PLoS ONE* **3**:e 3195.

Van Lancker Sidtis, D. 2006. Where in the brain is nonliteral language? *Metaphor and Symbol* **21**:213–244.

Virtue, S., Haberman, J., Clancy, Z., Parrish, T., and Jung-Beeman, M. 2006. Neural activity of inferences during story comprehension. *Brain Res.* **1084**:104–114.

Vollm, B.A., Taylor, A.N.W., Richardson, P., Rhiannon, C., Stirling, J., McKie, S., Deakin, J.F.L, and Elliott, R. 2006. Neuronal correlates of theory of mind and empathy: a functional magnetic resonance imaging study in a nonverbal task. *Neuroimage* **29**:90–98.

Vuilleumier, P., Armong., J.L., Driver, J., and Dolan, R.J. 2001. Effects of attention and emotion of face processing in the human brain: an event-related fMRI study. *Neuron* **30**:829–841.

Watkins, K.E., Smith, S.M., Davis, S., and Howell, P. 2008. Structural and functional abnormalities of the motor system in developmental stuttering. *Brain* **131**: 50–59.

Westbury, C.F., Zatorre, R.J., and Evans, A.C. 1999. Quantifying variability in the planum temporale: A probability map. *Cereb. Cortex* **9**:392–405.

Wise, R.J., Scott, S.K., Blank, S.C., Mummery, C.J., Murphy, K., and Warburton, E.A. 2001. Separate neural subsystems within "Wernicke's area." *Brain* **124**:83–95.

Wright, I.E., Rabe-Hesketh, S., Woodruff, P.W., David, A.S., Murray, R.M., and Bullmore, E.T. 2000. Meta-analysis of regional brain volumes in schizophrenia. *Am. J. Psychiatry* **157**:16–25.

Xu, J., Kemeny, S., Park, G., Frattali, C., and Braun, A. 2005. Language in context: emergent features of word, sentence, and narrative comprehension. *Neuroimage* **25**:1002–1015.

Yang, J-C.P., Park, K., Eun, S-J., Lee, M-S., Yoon, J-S., Shin, I-S., Kim, Y-K., Chung, T-W., Kang, H-K., and Jeong, G-W. 2008. Assessment of cerebrocortrical areas associated with sexual arousal in depressive women using functional MR imaging. *J. Sex. Med.* **5**:602–609.

Young, M.W., Robinson, I. H., Hellavell, D.J., DePauw, K.E., and Pentland, B. 1992. Cotard delusion after brain injury (case study). *Psychol. Med.* **21**:799–804.

Yovel, G., Tambini, A., and Brandman, T. 2008. The asymmetry of the fusiform face area is a stable individual characteristic that underlies the left visual field superiority for faces. *Neuropsychologia* **46**:3061–3068.

Zaehle, T., Geiser, E., Alter, K., Jancke, L., and Meyer, M. 2008. Segmental processing in the human auditory dorsal stream. *Brain Res.* **1220**:179–190.

Zaki, J., Ochsner, K.N., Hanelin, J., and Wager, T.D. 2007. Different circuits for different pain: Patterns of functional connectivity reveal distinct networks for processing pain in self and others. *Soc. Neurosci.* **2**: 275–291.

Zatorre, R.J. 2007. There's more to auditory cortex than meets the ear. *Hear. Res.* **229**:24–30.

Zatorre, R.J., Bouffard, M., Ahad, P., and Belin, P. 2002. Where is the 'where' in the human auditory cortex. *Nat. Neurosci.* **5**:905–909.

Zetzsche, T., Meisenzahl, E.M., Preuss, U.W., Holder, J.J., Leinsinger, G., Hahn, H., Hegeri, U., and Möller, H.J. 2001. In-vivo analysis of the human planum temporale: does the definition of PT borders influence the results with regard to cerebral asymmetry and correlation with handedness? *Psychiatry Res.* **107**: 99–115.

Introduction

The elusive functions of the frontal lobe continue to fascinate the neuroscientist and the neuropsychologist. The frontal lobe is impressively developed in humans and makes up more than a third of the entire cortical area (Damasio and Anderson, 1993). It controls the actions of our body through its motor areas. The frontal lobe appears to be responsible for shaping our attitudes and organizing our repertoire of behaviors. Functions that are hallmarks of human behavior, such as intentionality, self-regulation, and self-awareness, are thought to be under the executive control of the frontal lobe. In fact, the prefrontal cortex provides the capacity for judgment, which can constantly adapt behavior in order to optimize its outcome.

An ongoing controversy among researchers is whether the prefrontal area contains regions with discrete functions subservient to an overall executive module that provides an integrated output of the system, or that the entire prefrontal region is involved in this integrative function. The latter hypothesis requires that the neural modules of the prefrontal regions be highly dynamic. Evidence for both theories exists.

The truth is likely to have elements of both schemas, with specialization as well as versatility contributing to the proper functioning of this most fascinating of brain regions. Different competing, and not necessarily mutually exclusive, theories will be introduced throughout the chapter.

Subdivisions of the frontal lobe

The frontal lobe lies anterior to the central sulcus and is made up of three anatomically distinct regions: the dorsolateral aspect, the medial aspect, and the orbital (inferior) aspect. The motor cortex [Brodmann's areas (BA) 4, BA 6, BA 8, BA 44, and BA 45] makes up the posterior portion of both the dorsolateral and medial aspects. Broca's area (BA 44 and BA 45) and the frontal eye fields (BA 8) are considered by some to be part of the motor cortex. The frontal lobe anterior to the motor area, including the orbital cortex, is the prefrontal cortex (Figures 6.1, 6.2, and 6.3).

The motor cortex is responsible for the origin of the majority of the axons that make up the corticobulbar and corticospinal (pyramidal) tracts. The corticobulbar tract projects to the brainstem (the bulb is the lower

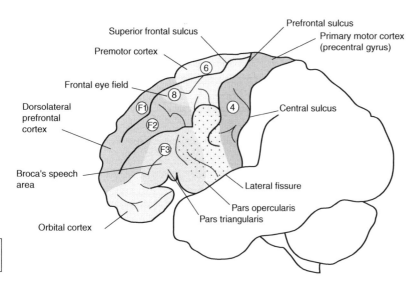

Superior frontal sulcus
Premotor cortex
Frontal eye field
Dorsolateral prefrontal cortex
Broca's speech area
Orbital cortex
Prefrontal sulcus
Primary motor cortex (precentral gyrus)
Central sulcus
Lateral fissure
Pars opercularis
Pars triangularis
6
8
F1
F2
F3
4

Figure 6.1. Lateral view of the frontal cortex indicating gyri, sulci, and functional areas. The prefrontal cortex is represented in this view by the dorsolateral prefrontal cortex and the orbital cortex. The remainder of frontal cortex seen here is motor cortex. F1, superior frontal gyrus; F2, middle frontal gyrus; F3, inferior frontal gyrus. Stippling indicates approximate location of frontal lobe mirror neurons.

brainstem). The corticospinal tract projects to the spinal cord. The motor cortex consists of the:

- Primary motor cortex.
- Premotor cortex.
- Supplementary motor area (SMA).
- Frontal eye field.
- Broca's speech area.

The prefrontal cortex is served by axons that arise from the mediodorsal (MD) thalamic nucleus and consists of the:

- Dorsolateral prefrontal cortex (DLPFC).
- Medial prefrontal cortex (MPFC).
- Orbitofrontal cortex (OFC).

The anterior cingulate gyrus is also served by the MD thalamic nucleus and is often included as part of the prefrontal cortex (Figures 6.3 and 12.1). Distinct clinical syndromes can be identified with lesions of each of the three prefrontal areas, but in practice there is often overlap in resulting symptomatology. The MPFC and anterior SMC may overlap in function.

The gray and white matter of the prefrontal cortex develop at different rates. The gray matter increases in volume until somewhere between 4 and 12 years of age after which it decreases gradually (Giedd *et al.*, 1999). Synaptic density decreases as gray matter volume increases (Huttenlocher, 1979), and white matter volume continues to increase beyond adolescence into early adulthood (Sowell *et al.*, 2001). It is believed that primary motor and sensory areas myelinate before association areas (Fuster, 2002).

Motor cortex

Primary motor cortex

The primary motor cortex (BA 4) corresponds with the precentral gyrus on the lateral surface of the cortex and extends medially into the longitudinal cerebral

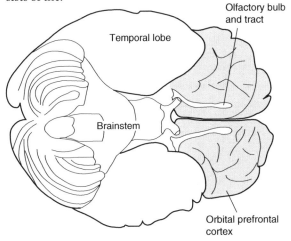

Figure 6.2. Inferior aspect of the frontal cortex.

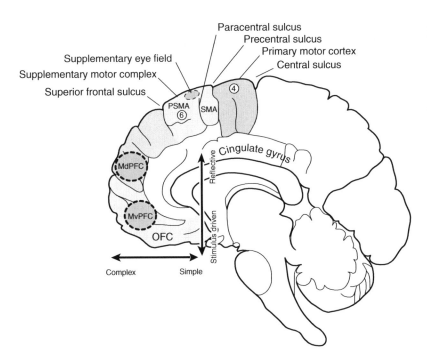

Figure 6.3. Medial view of the frontal cortex. The prefrontal cortex is represented in this view by the medial prefrontal cortex and the orbital prefrontal cortex, including the gyrus rectus. The premotor cortex and supplementary motor complex represent the motor cortex on the medial surface. SMA, supplementary motor area; PSMA, pre-supplementary motor area; MdPFC, dorsomedial prefrontal cortex; MvPFC, ventromedial prefrontal cortex; OFC, orbitofrontal cortex. The arrows represent two dimensions of a three-dimensional model of the prefrontal cortex. See text for details (Olsson and Ochsner, 2008).

fissure where it makes up the anterior paracentral lobule (Figures 6.1 and 6.3). About a third of the fibers that make up the corticospinal (pyramidal) tract arise from nerve cell bodies found in BA 4. The remainder of the pyramidal tract originates from cell bodies located in other areas of the cortex, including the premotor, supplementary motor, and somesthetic (parietal) cortex. Axons from BA 4 also terminate in the cranial nerve motor nuclei of the brainstem, the basal ganglia, the reticular formation, and the red nucleus. Projections from the red nucleus (rubrospinal tract) along with the corticospinal tract make up the major lateral descending motor system.

A pattern of the body is represented by neurons distributed across the primary motor cortex, producing a motor homunculus. The extent of each body part over the cortex corresponds with the degree of motor control over each of the represented parts. For example, the fingers, lips, and tongue are represented by large regions of cortex, whereas the toes are represented by a relatively small region. The primary motor cortex located along the midline controls the body below the waist. The primary motor cortex located on the lateral surface of the brain controls the muscles of the body found above the waist. Control exerted by the primary motor cortex by way of the pyramidal tract is greatest over the musculature of the hand. Note that in contrast to the legs, which function in locomotion, the face, head, and hands are more commonly used to transmit signals that express emotion.

A lesion of the primary motor cortex will result in paralysis of contralateral musculature. The affected muscles are flaccid at first; then, over the course of several days, reflexes become brisk and the muscles exhibit spasticity. Gross movement control reappears after several weeks or months, but fine movements, especially those of the hand, are usually lost permanently (Brodal, 1981).

Clinical vignette

A 65-year-old man, experienced a right hemisphere stroke that resulted in left arm paralysis. After discharge from the hospital he noted that his wife as well as other people around him were not as responsive to him as they were before the stroke. He found that just being angry or trying to look or sound angry had no effect on people. He had to explode in a rage to get his point across. His wife demanded that he see a psychiatrist. On examination the patient was found to have severe expressive aprosodia. He was totally unable to express anger, happiness, sadness, surprise, or even inquisitiveness.

Premotor cortex

The premotor cortex (BA 6 on the lateral surface; Figure 6.1) receives the majority of its input from the superior parietal cortex (Wise et al., 1997). The greatest number of axons that leave the premotor cortex terminate in the primary motor cortex. Approximately 30% of the axons in the corticospinal tract arise from neurons in the premotor cortex. The actions of premotor corticospinal neurons differ from primary motor corticospinal neurons in that premotor neurons control more proximal limb musculature.

A number of axons descend from the premotor cortex through the internal capsule to the reticular formation of the brainstem where they influence the reticulospinal tracts. The reticulospinal tracts are part of the major medial descending motor system that functions in support of body posture and locomotion through control of axial and proximal limb musculature.

Premotor areas are activated when new motor programs are initiated or when learned motor programs are modified. Premotor neurons begin to fire in anticipation of a movement. Just the presence of a learned cue can set off a burst of firing. The action of these neurons may represent a rehearsal or intent of a particular motor response. Premotor areas appear to be involved in the generation of a motor sequence from memory that requires precise timing (Halsband et al., 1993) and appear to play an important role in sensory conditioned motor learning. Patients with lesions of the premotor area exhibit deficits in visually guided movements and are unable to match sensory stimuli with previously learned movements (Halsband and Freund, 1990).

Passive viewing of faces has been reported to lead to activation of the right ventral premotor area, and imitative viewing to bilateral activation. This suggests that the right hemisphere may play a key role in the production of empathetic facial movements (Dimberg and Petterson, 2000; Leslie et al., 2004). Individuals who score high on empathy tests also demonstrate the chameleon effect (Sonnby-Borgström, 2002), that is, they unconsciously tend to mimic the facial expressions of the individual with whom they are speaking and even experience the mood of their interactive partner (Levenson et al., 1990).

Clinical studies suggest that the descending influence of the premotor cortex is over axial and proximal limb musculature. Unilateral lesions of the premotor cortex result in moderate weakness of contralateral shoulder and pelvic muscles. Forearm strength remains unaffected, but grasping movements are impaired when they are dependent on the supporting action of the shoulder. Movements are slow and there is a disturbance of their kinetic structure. Normal proximal-distal sequencing of muscle action is disturbed. Windmilling movements of the arms below shoulder level are normal in the forward direction but abnormal when attempted in the backward direction. Bicycling movements of the legs are unaffected (Freund and Hummelsheim, 1984).

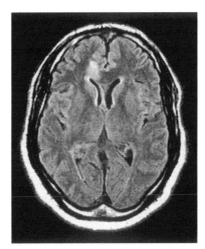

Figure 6.4.
Horizontal magnetic resonance image [fluid attenuated inversion recovery (FLAIR) sequence] showed an infarct in the region of the right supplementary motor area. (Reprinted with permission from Mendez and Clark, 2004.)

Clinical vignette

A 55-year-old right-handed man had an acute onset of hesitant, effortful speech. Examination showed predominant difficulty with articulatory fluency. His forward flow of speech was disrupted by speech sound repetitions and by lengthy pauses while preparing for the next utterance. He also had frequent vowel distortions and substitutions, fluctuating resonance, and a halting and harsh vocal quality. In contrast, his language abilities were preserved, including reading and writing. This patient had difficulty due to a right supplementary area lesion. Neuroimaging revealed a right hemisphere stroke of probable embolic origin involving the pericallosal branch of the right anterior cerebral artery (Figure 6.4). His deficit illustrates the disruption of complex motor routines for speech from a supplementary area lesion.

Mirror neurons

Mirror neurons were first observed in the premotor cortex of monkeys. The investigators were monitoring individual premotor neurons and found that if the monkey observed a particular grasping movement made by the investigator that neurons in the premotor cortex would fire even though the monkey made no movement. The same premotor neurons discharged if the monkey made a similar grasping movement. The investigator's movement that produced the effect was particular in that it was a goal-directed movement. Random arm/hand movements had no affect (Di Pellegrino et al., 1992; Gallese et al., 1996; Rizzolatti et al., 1996a). The human homologs of the monkey's mirror neuron areas are believed to be located in the pars opercularis of the inferior frontal gyrus (Petrides et al., 2005). However, several studies have not shown convincing mirror neuron activity in this region (Makuuchi, 2005; Williams et al., 2006; Jonas et al., 2007). The strict definition of "mirror neuron" requires that the neuron fires when the subject is observing an action and the same neuron fires when executing a similar action, e.g., grasping a

cup (Turella et al., 2009). A broader definition is a neuron that fires for "logically related actions" (Iacoboni and Mazziotta, 2007).

Since their discovery, mirror neurons also have been found in the anterior inferior parietal lobule in monkeys (Rizzolatti et al., 2001; Fogassi et al., 2005). A similar system is believed to exist in the human. Imaging studies have show activation in the inferior parietal lobule of the human as well as the ventral premotor area and posterior inferior frontal gyrus under test conditions designed to activate mirror neurons (Figures 4.2 and 6.1) (Rizzolatti and Craighero, 2004).

The mirror neuron system is believed to be a mechanism used by the brain to appreciate the actions of others. Activation of the mirror neurons provides a blueprint that can be used to imitate another's action (Iacoboni et al., 1999; Buccino et al., 2004). It is speculated that this system is useful in the motor sphere to learn new motor skills including language. Since only goal-directed movements are mirrored, this system is believed to support the understanding of the intent of another's movement. This is interpreted to mean that the system is a foundation for the concept of empathy, sympathy, and other aspects of emotional feeling. These emotions are important for developing appropriate social skills (Fabbri-Destro and Rizzolatti, 2008).

Supplementary motor area and supplementary motor complex

The supplementary motor complex (SMC) is found on the medial side of the frontal lobe along the longitudinal cerebral fissure (Figure 6.3). It corresponds approximately with BA 6 on the medial surface, although the exact boundaries are debated (Wise et al.,

The relationship between actual frontal lobe ictal activity and the exhibited psychopathology is complex, as exemplified by the following case reported by Boone and associates in 1988. A 13-year-old girl was admitted to a psychiatric hospital for deteriorating behavior. Before hospitalization she was becoming increasingly inattentive and was sexually active with a number of partners. She was becoming progressively more volatile and unpredictable with verbal and physical aggressiveness. She also exhibited pressured speech with periodic incoherent and bizarre output. She had one episode in which she cut the superficial skin over her wrists with a razor. Concurrent with the deteriorating behavior, spells developed during which she turned briefly to the right, stared and picked at her clothes. The episode was usually followed by urinary incontinence. Computed tomography and magnetic resonance imaging findings were normal. Electroencephalography demonstrated ictal activity of 2.5 Hz spike and slow wave complexes that originated primarily in the left frontal lobe but also occasionally in the right frontal regions.

1996). Two major subdivisions are recognized; the pre-supplementary motor area (pre-SMA) and the SMA proper (Picard and Strick, 1996; Nachev et al., 2008). A third subdivision, the supplementary eye field (SEF) lies at the junction of the pre-SMA and SMA close to the precentral sulcus (Figure 6.3). The SEF is considered an ocular motor extension of the SMA.

The SMC receives afferents from the primary somesthetic area of the parietal lobe as well as from the superior parietal lobule, the prefrontal cortex, and the cingulate gyrus. Afferent fibers from the thalamus arise from both the ventral anterior and ventral lateral nuclei, making the SMC a recipient of feedback from both the basal ganglia and the cerebellum.

Efferent fibers from the SMC include reciprocal, transcortical fibers to the premotor and primary motor areas. The SMA also provides projection fibers to the red nucleus and spinal cord. The SMA, but not the pre-SMA, makes a significant (~10%) contribution to the corticospinal tract. Many of the SMA axons, such as those from the primary motor area, make direct connections with motor neurons (Dum and Strick, 1996). In contrast, output of the pre-SMA and SEF is to the DLPFC. These two areas are believed to be involved in executive control in situations of response conflict (Nachev, 2006). Neurons in the SEF do not directly control saccades. They become activated when dealing with anticipation, errors and conflicts (Schall and Boucher, 2007). All parts of the SMC have connections with the basal ganglia. A group of special fibers from both the pre-SMA and SMA project directly to the subthalamic nucleus of the basal ganglia. These are called "hyperdirect" fibers. Activation of these fibers would rapidly "brake" any ongoing activity in the cortical-basal ganglia circuit (Frank et al., 2007).

The SMC becomes activated before the primary motor area (i.e., when the subject imagines performing an activity or intends to perform an activity) and is activated during complex motor subroutines. It is suggested that the SMC assembles a sequence of motor actions into a motor plan and is involved in the intentional preparation of movement (Grafton et al., 1992a). The SMC and anterior cingulate cortex became active in preparation for both internally generated and environmentally cued movements, indicating involvement with motor planning (Sahyoun et al., 2003). Activation of the pre-SMA has been reported to be more extensive for self-initiated movements as opposed to visually triggered movements (Deiber et al., 1999). This has led to the suggestion that the pre-SMA is specialized for internally guided rather than externally cued actions (Thaler et al., 1995). However, evidence indicates that the primary responsibility of the SMC is to use a time-linked blueprint to sequence potential action patterns (Tanji et al., 1985). The more anterior pre-SMA appears to function as a clearinghouse for cognitive and motivational information arriving from the prefrontal and cingulate areas before distribution to the more posterior SMA proper (Rizzolatti et al., 1996b). Activity in the pre-SMA is enhanced when an individual attends to the task to be performed ("attention to intention") (Lau et al., 2004). Deiber et al. (1999, 2005) reported that the SMA proper was activated when sequential rather than repetitive (fixed) movements were elicited.

The SMC assembles a new sequence of actions and becomes activated when a familiar motor sequence must be altered (Nakamura et al., 1999; Parton et al., 2007). The pre-SMA is activated when performing unfamiliar motor tasks, e.g., a pianist playing an unfamiliar piece of music (Parsons et al., 2005). In learning a new motor sequence, familiar sequences must be inhibited. Inhibition is also a product of the SMC. The SMA may be involved in procedural memory –the process responsible for acquisition and recall of motor programs (e.g., how a novice learns to grip and swing a golf club). Blood flow studies suggest that the SMA acts as an executor during the acquisition and articulation of new motor skills (Grafton *et al.*, 1992b). It may be involved in more fundamental processes such as preattentive inhibition of incoming irrelevant or redundant sensory input (i.e., sensory gating) (Grunwald *et al.*, 2003).

Clinical deficits resulting from surgery (tumor resection) or anterior cerebral artery infarction produce a lesion of the SMC. Either or both anterior cerebral arteries may be involved. The surrounding structures that are affected may include the dorsomedial prefrontal area, the anterior corpus callosum, and the cingulate gyrus (Chapter 12). Such a lesion of the SMC can result in motor neglect (Laplane *et al.*, 1977; Krainik *et al.*, 2001). Motor neglect is characterized by underutilization of the contralesional side, without defects of strength, reflexes, or sensibility. More severely affected patients may present with akinetic mutism. In this case, the patient may be mute or exhibit markedly reduced speech. Akinetic mutism is accompanied by akinesis or weakness, especially on the right side. Comprehension remains normal and speech may return, however, spontaneous and propositional speech is reduced. Initial effects are profound, but rapid recovery ensues over several months, with speech defects recovering more slowly. Recovery may appear complete in several years. Even after this time, however, mistakes may be observed in repeated complex movements of the hand (alternating supination and pronation), with the hand hesitating to reverse movement (Bleasel *et al.*, 1996; Nagaratnam *et al.*, 2004). The alien hand sign has been reported in some cases (Chapter 14; Feinberg *et al.*, 1992).

Frontal eye field

The traditional frontal eye field is found on the dorsolateral frontal cortex and corresponds with BA 8 (Figures 2.3 and 6.1). The portion of the frontal eye field actually involved with generating eye movements appears to be localized deep within the junction of the precentral sulcus and the superior frontal sulcus (Rosano *et al.*, 2003). The frontal eye field contributes to voluntary eye movements but is not necessary for initiation of all types of eye movements. The frontal eye field projects to the superior colliculus, to the caudate nucleus, and to the paramedian pontine reticular formation (PPRF), which is the pontine center for lateral gaze and to the midbrain (rostral interstitial nucleus of the medial longitudinal fasciculus (riMLF), which is the midbrain center for vertical gaze).

There are basically two important cortex-generated eye movements. The saccade is a fast eye movement that functions to reset eye position onto a new target. Visual signals from the retina to the cortex are inhibited during a saccade. The second eye movement is pursuit. Pursuit eye movements occur once the target of interest is positioned on the fovea. Pursuit allows the eye to track a moving object.

Saccadic eye movements are the only voluntary conjugate eye movements (Buttner-Ennever, 1988). The posterior parietal cortex plots the position and movement ("where") of all visual targets simultaneously and provides this information to the brainstem (superior colliculus). The parietal and temporal cortex also provide the frontal eye field with information about the identity ("what") of each of the targets. The frontal cortex acts as the executive and selects one target out of all the available visual targets. It then generates and triggers a saccade to move the eyes onto the selected target. An intimate relationship exists between the function of the DLPFC and the frontal eye field in the voluntary control of eye movement, which is one of the highest orders of cognitive processing in primates including humans (Goldberg and Bruce, 1986).

The supplementary eye field, DLPFC, and anterior cingulate gyrus also play a role in eye movements. Their individual contributions are unclear but it is thought they play a central role in planning eye movements in response to target location information received from the parietal lobe (Johnson and Everling, 2008; Medendorp *et al.*, 2008). The anterior cingulate gyrus becomes activated when task demands increase (Johnson and Everling, 2007). It is suggested that the DLPFC functions to add excitatory drive to either fixation or inhibitory neurons in the superior colliculus, which acts to suppress saccade-related neurons (Kaneda *et al.*, 2008). Eye tracking dysfunction (ETD) appears to be a genetically determined trait marker of schizophrenia. One hypothesis suggests that ETD reflects dysfunction of the DLPFC (Gooding and Talent, 2001).

Saccade eye movements

Saccades are fast eye movements used to reset the eyes onto a new target. Generation of a saccade relies on basic, largely brainstem circuitry coupled with oversight from the parietal and frontal lobes. Two major classes of saccades are those that are triggered automatically by the sudden appearance of an external visual target and those that are triggered internally.

89

Internally triggered saccades may be produced on command (i.e., voluntarily) to a remembered location even in the dark. Saccades can be measured in terms of latency, velocity, and accuracy. Two saccade tasks can reveal information about basic saccade circuitry and oversight control. In both tasks the subject fixates on a central target. A prosaccade is generated to a peripheral target when the central target is extinguished and peripheral target appears. A prosaccade is a test of the basic saccade circuitry. An example of a more complex saccade paradigm is the antisaccade. An antisaccade tests for function of the oversight controls, especially that of the frontal lobe. To prepare for an antisaccade the subject is instructed to note the location of the peripheral target when it appears but to inhibit a saccade to its location. The subject is instructed to not look at the target when it appears, but to generate a saccade to a location equidistant and in the direction opposite to the peripheral target.

It has been recognized for some time that patients with schizophrenia have abnormalities in eye movement control (Diefendorf and Dodge, 1908). Saccadic eye movements have been the focus of study and some abnormalities have been documented.

Testing of schizophrenia patients using basic tests such as the visually guided prosaccade tasks that measure saccade latency, average and peak velocity, gain, and final eye position in most cases has revealed these to be within normal limits (Krebs *et al.*, 2001; Thampi *et al.*, 2003). However, more sophisticated tests such as the antisaccade task have revealed an error rate of 20%–75% among schizophrenia patients (Gooding and Basso, 2008). Test results indicate patients understand instructions and are motivated (Gooding and Talent, 2001; Polli *et al.*, 2008). Schizophrenia patients make a large number of glances to the peripheral target instead of generating a saccade in the direction opposite (Harris *et al.*, 2006). They consistently produce fewer correct responses and make significantly more directional errors when generating a saccade away from the target (Reuter *et al.*, 2005; Radant *et al.*, 2007). It is interesting to note that some components of antisaccade performance are reported to improve in patients taking risperidone and nicotine (Burke and Reveley, 2002; Hutton, 2002; Larrison-Faucher *et al.*, 2004). Antisaccade task errors also are reported in individuals with schizotypal traits and/or symptoms (Ettinger *et al.*, 2005; Gooding *et al.*, 2005; Holahan and O'Driscoll, 2005).

Fewer saccade studies have been reported on other psychiatric patient populations. Results of studies involving adult patients with attention-deficit hyperactivity disorder, bipolar disorder, obsessive-compulsive disorder (OCD), and major depression have been equivocal. In general, results of visually guided prosaccade tasks have been unremarkable. An increase in errors is more often reported in the antisaccade task (Maruff *et al.*, 1999; Gooding *et al.*, 2004; Carr *et al.*, 2006; Winograd-Gurvich *et al.*, 2006).

These findings suggest that in all groups tested the basic saccade generating circuitry is intact. The antisaccade task places demands on higher order eye movement control systems. It is hypothesized that antisaccade task errors represent dysfunction in the DLPFC (McDowell and Clementz, 2001; Gooding and Basso, 2008). Greater error rates have been reported in subjects with reduced gray matter volume in the right medial superior frontal cortex, including the frontal eye field and supplementary eye field (Bagary *et al.*, 2004; Tsunoda *et al.*, 2005). It is further suggested that antisaccade errors in schizophrenia represent impairments in working memory, including elements of inhibition (Hutton *et al.*, 2004).

Broca's speech area

Broca's speech area occupies BA 44 and BA 45 on the inferior frontal gyrus and consists of the pars opercularis and pars triangularis (Figures 2.3 and 6.1). It is considered to be part of the prefrontal cortex and consists of both heteromodal prefrontal cortex and premotor cortex. This region is specialized on the dominant side of the cortex for the production of speech. The major input to this region is from Wernicke's area by way of the arcuate fasciculus. Wernicke's area corresponds with the posterior region of the superior temporal gyrus (BA 22). Fibers that originate from cells in Broca's area project to the facial region of the primary motor cortex which directly controls the muscles of speech. The area comparable to Broca's on the nondominant cortex is responsible for the emotional/melodic component of speech (Joseph, 1988).

Broca's speech area is activated during the production of both overt and covert speech as well as when an individual imitates another person's speech (Figure 6.5; Smith *et al.*, 1992; Sukhwinder *et al.*, 2000). Evidence indicates that this region is active during inner speech in normal subjects and may be critical in verbal hallucinations experienced by patients with schizophrenia (McGuire *et al.*, 1993, 1996). Impairment in verbal fluency ("Say as many words beginning with 's' in the next 30 seconds") is seen in patients with lesions in

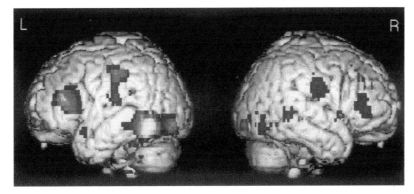

Figure 6.5. Functional magnetic resonance images demonstrating greater activation to words than to consonant letter strings during a nonlinguistic visual feature detection task. The images illustrate a left hemisphere language network for reading, probably including temporal-occipital visual word form and lexical regions, an inferior parietal phonological encoding region, and Broca's area in the inferior frontal lobe. The right hemisphere also participates but to a much smaller degree than the left hemisphere. See also color plate. (Reproduced with permission from Price *et al.*, 1998.)

Broca's area as well as in other regions of the DLPFC. Broca's area is involved in word retrieval as well as in verbal fluency (Caplan *et al.*, 2000). Verbal fluency activates left BA 44 and BA 45, whereas semantic processing preferentially activates only BA 45 (Amuts *et al.*, 2004).

A lesion of Broca's area on the dominant side results in an inability to produce speech (motor or expressive aphasia). The patient retains the ability to understand the written and spoken word. With recovery, the patient learns to speak with difficulty producing only key nouns and verbs and leaving out modifying adjectives and adverbs. The same cortex on the non-dominant side is believed to be responsible for the musical intonation of speech (prosody). A lesion on the nondominant side results in expressive aprosodia in which the patient is unable to effectively modulate speech (i.e., speech becomes monotone without facial expressions).

Depression often accompanies Broca's and other nonfluent aphasia. Some of the depression is a result of left hemisphere damage, not just a reaction to the psychosocial loss (Benson and Ardila, 1993). Severe depression correlates with deep left frontal lesions, especially if the lesion includes the anterior limb of the internal capsule (Starkstein *et al.*, 1987). Blood flow to Broca's area is decreased in patients with post-traumatic stress disorder (PTSD) when provoked (Figure 11.8; Rauch *et al.*, 1996). A significant volume reduction was reported in only BA 44 and 45 on both the left and right side in patients with schizophrenia when the entire prefrontal cortex was compared (Buchanan *et al.*, 1998).

Clinical vignette

A 67-year-old right-handed man with frontotemporal dementia (FTD) was hospitalized with a gradual personality change. He sold his successful business, stopped paying the bills, and ran up large debts on merchandise from a television home shopping network. He became impulsive and disinhibited, fondled his wife in public, sexually propositioned his daughters, and uttered uncharacteristic racial slurs at social gatherings. At the same time, he became distractible and hyperactive, with compulsive behaviors such as repeatedly pulling the hair of his arms (trichotillomania) and exhibited hyperoral behavior such as overeating. The patient met the criteria for FTD, probably of a familial nature. His family history was positive for a similar dementing illness in his father and in a paternal grandparent. Single photon emission tomography scans showed extensive hypoperfusion in both frontal lobes, more extensive in the right hemisphere (Figure 6.6). His initial personality changes including poor judgment, disinhibition, and inappropriate behaviors, were consistent with involvement of the orbital prefrontal cortex.

Prefrontal cortex

The prefrontal cortex is loosely defined as the cortex that receives of fibers from the MD nucleus of the thalamus. It is divided into a dorsolateral region (Figure 6.1), an orbital (inferior) region (Figure 6.2), and a medial region (Figure 6.3). All three regions receive fibers from the MD thalamic nucleus, which relays information from the temporal cortex, the pyriform cortex, and the amygdala. It also has direct, reciprocal connections

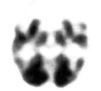

Figure 6.6. The patient's 18-flurodeoxyglucose positron emission tomography scan showed prominent hypometabolism of the frontal lobes. Note the near absence of activity in the anterior part of the brain. (Reprinted with permission from Mendez *et al.*, 1997.)

with the amygdala. The orbital and dorsomedial subdivisions of the prefrontal cortex are included as part of the limbic association cortex. The dorsolateral region functions in the cognitive sphere dealing with perception, memory and motor planning. The orbital and medial regions function in support of social and emotional behavior. Prefrontal output to the basal ganglia and to the frontal motor regions (BA 6 and BA 4) also indicates a significant role of the prefrontal cortex in motor behavior. Output from the prefrontal cortex

Clinical vignette

A 17-year-old female student, was involved in competitive piano and ballet. Her grades were consistently outstanding. She had no personal or family history of psychiatric problems. She was out with friends on a Saturday night when she was involved in an accident. She fell off the back of a pickup truck and landed on her head. At the accident scene she was alert and oriented but felt dazed. In the emergency room, computed tomography and neurological examinations were normal. She was observed for two hours and discharged. The patient's mother was told that her daughter was fine and that she should return to school and full activity on Monday. For the following few weeks, the patient was unable to perform either piano or ballet at school, although she had no problem practicing at home. Her grades deteriorated. She became depressed and attempted suicide. Neuropsychological testing showed that the patient had a problem performing in the presence of interference (i.e., difficulty in maintaining a mental set). This is evidence of damage in the prefrontal region. The patient responded well to antidepressant therapy. Her frontal lobe deficit resolved spontaneously over time with continued nonpressured practice.

to the limbic system takes both direct and indirect routes. The indirect route exits via the cingulate gyrus and these prefrontal fibers distribute to many cortical regions throughout their long course around the corpus callosum.

Prefrontal neurons respond in situations that reflect learned associative relationships between goal-relevant tasks. They appear to form ensembles that represent commonalities across past experiences that have proven to be effective in achieving a particular goal (Miller, 2000). Prefrontal areas are involved in storage and retrieval related to sequential and temporal aspects of planning (Goel *et al.*, 1997). This planning and the ability of the prefrontal cortex to rearrange the sequence and complexity of planning have earned the prefrontal cortex the title "organ of creativity" (Fuster, 2002).

An increase in blood flow in the frontal lobes has been associated with introversion. Extraverts show lower blood flow in the frontal lobes and hippocampus. These findings suggest that introverts are engaged in frontally based cognition, including remembering events from their past, making plans for the future, or solving problems (Johnson *et al.*, 1999).

Patients with lesions in the left frontal cortex demonstrate a higher frequency of depression than patients with more posterior lesions or patients with either anterior or posterior right hemisphere lesions (Morris *et al.*, 1992; Starkstein and Robinson, 1993). Glucose metabolism studies in both teenagers and adults with a history of attention-deficit hyperactivity disorder show decreased metabolism in the left anterior frontal areas (Zametkin *et al.*, 1990; Ernst *et al.*, 1994).

The inhibition of glutamatergic transmission in the prefrontal lobes correlates with cognitive dysfunction seen in patients with schizophrenia. It is hypothesized that this inhibition is responsible for dysregulation of dopamine in the corpus striatum (Breier, 1999).

Generalized, bilateral damage to the prefrontal lobes can produce severe behavioral changes. Characteristically these patients become apathetic and exhibit disinhibition of impulsive behavior. They appear unconcerned (abulia) and exhibit slowness and lack of spontaneity in speech and slowness in thought and in emotional expression. The movements of frontal lobe patients are slow (bradykinesia), and they exhibit a slow, uncertain "magnetic" gait (frontal ataxia or gait apraxia). In contrast, their behavior may change, and they may become irritable and euphoric.

An intriguing prefrontal syndrome called the environmental dependency syndrome (EDS) has been described (Lhermitte, 1986). Two patients with focal unilateral frontal lobe lesions were observed in a doctor's office, in a lecture room, in a car, in a garden, and while visiting an apartment. In each situation the patients assumed behavior appropriate to the environment, including treating the physician as a patient while in the doctor's office. The patients' behavior was striking, as though implicit in the environment was an order to respond to the situation in which they found themselves. EDS implies a disorder in personal autonomy.

The orbitofrontal region like the anterior temporal region (Chapter 4) is in close proximity to bony protrusions. Both are vulnerable to injury, particularly when rotational acceleration is imparted to the freely moving head (Levin and Kraus, 1994). The injury may include white matter damage that may be diffuse and not detectable using structural imaging. Orbitofrontal damage alone or combined with temporal pole damage can result in complex behavioral changes. The orbital prefrontal cortex may be damaged by trauma or tumors (e.g., meningiomas). Since lesions in this area impact complex psychological functions, neuropsychological impairment may go unnoticed for years. Subtle personality changes may be the only early clue before the eventual development of signs of increased intracranial pressure, including seizures in the case of a space-occupying lesion. Extensive orbital cortex damage blunts emotional reactions, and the patient may sit quietly and silently. If sufficiently stimulated, animals and humans respond in an irritable and aversive manner (Butter *et al.*, 1968). Social responses are lacking or inappropriate. Human mothers with orbital lesions neglect or beat their children or both without provocation (Broffman, 1950). Monkeys with orbital lesions separate themselves from their social group (Myers *et al.*, 1973).

The pseudopsychopathic subject usually has sustained an orbital prefrontal lesion. The patient's attention is easily distracted by irrelevant stimuli. There is also excessive and aimless motility, disinhibition and hypomanic stance. Paranoid tendencies may develop. The pseudodepressed subject often has sustained a lesion to the dorsomedial prefrontal region. There is general decrease of awareness, and a state of apathy with basic lack or weakness of drive. In extreme cases, this can lead to an akinetic-abulic syndrome and mutism.

Clinical vignette

A 52-year-old woman presented with a personality change over 2–3 weeks characterized by disinterest, disengagement, and decreased ability to solve problems. She was a school teacher and could no longer plan her lessons, process feedback from her students, or follow-through on her assignments. Her general and neurological examinations were normal except for mental status testing which showed decreased verbal output, diminished motor initiation, lack of concern, and poor sequencing and set-shifting abilities. Magnetic resonance imaging (MRI) showed an enhancing dural mass over the left cerebral convexities with effacement of the sulci in both frontal lobes (see Figure 6.7). Biopsy of the lesion revealed changes consistent with dural neurosarcoidosis. The patient's personality changes resulted from pressure of the neurosarcoid mass on her dorsolateral prefrontal cortex. She was treated for neurosarcoidosis with corticosteroids (prednisone). One month after initiation of therapy, a second MR scan showed decreases in the dural lesion, and repeat neuropsychological testing showed coincident improvements in all measures of frontal function.

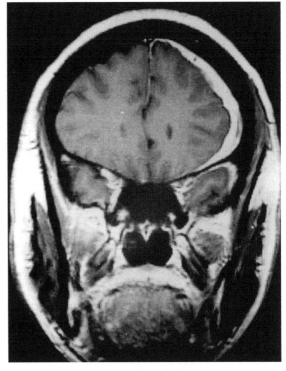

Figure 6.7. Magnetic resonance imaging demonstrating dural mass over left cerebral convexities resulting in dorsolateral frontal personality changes (Mendez and Zander, 1992).

A 59-year-old man who was admitted to a psychiatric hospital in a floridly hypersexual state. He had a history of subfrontal meningioma that was surgically removed two years before presentation. The patient reported that after the surgery his desire for sexual activity increased from once a week to as much as three to four times a day. Intercourse frequently lasted more than an hour in duration and he had difficulty in achieving orgasm. Other than an absence of olfaction, his neurological exam was normal. A recent CT scan revealed bilateral basal medial frontal lucencies consistent with old infarctions (Miller *et al.*, 1986).

Dorsolateral prefrontal cortex

The DLPFC extends between the longitudinal cerebral fissure above and the lateral fissure below on the lateral surface of the brain centered in BA 46. It receives input from the motor cortex as well as from the multimodal temporoparietal junction area. In contrast to the orbital cortex, the connections of the DLPFC place it in a position to evaluate and regulate information from the somatic sensory system that can be used by the motor cortex to produce a response. The DLPFC has been described as a place "where past and future meet." It looks backward in time to create memories from sensory input. It looks forward in time to assemble a motor plan of action (Fuster, 1995).

The DLPFC is heavily involved in working memory. Working memory is the act of bringing to mind and processing limited amounts of information, for example, reading and recalling a telephone number or solving a math problem "in your head" (Baddeley, 1992; Goldman-Rakic, 1997). Studies indicate that the events that take place in the DLPFC make up what is considered working memory (Goldman-Rakic, 1996). Brodmann's areas 6, 8, and 9 become preferentially activated when a working memory task must be continuously updated and revised for temporal sequence (Wager and Smith, 2003).

Two components of working memory are recognized. The short-term component operates on the order of seconds. The second represents executive processing and operates on information retrieved from storage. Different frontal regions are associated with the storage of different kinds of information. Use of verbal material activates Broca's area and left supplementary and premotor areas. Use of spatial information activates the right premotor area. Two forms of executive processing are selective attention and task management. Both activate the anterior cingulate and dorsolateral prefrontal cortex (Smith and Jonides, 1999). Working memory and attention are closely related. For example if we anticipate a friendly face within a crowd of strangers, we must hold the visual memory of the familiar face at the ready as we attend to the different individuals in the crowd.

The DLPFC samples and regulates the flow of information to the motor cortex by way of direct connections with the motor cortex and indirect connections with the mediodorsal and reticular nuclei of the thalamus. The reticular thalamic nucleus regulates and directs sensory information to the cortex (Yingling and Skinner, 1977). In contrast, the projections from the orbital prefrontal region to the motor cortex regulate arousal and control the degree to which the limbic system influences motor behavior. The DLPFC monitors and adjusts behavior. The more superior portions of the DLPFC direct behavior in terms of sequential or temporal cues (Knight *et al.*, 1995). More inferior portions regulate behavior in terms of spatial cues. Neurons involved with memory (~40% of total) decrease their firing rate over time after a stimulus. In contrast, neurons involved with encoding a motor response (~60% of total) increase their firing rate as the time to act approaches (Quintana and Fuster, 1992).

Symbolic representations retrieved from long-term memory as well as from current sensory cues are "sketched out" in the DLPFC as a function of working memory (Figure 6.8). Working memory allows the representations to be manipulated and associated with other ideas along with incoming information in order to guide behavior. There appears to be no one locus of a central executive processor. Instead, visuospatial processing takes place throughout the DLPFC. The working memory for faces and objects takes place in more lateral and inferior regions of the prefrontal cortex. Semantic encoding and verbal representations are found in more inferior, insular, and anterior prefrontal regions (Goldman-Rakic and Selemon, 1997). Activity in the left inferior prefrontal cortex correlated with retrieval of words and was more active for remembered versus forgotten words. The more active the region, the better is the memory performance (Reynolds *et al.*, 2004).

A second hypothesis recognizes a similar dorsoventral gradient, but distinguishes between types of processing rather than material types. In this second

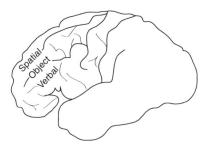

Figure 6.8. The approximate location of working memory for visuospatial processing (spatial), for features of faces or objects (object), and for semantic encoding and verbal processes (verbal), on the prefrontal cortex. Compare with Figure 6.10.

view the superior frontal cortex is involved in monitoring and manipulation of information whereas the more ventral dorsolateral cortex is responsible for rehearsal during short-term storage (Owen, 2000). More recent evidence supports this second hypothesis (Wager and Smith, 2003).

Goal-directed behaviors related to short-term planning (e.g., hammering) activates the left middle frontal gyrus, supramarginal gyrus, inferior temporal gyrus, and middle occipital gyrus. Activity in BA 46 has been found to be associated with willed actions including finger movements and freely generated words. It is hypothesized that activation of the DLPFC reflects selection of a single action out of a number of potential actions (Lau et al., 2004).

Lesions of the dorsolateral area cause abnormalities in complex psychological functions that are classified as executive function deficits. The patient demonstrates difficulties in planning, feedback, learning, sequencing, establishing, maintaining, and changing a set behavior. The ability to organize events in temporal sequence is most affected. Perseveration, stimulus-bound behavior, and echopraxia may be seen (Sandson and Albert, 1987). The Wisconsin Card Sorting Test is valuable in evaluating the status of the dorsolateral area (Drewe, 1974). Blood flow to the DLPFC increases during the performance of the Wisconsin Card Sorting Test. This increase is not seen in schizophrenia patients (Weinberger et al., 1986). Performance on this test is more adversely affected with high dorsolateral or dorsomedial lesions (Milner, 1995). The patient may present with a general disinterest, apathy, shortened attention span, lack of emotional reactivity, and difficulty in attending to relevant stimuli. The patient often finds comfort in following established routines and thought processes (Fuster, 1996). A reduction in verbal fluency may be seen if involvement of the left dorsolateral area

is significant. Verbal fluency is reduced in patients with Parkinson disease (Gurd and Ward, 1989). It is believed this is a result of impaired dopaminergic projections to the DLPFC in this population (Amuts et al., 2004).

Patients with dorsolateral lesions are able to order words within a sentence but fail to properly sequence words when describing a plan of action. Prefrontal lesions seem to produce impairments in long-term planning whereas inferior parietal lesions produce impairments in short-term sequence execution (Sirigu et al., 1998). Lesions of the left dorsolateral area affect semantic speech that requires searching within a category (e.g., naming fruits or cars) (Gurd et al., 2002). In contrast, over-learned sequence speech (e.g., naming days of the week) does not activate the DLPFC but does activate Broca's area on the left (Bookheimer et al., 2000).

Anderson et al. (2004) reported that subjects successful in repressing unwanted nonemotional memories showed bilateral dorsolateral prefrontal cortical activation coupled with right hippocampal deactivation. The degree of hippocampal deactivation correlated with the magnitude of repression. These results support the concept of an active process of repression. In another study, successful suppression of emotional memories also showed bilateral prefrontal activation but was coupled with suppression of activity in the amygdala (Ochsner et al., 2002).

Ventrolateral prefrontal cortex

The ventrolateral prefrontal cortex (VLPFC) includes BA 44, BA 45 and the lateral aspect of BA 47. This includes pars opercularis, pars triangularis, and pars orbitalis, and Broca's speech area (Figure 6.1). The left VLPFC and is involved with semantic processing and is better understood. The right VLPFC is linked to emotional aspects of faces (Marumo et al., 2009). The left VLPFC is important in the control of memory and provides multimodal integration and executive function that underlies goal-directed behavior. It receives semantic memory information from the lateral and inferior temporal areas (Zhang et al., 2004; Croxson et al., 2005). The information received can be the result of a bottom-up flow or it may be selected in a top-down manner by the VLPFC. If the currently available data are insufficient, the anterior portion of the VLPFC can call for additional information from the temporal cortex in a top-down manner. The VLPFC acts to interpret information using a competitive selection process that may activated even before completion of the retrieval stage. This indicates that processing in the VLPFC is in parallel rather than in series with other cortical areas (Badre *et al.*, 2006). It uses a two-stage process. The first operates in a top-down manner to provide controlled access to memory. The second is a post-retrieval selection process, which acts to resolve competition between simultaneously active representations (Badre and Wagner, 2007).

The VLPFC and amygdala are part of a network that monitors and selects a response to threat (Hariri *et al.*, 2003). In this report, adolescents with generalized anxiety disorder compared with controls, exhibited greater activation of the right ventrolateral prefrontal cortex in response to images of angry faces and showed attentional bias away from the angry faces. The authors stated that the VLPFC may be involved in the manifestation of anxiety symptoms and through connections with the amygdala may regulate responses to anxiety-provoking stimuli, thereby reducing the severity of symptoms (Monk *et al.*, 2006).

Orbitofrontal cortex

The OFC is defined as the ventral surface of the frontal lobe from the gyrus rectus on the ventral surface to the ventrolateral convexity laterally, and from the limen of insula posteriorly to the frontal pole. This includes BA 11, BA 12, and the medial portion of BA 47. Brodmann's area 13 is often included although it is usually designated to be part of the insula. Its inclusion as part of the OFC underscores the close relationship of the OFC and anterior insula. Some authors include BA 24, BA 25, and BA 32, however, these areas are more often recognized as MPFC or as part of the anterior cingulate gyrus including the subgenual anterior cingulate gyrus (Phillips *et al.*, 2003).

The OFC receives input from the temporal association cortex, amygdala, and hypothalamus, making it the highest integration center for emotional processing. It also receives inputs from the visual system, taste, olfaction, and somatosensory regions. The secondary taste cortex is localized to the posterior, lateral part of the orbitofrontal cortex (Rolls, 1990). A smell (olfactory) region medial to the taste region is also described (Rolls *et al.*, 2003a). Visual input seems to reach this region via temporal lobe structures. Somatosensory and auditory inputs also arrive from the primary sensory regions. The insula is similarly connected to the OFC. The more posterior regions of the OFC receive strong input from the amygdala (Price *et al.*, 1991).

In a general sense, the OFC is concerned with the appreciation of emotions of either one's self or of others in terms of positive or negative reward. Activity is reported to be associated with anticipated regret (Coricelli, *et al.*, 2005). Thinking about feelings of others (emotional perspective taking) also produces activation of the OFC (Hynes *et al.*, 2006). There appear to be differences in function between the medial and lateral OFC. The medial OFC is more often activated during the anticipation of reward (Cox *et al.*, 2005; Galvan *et al.*, 2005; Ursu and Carter, 2005; Kim *et al.*, 2006), when viewing attractive faces (O'Doherty *et al.*, 2003; Ishai, 2007; Winston *et al.*, 2007), or when enjoying chocolate (Small *et al.*, 2003). On the other hand the lateral OFC is more activated during the absence of reward (Markowitsch *et al.*, 2003; Ursu and Carter, 2005), experiencing an unpleasant smell or touch (Rolls *et al.*, 2003a, b), when viewing aversive pictures (Nitschke *et al.*, 2006), and when eating chocolate to excess (Small *et al.*, 2003).

A primary role of the OFC is the acquisition of appropriate behaviors and the inhibition of inappropriate behaviors based on reward contingencies (Elliot *et al.*, 2000, 2004). The medial OFC is related to cognitive and emotional processes and the sense of reward when making the correct choice. Choosing between small, likely rewards and large, unlikely rewards activates the OFC (Rogers *et al.*, 1999), which modulates behavioral and visceral responses to emotionally provoking stimuli. Its close ties with the olfactory and taste cortices put it in a position to evaluate and select food items. It can establish and recall the rules that lead to visceral/emotional reward, and it calculates risk/reward ratios when selecting behaviors. This function is expanded beyond food selection to include many aspects of social behavior. The OFC evaluates the emotional salience of stimuli and selects behavioral responses based on the level of reward provided by the response. It has the ability to redirect behavior if the level or probability of reward changes (Rolls and Grabenhorst, 2008). The medial OFC plays a key role in the circuitry of positive emotion. Lateral OFC regions are more involved with inhibiting the more familiar response when the novel, less familiar response produces a reward (Zald and Kim, 1996). A particular feature of the OFC is suppression of distracting internal and external signals during the performance of current behavior (Fuster, 1996). Olfactory signals converge with taste signals in the OFC to create the representations of flavor. Other sensory signals converge with flavor in the OFC and visual-to-taste associations occur here as well (Rolls, 1997). This is reflected by its activation in response to pleasant and painful touch, rewarding and aversive taste and by odor (Rolls, 2000).

The OFC receives information about faces. Face-responsive neurons of the orbitofrontal region may convey information about which face is being seen (Rolls *et al.*, 2005). Attractive faces have been shown to produce activation of the medial OFC, which is enhanced by a smiling expression (O'Doherty *et al.*, 2003). Some of the OFC face-responsive neurons seem to be sensitive to facial expressions and movements. In one study, individuals showed greater activation in the medial OFC to more attractive than less attractive faces. Homosexual individuals showed greater activation to attractive same-sex faces and heterosexual individuals showed greater activation to attractive opposite-sex faces (Ishai, 2007). These findings relate to the function of social reinforcement since facial expressions are crucial for conveying social approval or disapproval. It is likely that most of the associations developed in this region occur in a subconscious or unconscious (automatic) fashion. This area plays a role in reexperiencing emotions. Most patients with lesions here find it difficult to reexperience emotions with the exception of fear and have difficulty in attaching emotional tone to images (Bechara *et al.*, 2000).

The OFC plays a dominant role in mediating arousal (Joseph, 1996). It is also postulated to regulate the experience of anxiety (Gray, 1987). Inhibitory control over emotion and social behavior arises from the orbital and MPFC. Inhibition can help prevent distraction and support the focusing component of selective sensory attention (Fuster, 2002).

Acts of imagined social embarrassment produced significant activation of the left OFC (BA 10 and BA 47) (Berthoz *et al.*, 2002). The same region has been reported to be activated on viewing angry faces (Blair *et al.*, 1999; Kesler/West *et al.*, 2001). Activity was seen to increase bilaterally when a sample of mothers were asked to view pictures of their own 3–5-month-old infants over activity compared with viewing pictures of other 3–5-month-old infants (Nitschke *et al.*, 2004). In other studies, male and female subjects viewing erotic film excerpts showed increased bilateral activity in the MPFC and OFC as well as ventral striatum (nucleus accumbens) and amygdala (Redoute *et al.*, 2000; Karama *et al.*, 2002).

Lesions in the orbital region result in a syndrome that is characterized by disinhibition, which varies from lack of social tact to the commission of antisocial acts. Patients with OFC lesions are emotionally labile, irritable, and impulsive. They appear to no longer recognize the inappropriateness of their actions. This may be in part because the patient is impaired in the ability to interpret and respond to emotional voice or face expressions (Hornak *et al.*, 2003; Shaw *et al.*, 2005). The patient with an OFC lesion may be hyperactive, even hypomanic, especially if the lesion involves the posterior OFC. Although overt sexual aggression is rare, sexual preoccupation and improper sexual comments are frequent. They may lose interest in personal appearance and hygiene, eat excessively and show lack of concern for others (Fuster, 2008). Symptoms may appear sporadically, often accompanied by irritability, distractibility, and childish behavior (puerilism) (Clark and Manes, 2004). Disinhibition from normal social controls is often seen with the patient exhibiting inappropriate social behavior. They may engage in risky and dangerous behavior suggesting they are unable to balance risk against reward. Patients are easily distracted, and often they are unable to complete tasks because they are distracted by ordinarily insignificant stimuli. Patients with OFC lesions have been compared with drug users. They choose instant reward over waiting, and they have great difficulty in decision making in part because they are unable to anticipate the possible negative consequences of their immediate actions. They also tend to take risks whether or not the outcome produces positive reward. Lesions early in life have greater effects.

Apathy can be seen following a lesion involving the OFC although apathy is more commonly associated with an extensive lesion involving the lateral aspect. Depressed mood can result from lesions involving the anterior and lateral surfaces, especially left-sided lesions. Apathetic or depressed patients will avoid social contact.

Medial prefrontal cortex, default brain network, and the social brain

The MPFC includes BA 10 on the medial aspect, anterior cingulate (BA 24 and 32) and BA 8 and BA 9 of the prefrontal cortex on the medial aspect (Buckner *et al.*, 2008). Some authors include BA 25, which is also identified as the infralimbic, subgenual cingulate gyrus. Major connections of the MPFC are with the posterior cingulate gyrus, retrosplenial area, superior temporal gyrus and hippocampal formation. It is closely linked with the anterior insula, temporal pole, medial temporal lobe and hippocampus, inferior parietal lobe and amygdala. These connections relate it to long-term memory as well as to emotions processed through the limbic system.

The default brain network includes the MPFC and is a group of interconnected structures that become active when the brain is at rest. The precuneus, retrosplenial cortex and posterior cingulate form a posterior core and are sometimes referred to as the "posteromedial cortex" (Cavanna and Trimble, 2006).

The default brain network is tonically active during a resting, mind-wandering, baseline state (Mason et al., 2007). When questioned, subjects report that while resting, they are remembering the past, envisioning future events, and considering the thoughts and perspectives of other people (Buckner and Carroll, 2007). The medial temporal lobe subsystem is activated during retrieval of episodic memories that may provide "the building blocks of mental exploration" (Wagner et al., 2005; Buckner et al., 2008).

The MPFC is believed to be involved in reasoning about the contents of other person's thoughts (mentalizing) as they relate to the self (Gallagher and Frith, 2003). Other components of the mentalizing network include the temporal poles, posterior superior temporal sulcus, and the ventral striatum. The MPFC appears to involve analysis and appreciation of the mental self as well as the mental status of others (Uddin et al., 2007). It is activated in response to information about another person that is socially or emotionally relevant. It became activated in individuals hearing socially relevant adjectives such as "curious" or "friendly" but abstract adjectives such as "celestial" or words referring to body parts ("liver") or object parts ("pedal") (Mitchell et al., 2006).

The MPFC along with the anterior cingulate gyrus, amygdala, insula, superior temporal sulcus, and temporoparietal junction has been described as the "social brain" (Figure 6.9; Frith, 2007; Blakemore, 2008) (see also social brain in Chapter 5). The social brain allows us to interact with other people. The MPFC and adjacent subgenual cingulate gyrus are activated when subjects think about mental states of self or others in a social situation (mentalizing) (McCabe et al., 2001). Thinking about the feelings of others activates the OFC (Hynes et al., 2006). The amygdala in a social context, pre-judges faces, facial expressions, etc., based on previous experience with similar faces. The temporal pole brings together and stores facts about people and social situations in which they have been found in the past.

This recollection is applied to the current social situation and recalls feelings (e.g., confidence, embarrassment, etc.) related to similar past situations (Damasio et al., 2004). Mirror neurons located in many areas of the brain allow us to experience feelings of others as they move, feel pain, pleasure, etc. (Wicker et al., 2003; Rizzolatti and Craighero, 2004; Jackson, et al., 2005). We even tend to imitate their actions, e.g., yawn when they yawn (Chartrand and Bargh, 1999). Much of this is brought together in the posterior superior temporal sulcus and temporoparietal junction. It is here that body, limb and eye movements of other are evaluated. The movement trajectory or direction of gaze is determined and we take the perspective of the other person, (e.g., What are they are looking at? What are they afraid of?) (Pelphrey et al., 2004; Frith 2007). All of this is used to judge risk and reward of alternative behaviors we might select to be successful in a social situation.

The MPFC may be subdivided into a ventral and dorsal part. Some authors include portions of the anterior cingulate gyrus in both parts (Phillips et al., 2003), and both not only respond to environmental stimuli but also operate in a top-down manner to determine self-relevance.

Dorsomedial prefrontal cortex

The dorsomedial component of the prefrontal cortex (MdPFC) lies within an arc that extends from the SMC downward to the orbital component of the prefrontal cortex (Figure 6.3). It contains portions of BA 9, BA 10, and BA 32. It is dorsal and anterior to much of the cingulate gyrus, but many authors include the anterior cingulate gyrus as part of the MdPFC (Figures 2.3, 6.3, and 12.1). This entire region is mainly supplied by the anterior cerebral artery. Aneurysms of this artery are a common cause of medial frontal lobe damage. The involved cortex may include the supplementary motor area as well.

The MdPFC has particularly strong connections through a network that involves the anterior and posterior cingulate gyri (Gusnard et al., 2001). It is also the target of signals from the anterior insula. This network has a high baseline activity and is believed to be active independent of external stimuli (Fransson, 2005). In fact, sensory input is missing (Price, 2007). It is thought that the role of the MdPFC is to engage in introspection. It has shown to be activated when reflecting on the intentions behind and consequences of actions, and when forgiving the transgressions of others (Farrow

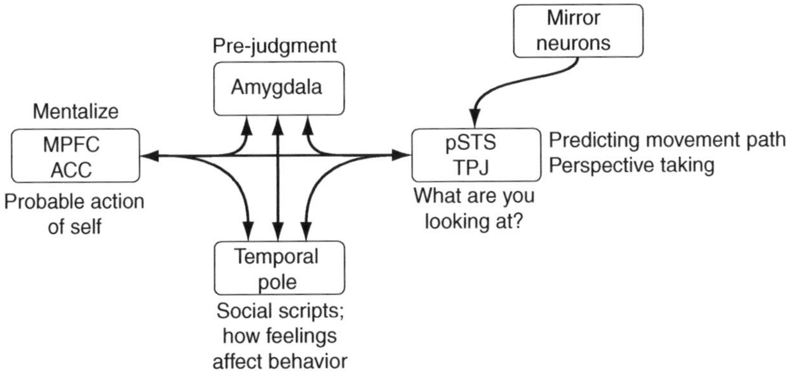

Figure 6.9. The social brain. The amygdala stores expectations based on past experience (pre-judgment). The mirror neurons from various areas of the brain react to actions of others reflecting their movements and sensations. The posterior superior temporal sulcus (pSTS) and temporoparietal junction (TPJ) monitor others to determine social importance of their gaze and movements. The medial prefrontal cortex (MPFC) and subgenual cingulate cortex (sgACC) account for mentalizing, i.e., thoughts and emotions of self and others and how these may impact on actions taken by self or other. The temporal pole helps to apply general knowledge of social situations to the current social situation. (After Frith, 2007.)

et al., 2001; Gallagher et al., 2002). The introspection involves recollection, self-reflection, and evaluation (Schmitz and Johnson, 2007).

The MdPFC is important in motivation and the initiation of activity (Figure 6.10). It is sensitive to gaze and was activated when subjects evaluated the emotional aspect of gaze (Wicker et al., 2003). A more ventral area appeared to be involved in emotion processing. The MdPFC is often activated by theory-of-mind tasks (Happé et al., 1996; Brunet et al., 2000).

The MdPFC regulates our own emotional responses in two ways. First, it can allow one to focus on the behavior of another and evaluate other's intentions or feelings. The MdPFC evaluates the social situation and determines the meaning of others' intentions or feelings. Simply estimating the feelings or intentions of others has been shown to interrupt amygdala-mediated negative judgments of them. Second, the MdPFC allows one to focus on one's own involvement in an emotionally charged situation and to imagine one's position from the point of view of a third emotionally detached person. It is speculated that this activity may also modulate stimulus-driven amygdala activity (Olsson and Ochsner, 2008).

The MdPFC also responds to interoceptive and exteroceptive stimuli, especially those involved in social situations. The MdPFC is activated during the perception of pain in one's self and in others. It responds to information that represents a more complex, three-place (triatic) scenario: 'You, me, and this' (Saxe, 2006). That is, the MdPFC monitors others' actions, sensations, and personalities as well as our own social

responses to a particular context or situation (Winston et al., 2002; Cunningham et al., 2004; Iacoboni and Dapretto, 2006; Todorov, et al., 2006). It appears to play a unique role in the perception of others' perception of the self (Ochsner et al., 2005). Brunet et al. (2003) found that the MdPFC of control subjects was activated bilaterally when viewing images of people, whereas schizophrenia patients viewing the same images showed no activation of either side of the MdPFC.

Social/emotional cognition has been organized in a three-dimensional pattern in the prefrontal cortex (Figure 6.3) (Olsson and Ochsner, 2008). Along a medial–lateral axis, midline cortical areas are interconnected with visceral centers including the amygdala and striatum. Midline areas are concerned with internal states. Lateral areas are concerned with externally generated representations and are interconnected with visuospatial centers.

The anterior–posterior axis involving the midline prefrontal and cingulate cortices follows the degree of complexity of the mental state. Less complex representations are processed beginning in the anterior cingulate cortex. As processing proceeds anteriorly along the axis, representations become more complex providing awareness of, and judgments about, the meaning of affective mental states. The third prefrontal cortex dimension extends from the inferior surface where stimulus-driven processes take place to superior regions where reflective speculation of mental state can occur.

The MdPFC along with the thalamus was activated when a group of 12 women were asked to recall recent

99

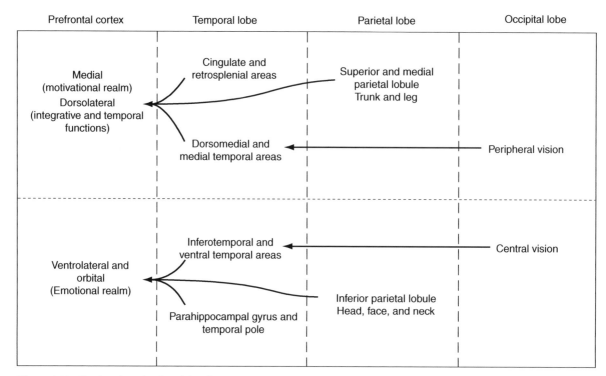

Figure 6.10. The dorsolateral and medial prefrontal areas receive input from dorsal temporal and superior parietal lobes and portions of the occipital lobe that mediate peripheral vision. This dorsal system appears to function in the motivational and planning realm, closely associated with the trunk and lower limb, and with the location of an object in space (where). The ventrolateral and orbital prefrontal areas receive input from inferior temporal and inferior parietal lobes and portions of the occipital cortex that mediate central vision. This ventral system appears to function in the emotional realm, closely associated with the head, face and neck, and with the identification of an object (what). (After Pandya, D.N., and Yeterian, E.H. 1990. Prefrontal cortex in relation to other cortical areas in rhesus monkey: Architecture and connections. In: H.B.M. Uylings, C.G., Van Eden, J.P.C., DeBruin, M.A., Corner, and M.G.P., Feenstra (eds.) The Prefrontal Cortex: Its Structure, Function and Pathology. Amsterdam: Elsevier, pp. 63–94.)

emotional events. Additional brain areas were activated when they viewed an emotion-evoking filmstrip. Activation was independent of the nature of the emotion –happiness, sadness, disgust. A similar experiment revealed activation in the MdPFC and cingulate cortex, but only on the right side (Teasdale *et al.*, 1999). The authors suggested that the MdPFC and thalamus are important in the appreciation of emotion in the absence of concurrent sensory input (Lane *et al.*, 1997; Reiman *et al.*, 1997).

The patient with a lesion of the MdPFC is apathetic. The area affected may include parts of the SMC. He or she exhibits a lack of spontaneous movement. Immediately after the onset of the lesion, the patient often presents with akinetic mutism. Paresis of the lower limb may be seen if the lesion extends posteriorly to infringe on the primary motor cortex. The patient often fails to respond to commands. Incontinence is frequently seen, and the patient appears indifferent to the problem.

Ventromedial prefrontal cortex

The ventromedial prefrontal cortex (MvPFC) is located inferior to the MdPFC and occupies portions of BA 10, BA 12, and BA 32 (Figure 6.3). It may extend posteriorly to include portions of the infralimbic, subgenual anterior cingulate gyrus (BA 25). A key difference from the MdPFC is that the MvPFC receives input from all sensory modalities. It functions in basic stimulus-reinforcement association learning involving social/emotional cues. It has connections with the ventral anterior cingulate gyrus, insula, amygdala, and nucleus accumbens. These structures function to identify valence and emotional tone of both interoceptive and exteroceptive stimuli. The role of the MvPFC with respect to these other structures is to determine the degree to which these stimuli are relevant to the self. It may use past experience to predetermine self-relevance to current or anticipated stimuli (Schmitz and Johnson, 2007). It responds when an individual experiences empathy, a component of social cognition

(Saxe, 2006). One report showed that the MvPFC, along with the bilateral temporoparietal junction, was activated when subjects were asked to take the perspective of another in a situation containing either emotional or cognitive content. Activation was more intense in the OFC and MvPFC to scenarios containing emotional content (Hynes *et al.*, 2006). It was concluded the MvPFC is involved with perspective-taking in situations involving empathetic and sympathetic aspects of emotion, especially in situations that require more conscious and effortful reasoning (Hynes *et al.*, 2006). It may support a process in which we use our own thoughts, feelings and desires as a proxy for those of other people in order to infer the other's mental state: "You and me" (Jackson *et al.*, 2006; Jenkins *et al.*, 2008).

Finally, the MvPFC has been proposed to be where the capacity to develop theories of the mind resides. Human social behavior is characterized by the unique capability to make inferences regarding others' mental states, needs, feelings, and intentions (so called theory-of-mind) (Happaney *et al.*, 2004). More recent data indicate that cognitive and affective theory-of-mind may be mediated by different regions. While the MvPFC may be mediating affective theory-of-mind, a wider region of the prefrontal cortex including the dorsolateral cortex may be necessary to develop a cognitive theory-of-mind (Shamay-Tsoory and Aharon-Peretz, 2007).

Based on the nature of the connections of the MvPFC with sensory input and output to autonomic-visceral control, and to other limbic as well as other frontal cortical regions, a hypothesis known as the "somatic marker hypothesis" was advanced by Antonio Damasio (1994) to shed light on the process of decision making by humans. The somatic marker hypothesis suggests that structures in the MvPFC hold representations of the associations between certain complex situations and the visceral sensations or emotions previously linked to that situation. The actual memories are not held here thus damage to this region will not affect the memories themselves but will affect the link between them. When an individual experiences a situation similar to one experienced in the past, the ventromedial region is activated and the visceral/emotional memory tied to the previous situation is recalled. The recall may be an actual visceral reexperience of emotions and feelings or just a cognitive representation. This evocation process functions as a constraint over the process of reasoning

dealing with multiple options and response choices. Certain choices can be either eliminated or endorsed, thus decreasing the number of choices available. In the absence of this hypothesized process, options and outcomes become more equalized and the process of choosing will depend entirely on logical processes. This strategy would be slower and may fail to take into account previous experience.

Patients with damage to the MvPFC present with severe impairment of social and personal decision making (Damasio, 1994). These patients have largely preserved intellectual abilities. Patients may have difficulty planning their workday as well as difficulty choosing suitable friends, partners, or activities. Their choices are not personally advantageous, rather they are inadequate and usually lead to financial losses, losses in social standing, and losses to family and friends.

Individuals with lesions involving the MvPFC score abnormally low on self-rating scales of emotional empathy but not on scales of cognitive empathy. Degeneration of the MvPFC in the frontal variant of frontal temporal dementia correlates with a rapid drop in empathetic concern (Lough *et al.*, 2006).

Prefrontal networks

There are two networks associated with the prefrontal cortex. Both act to regulate emotional behavior and interact with each other. The "orbital prefrontal network" (ventral system) is centered in the OFC. The orbital network receives input from the sensory association cortex of the parietal and temporal lobes as well as olfactory and taste cortices that make up the posterior orbital cortex. The network also includes the insula, amygdala, and ventral striatum (nucleus accumbens). Taken together this network can be interpreted historically to provide a basis for assessment of food (flavor, appearance, texture). The orbital prefrontal network is recognized to evaluate sensory stimuli, identify emotionally salient components, and in response, generate an appropriate affective state. It also signals other areas (hypothalamus and brainstem) to activate appropriate autonomic responses. The orbital system forms a cortico-striatal-thalamic-cortical loop, with connections with the ventromedial putamen and lateral caudate nucleus (Price, 2007; Saleem *et al.*, 2008). This system integrates sensory and emotional aspects and assigns characteristics such as reward, aversion, and relative value to sensory input (Drevets *et al.*, 2008). Of particular interest is its close connection with the dorsolateral and ventrolateral prefrontal cortices. It is proposed that the orbital prefrontal network provides for a top-down, effortful, voluntary regulation of emotional behavior (Ochsner and Gross, 2007; Phillips *et al.*, 2008).

The DLPFC bilaterally along with the right anterior cingulate gyrus and right parietal cortex is believed to function in support of voluntary suppression of attention to the emotionally salient stimulus or inhibition of the emotional response. The actions are hypothesized to be carried out through pathways involving the OFC.

The "medial prefrontal network" (dorsal system) is centered in the medial prefrontal cortex. It receives input from the region of the superior temporal gyrus that lies anterior to Heschl's gyrus as well as from the posterior superior temporal sulcus. The medial network includes the hippocampus, DLPFC, and dorsal anterior cingulate gyrus, and has close links with the amygdala and insula (Price, 2007; Saleem *et al.*, 2008). Unlike the orbital network, the medial network receives little sensory input. It sends fibers to the hypothalamus and midbrain, including the periaqueductal gray. The medial prefrontal network integrates visceromotor information and provides for the automatic control of emotion. Automatic control acts by either disengagement of attention away from the emotional stimulus or by reassignment of emotional salience (Phillips *et al.*, 2003, 2008).

The medial prefrontal cortex is central to the "medial prefrontal network." It receives input from the region of the superior temporal gyrus as well as the posterior superior temporal sulcus. The medical prefrontal network includes the DLPFC and cingulate gyrus. It is closely connected with the amygdala, hypothalamus and insula (Price, 2007; Saleem *et al.*, 2008). Unlike the orbital network, the medial prefrontal network receives little sensory input. It is activated during self-referential processing (i.e., appraisal of stimuli as they relate to one's own person). The DLPFC and posterior cingulate gyrus are coactivated. Activation of the cingulate gyrus may represent retrieval of autobiographical memory. Coactivation of all three provides for conflict monitoring between the current self and an inner standard. Interaction with the DLPFC suggests cognitive control that allows for directing attention elsewhere or by reassigning of emotional salience (Phillips *et al.*, 2003, 2008). Connections from the MPFC to the amygdala and hypothalamus allow for autonomic expression of emotions (e.g., blushing).

Behavioral considerations

Blood flow to the brain is decreased in major depression in elderly patients to about the same extent as in Alzheimer disease (Baxter *et al.*, 1985). Reductions are particularly evident in the parietal, superior temporal, and frontal cortices (Sackeim *et al.*, 1990). Positron emission tomographic scanning in patients with major depression reveals decreased metabolism in the DLPFC. Both blood flow and metabolism have been reported to be decreased in the DLPFC in patients with primary depression (Baxter *et al.*, 1989; Bench *et al.*, 1992; Dolan *et al.*, 1992). Increases in hypometabolism and hypoperfusion to normal levels have been reported following successful drug therapy but not after unsuccessful drug therapy (Mayberg, 1997). The dorsolateral prefrontal cortex is usually easy to evaluate by computed tomography (CT) and is the region of the prefrontal lobe sampled by routine electroencephalography (EEG). Depressed patients exhibit hypometabolism in the left anterolateral prefrontal cortex (Baxter *et al.*, 1989).

Patients with schizophrenia showed abnormal prefrontal activation, particularly in response to tasks that require executive function such as working memory (Manoach *et al.*, 2000). Pfefferbaum *et al.* (2001) found that alcoholic subjects, showed diminished activation of BA 9, BA 10, and BA 45 when compared with normals in a visual spatial task requiring working memory. At the same time the alcoholic subjects showed increased activation in BA 47, suggesting they were using the more inferior "what" stream and declarative memory as compared with the more dorsal "where" stream used by the controls. Subjects at high risk for alcoholism showed decreased bilateral activation of BA 40 and 44 and the inferior frontal gyrus when compared with low risk subjects (Rangaswamy *et al.*, 2004).

Information processing in the dorsolateral prefrontal lobes of schizophrenic patients is deficient. This correlates with the finding that an abnormally high density of neurons is found in the prefrontal cortex of brains of patients with schizophrenia (Figure 6.11). The increased density corresponds with a slight, nonsignificant decrease in cortical thickness (Selemon *et al.*, 1995). The left dorsolateral region has been shown to have decreased cerebral blood flow corresponding with psychomotor poverty seen in schizophrenia (Liddle *et al.*, 1992). Negative symptoms of schizophrenia correlate with a decrease in glucose utilization in the frontal and parietal cortex (Tamminga

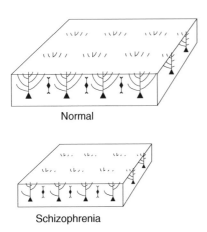

Normal

Schizophrenia

Figure 6.11. An increase in density is seen in prefrontal neurons in postmortem tissue of schizophrenia patients. (Reproduced by permission from Selemon, L.D., Rajkowska, G., and Goldman-Rakic, P.W. 1995. Abnormally high neuronal density in the schizophrenic cortex. A morphometric analysis of prefrontal area 9 and occipital area 17. Arch. Gen. Psychiatry 52:805–818.)

et al., 1992). Thought disorder in schizophrenia may represent the breakdown of working memory and is hypothesized to correlate with abnormalities in the DLPFC (Goldman-Rakic, 1996). It has been hypothesized that the increased density is due to a reduction of the neuropil, suggesting a decrease in the number of synapses (i.e., excessive synaptic pruning; Glantz and Lewis, 1993; Tamminga, 1999).

Synaptic pruning in the frontal cortex is seen normally in adolescence, preceded somewhat by cell death (Huttenlocher, 1979). More efficient word processing may be the natural result of pruning. Excessive synaptic pruning is hypothesized to result in the hallucinated speech of schizophrenia (Hoffman and McGlashan, 1997). Protection provided by estrogens may account for later age of onset of schizophrenia in women (Seeman, 1997).

A decrease in interstitial neurons found in the white matter of the middle frontal gyrus of the DLPFC of schizophrenics has been reported (Akbarian *et al.*, 1996), and it was suggested that this decrease reflects an abnormal migration pattern during the second trimester of pregnancy.

There is no longer any doubt that the intactness of prefrontal function is essential for our normal function in society. Through the integration of sensory input, emotional tone, and motivation of cortical, subcortical, and limbic sources, the prefrontal cortex critically intervenes in the initiation and guidance of behavior.

Other behavioral considerations

Schizophrenia

An increased number of axospinous synapses (225%) and a decrease in axodendritic synapses (-40%) has been reported for the frontal lobe in schizophrenia (Aganova and Uranova, 1992). Increased neuron density has been observed in the prefrontal cortex (Figure 6.11) and a decrease in GABAergic axon terminals reported in the dorsolateral prefrontal cortex (Woo *et al.*, 1998). Abi-Dargham *et al.* (2002) reported that dopamine D_1 binding was increased in the prefrontal cortex and correlated with poorer working memory performance.

Pathology in the prefrontal region in schizophrenia predicts increased dopamine release in the striatum (Bertolino *et al.*, 2000; Meyer-Lindenberg *et al.*, 2002). This may occur through activation of corticostriatal glutamatergic pathways (Carlsson and Carlsson, 2006). It is speculated that dopamine release in the striatum conveys assignment of positive or negative valence to otherwise neutral cues (Schultz, 2006; Kéri, 2008).

It is theorized that positive symptoms of schizophrenia are caused by an overactivity of the mesolimbic system or an excessive number of D_2-like dopamine receptors. (D_2-like receptors include D_2-, D_3-, and D_4-receptor subtypes; Chapter 3.) This is because all clinically effective antipsychotic drugs are antagonists of D_2-like dopamine receptors (Nestler, 1997). The negative symptoms may be due to a loss of function of the mesocortical system. It is hypothesized that there is an increase in activity of the mesolimbic system, which responds to antipsychotic drugs (D_2-like receptors); and a decrease in activity in the prefrontal area, which does not respond to antipsychotic drugs.

It is postulated that the greatest development of the dopamine system in evolution is the increased abundance of D_1 receptors in the prefrontal cortex (Lidow *et al.*, 1991). Investigators propose that dopaminergic transmission in the prefrontal cortex modulates neuronal circuitry in a manner that augments significant incoming signals while attenuating irrelevant incoming noise (Winterer *et al.*, 2006). There are reduced numbers of the D_1-like dopamine receptors, which include D_1- and D_5-receptor subtypes in the prefrontal cortex of patients with schizophrenia. Dopamine is believed to be important in working memory largely through action on the D_1-like receptors. The reduced number of D_1-like receptors may underlie cognitive deficiencies common to schizophrenia patients.

Reduction in the density of D_1-like receptors which are found on the dendrites of pyramidal cells may be responsible for the reduction in cortical thickness (Selemon *et al.*, 1995).

Overactivity of the MPFC and posterior cingulate gyrus has been reported in patients with schizophrenia at rest, suggesting excessive introspection. Positive symptoms (hallucinations, delusions, and confused thoughts) were found to correlate with increased activity in the medial prefrontal cortex and posterior cingulate gyrus (Garrity *et al.*, 2007; Harrison, *et al.*, 2007; Zhou *et al.*, 2007).

Ventrolateral prefrontal cortex metabolic activity in schizophrenic patients was not different from controls when examined during working memory tasks (Manoach *et al.*, 2000; MacDonald and Carter, 2003). However, when presented with working memory or executive tasks there was hypoactivation in the dorsolateral prefrontal cortex accompanied by increased activation in the anterior cingulate and left frontal pole relative to controls (Hazlett *et al.*, 2000; Glahn *et al.*, 2005; Ragland *et al.*, 2007). During episodic memory recall both decreased and increased activity were reported. The literature remains confusing. Some authors found that hypoactivity in the left prefrontal area was predominant (Hofer *et al.*, 2003; Reichenberg and Harvey, 2007). Decreased activity during episodic memory encoding was more likely, especially on the right (Barch, 2005). Differences in results between studies conducted under different conditions suggest that frontal activity is inefficient (Keshavan *et al.*, 2008).

In one study, when viewing images of people the DMPFC of control subjects was activated bilaterally. Schizophrenia patients viewing the same images showed no activation of either side of the DMPFC (Brunet *et al.*, 2003).

Depression

A significant decrease has been reported in glial density and glial number in the OFC of patients with a history of major depression or bipolar disorder. Neuron cell size but not number was reduced (Torrey *et al.*, 2000; Cotter *et al.*, 2002). Decreased glial density and reduced neuron size has been observed in the dorsolateral (BA 9) as well as the orbitofrontal cortices (Rajkowska *et al.*, 1999, 2001).

Imaging studies have shown that decreased activity in the prefrontal cortex of patients with unipolar or bipolar depression compared with controls is one of the most consistent findings. The superior, middle, and inferior gyri of the DLPFC are particularly affected (Ketter *et al.*, 2001; Brooks *et al.*, 2009). The effect may appear bilaterally (Ketter *et al.*, 2001) or on either the right or left side (Cohen *et al.*, 1989). Depressed patients exhibit hypofrontality, with the effect more marked in the medial orbital region than in the dorsolateral region (Ho *et al.*, 1997). Decreased blood flow to the medial frontal pole appears to be the critical abnormality in depression-related cognitive impairment (depressive pseudodementia; Figure 6.12) and may be associated with emotional states such as withdrawal and apathy (Dolan *et al.*, 1992; Ho *et al.*, 1997). Activity in the MdPFC is reduced (Drevets *et al.*, 2002) and the size of the neurons and density of the glial is also reduced in the unmedicated, depressed condition (Uranova *et al.*, 2004).

In contrast, increased metabolism in the frontal lobes has also been reported (Drevets *et al.*, 2002; Ketter and Drevets, 2002). Activity in the orbital prefrontal cortex, VLPFC, and insula has been reported to be abnormally increased in unmedicated depressed patients while resting (Drevets, 2001, 2003). Activity

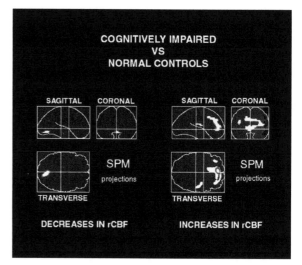

Figure 6.12. Statistical parametric maps (SPM) showing significant (p<0.05 Bonferroni corrected) decreases (left) and increases (right) in relative cerebral blood flow. The light areas represent mathematical differences between patients with depression-related cognitive impairment and control subjects. The pixels at which there is a significant change have been projected onto sagittal, coronal, and transverse renderings of the standard brain volume of Talairach and Tournoux. (Reproduced by permission from Dolan, R.J., EBench, C.J., Brown, R.G., Scott, L.C., Friston, K.J., and Frackowiak, R.S.J. 1992. Regional cerebral blood flow abnormalities in depressed patients with cognitive impairment. J. Neurol. Neurosurg. Psychiatry 55:768–773.)

in these regions decreased with antidepressant therapy (Drevets *et al.*, 2002). Alterations in activity in other areas has also been reported, including in the anterior cingulate gyrus, amygdala, insula, and ventral striatum (Drevets *et al.*, 1997; Kimbrell *et al.*, 2002). In one report, activity was increased in subjects with anxiety disorders during induced anxiety and obsessional states (Charney, 2002), and in another it was decreased in subjects under antidepressant treatment (Drevets and Raichle, 1998).

Metabolism was increased throughout the brain during nonrapid eye movement (non-REM) sleep in major depression (+30%), which supports the hyperarousal theory of depression. Regional increases have been seen in the occipital, temporal, parietal, and frontal lobes. By comparison, an increase in blood flow has been reported during transient sadness in healthy individuals (Mayberg, 1997) and in patients with simple phobia during provocation (Rauch *et al.*, 1995). Increased activation of the medial prefrontal network correlates with increased self-focus and cortical control (Lemogne *et al.*, 2009). A large decrease in perfusion was reported in the inferior frontal lobe of a woman who developed catatonia during a depressive episode (Galynker *et al.*, 1997).

Patients with depression and Parkinson disease or Huntington disease have diminished metabolism in both the orbital prefrontal cortex and the caudate nucleus. Depression has been diagnosed in 60% of patients with anterior frontal lesions (Cummings, 1993). This is consistent with a neuropsychiatry principle that suggests a contingent but not an obligatory anatomical relationship for specified behavioral syndromes. Left anterior lesions increase the patient's vulnerability to depression, but the occurrence of depression may also require environmental or psychosocial factors. This is in contrast to most neurological syndromes, in which an obligatory relationship is typical (Cummings, 1993). Decreased left prefrontal activity on positron emission tomography is consistently found in actively depressed patients. The decrease is more pronounced if the patient reports being more depressed on the day of scanning (Ketter *et al.*, 1994).

Bipolar disorder

Depressed bipolar disorder patients showed decreased metabolism in the DLPFC, lateral OFC, anterior insula, and ventral striatum; this is greater on the left than on the right (Martinot *et al.*, 1990; Ketter *et al.*,

2001; Brooks *et al.*, 2009). The anterior cingulate gyrus has also been reported to exhibit reduced metabolism in patients with bipolar disorder and major depressive disorder (Drevets *et al.*, 1997, 2007; Brooks *et al.*, 2009). The reduced metabolism in the subgenual anterior cingulate gyrus was accompanied by reduced gray matter volume and a reduction in glia but no loss of neurons (Ongür *et al.*, 1998). The neuron density appeared increased because of the loss of neuropil. The loss was observed early in the illness and in young adults at high familial risk (Hirayasu *et al.*, 1999; Botteron *et al.*, 2002; Boes *et al.*, 2007). The posterior subgenual anterior cingulate gyrus (infralimbic cortex) has been reported to exhibit an increase in gray matter after two years of naturalistic treatment (Coryell, *et al.*, 2005; Drevets and Savitz, 2008).

A reduction in activity has been reported in the right OFC during mania compared with controls (Rubinsztein et al, 2001; Blumberg *et al.*, 2003; Elliot *et al.*, 2003). Patients with the longest duration of mania episode showed the least right orbitofrontal activity (Altshuler *et al.*, 2005a). Greater activity in the amygdala in manic versus controls was observed during a task that normally activates the amygdala (Altshuler *et al.*, 2005b).

An anterior network that includes reciprocal connections between the right OFC and the amygdala bilaterally has been proposed to be dysfunctional in bipolar disorder. Reduced right orbitofrontal activity may result in impulsivity or unstable mood through dysregulation of the inhibitory prefrontal-amygdala circuit (Strakowski, 2002; Blumberg *et al.*, 2003; Altshuler *et al.*, 2005a). There is evidence that tracts in the OFC are reduced in volume (Kieseppa *et al.*, 2003; Adler *et al.*, 2004). However, it was not clear to the researchers if these tracts connect with the amygdala.

Obsessive-compulsive disorder

Reduced volume of the OFC is the most consistent reported morphological finding in OCD (Choi *et al.*, 2004; Kang *et al.*, 2004; Atmaca *et al.*, 2006, 2007; Menzies *et al.*, 2008). An increase in gray matter density has been reported in the left OFC (Kim *et al.*, 2001). Metabolism was found to be increased in the OFC along with the whole cerebral hemispheres, caudate nuclei, and cingulate gyri in patients with OCD (Figure 12.9; Baxter, 1992; Swedo *et al.*, 1992; Rauch *et al.*, 1994). The increase may be in response to reduced striatal inhibition and therefore reflects an attempt on the part of the OFC to inhibit obsessions and compulsions (Baxter et al., 1990). The increased metabolism in the OFC has been shown to be accompanied by a similar increase in the bilateral anterior cingulate gyrus. A significant decrease in OFC metabolism was seen after successful drug treatment, and the decrease in the right OFC region correlated directly with two measures of OCD improvement (Swedo et al., 1992).

van den Heuvel et al. (2005) found that increased activity at rest was replaced with decreased activity compared in the premotor cortex, anterior cingulate gyrus, DLPFC, precuneus, lateral parietal cortex, and putamen when subjects were presented with a task requiring planning aspects of executive function. This is believed to reflect a decreased responsiveness in DLPFC-striatal circuits in OCD. The OFC is a component of the orbitofronto-striatal loop. This loop has been proposed to be dysfunctional in OCD (Menzies et al., 2008). Models of OCD reflect results of studies showing changes in activation of prefrontal areas in response to activity in the caudate nucleus of the striatum (Chapter 7).

Posttraumatic stress disorder

The medial prefrontal cortex has been found to be less active in patients with PTSD in several studies (Semple et al., 2000; Shin et al., 2001; Bremner, 2002) but not in others (Mirzaei et al., 2001; Osuch et al., 2001; Pissiota et al., 2003; Lindauer et al., 2008). PTSD is characterized by abnormal reactions to fear-provoking stimuli. Some patients exhibit hyperactive responses in the autonomic and emotional spheres. Others exhibit dissociative phenomena, including emotional numbing, psychogenic amnesia, psychogenic amnesia, depersonalization and derealization symptoms (Falconer et al., 2008). Individuals who exhibit a hyperarousal PTSD response to traumatic narratives, with increased autonomic and emotional responses, have reduced activity in the medial prefrontal cortex and anterior cingulate gyrus compared with controls (Lanius et al., 2001). Patients with PTSD who exhibit a dissociated response exhibit increased activity in the medial prefrontal cortex and anterior cingulate gyrus. It is hypothesized that the areas activated in dissociative PTSD reflect increased emotional regulation and inhibition of the limbic emotional networks (Lanius et al., 2002). Liberzon and Sripada (2008) suggest the MdPFC allows heightened reactivity to salient emotional stimuli and fails to reevaluate the reaction. In their model the MvPFC fails to reduce conditioned fear. Transcranial magnetic stimulation focused on

the right dorsolateral prefrontal cortex was reported to have a therapeutic effect on ten patients with PTSD (Cohen et al., 2004).

Borderline personality disorder

The three main symptoms of borderline personality disorder (BPD) are impulsivity, emotional instability, and disturbed interpersonal relationships. Brain areas showing reduced metabolism and volume reductions in BPD patients include the orbital prefrontal cortex, cingulate gyrus, hippocampus, and amygdala (Soloff et al., 2000; Rusch, et al., 2003; Schmahl et al., 2003). Volume reductions in the left OFC (24%) and amygdala (23%–25%) were found to correlate and led to a fronto-limbic hypothesis (Tebartz et al., 2003) which included the suggestion that the reduced volumes correlated with impulsivity and aggressive behavior (Soloff et al., 2003; Tebartz et al., 2003). A decrease in metabolism seen in the DLPFC of patients with BPD is speculated to correspond with chronic feelings of depersonalization and unreality (De La Fuente et al., 1997).

Decreased serotonin synthesis capacity has been observed in the posterior superior temporal gyrus, anterior cingulate gyrus and in the medial frontal cortex (BA 10) (Leyton et al., 2001). Reduced activity in the OFC is hypothesized to associate with impulsive-aggressiveness in BPD (Soloff et al., 2003). Reduced OFC serotonin levels may also be a contributing factor (Siever et al., 1999). Smaller volume and reduced metabolic activity reported in the amygdala may be responsible for impaired emotional processing and emotional instability (Lyoo, 2005).

In subjects with BPD, increased metabolism was observed in the right VLPFC and left medial prefrontal cortex along with the amygdala bilaterally when viewing emotionally aversive images as well as sad, neutral and fearful faces, but not happy faces (Donegan et al., 2003; Herpertz et al., 2001). A task requiring response inhibition produced increased activity in the prefrontal in control subjects. When challenged with the same task BPD patients exhibited more widespread activity that extended to the inferior, middle, superior frontal gyri, and anterior cingulate cortex (Vollm et al., 2004).

Siever et al. (1999) suggested that serotonergic modulation decreased in BPD patients as a result of reduced metabolic response to administration of a serotonin-releasing agent (D,L-fenfluramine) compared with controls. This was localized to the medial

OFC (BA 9, BA 10, and BA 11). It was suggested that the decreased activity is associated with impulsive-aggressiveness (Soloff et al., 2003).

Autism spectrum disorders

Consistent frontal lobe structural abnormities in autism are lacking. However, behavioral studies have indicated a link between frontal lobe hyperplasia and autism. Frontal lobe size was found to correlate inversely with cerebellar vermis size in a group of 42 autistic boys (3–9 years) (Carper and Courchesne, 2000). At the microscopic level, abnormal minicolumn structure in the frontal lobe was reported (Casanova et al., 2002).

One theory of autism suggests some symptoms are due to impaired theory-of-mind (Penn, 2006). Theory-of-mind structures include the MPFC. Some theory-of-mind tasks result in abnormal frontal lobe activation in subjects with autistic spectrum disorder (ASD) (Castelli et al., 2002). Joint attention, the ability to follow the gestures of others, share interest in objects, and appropriately shift gaze during interaction with others has been reported to be dysfunctional in children with autism (Whalen and Schreibman, 2003). These tasks rely on normal function of the OFC, medial prefrontal cortex and DLPFC areas (Henderson et al., 2002). Working memory, also associated with the DLPFC, is impaired in ASD (Luna et al., 2002).

Autism and Asperger syndrome are suggested to involve dysregulation of the limbic-orbitofrontal circuitry (Bachevalier and Loveland, 2006). Several regions in the default brain network are affected in ASD. The volume of the MdPFC is reported to be reduced (Abell et al., 1999; McAlonan et al., 2005). Compared with control subjects, activity in the default network has been reported to be significantly reduced in individuals with ASD. More serious social impairment correlated with greater atypical activity in the vMPFC and posterior cingulate gyrus (Kennedy et al., 2006).

It is speculated that the difficulty that autistic children have in relating to other people may reflect a dysfunction in their mirror neuron system. Neurophysiological and brain imaging studies have provided some evidence in favor of this hypothesis (Dapretto et al., 2006; Oberman and Ramachandran, 2007). Autistic children appear to have a functioning fusiform face area and mirror neuron system (Calvo-Merino et al., 2005). However, they appear to be sensitive to only individuals with whom they are familiar,

(e.g., parent, guardian, sibling). They show improvement in eye contact, physical contact, and social interaction skills when interacting with a familiar as opposed to an unfamiliar individual (Knott et al., 1995; Oberman et al., 2008).

Frontotemporal dementia

The pathology in frontotemporal dementia (FTD) is more localized to the frontal and anterior temporal regions than in Alzheimer disease. Consequently, more behavioral disturbances (e.g., disinhibition, hypersexuality, irritability, depression, apathy) are seen in association with FTD than in Alzheimer disease.

Seizures

Frontal lobe seizures are particularly difficult to diagnose, but they are common and are usually secondary to head trauma. They can be brief, odd, or misleading, and can be misinterpreted as pseudoseizures. Extensive connections of the orbital prefrontal cortex to limbic structures (mainly amygdala and hippocampus) via the uncinate fasciculus help in understanding the difficulty in differentiating between ictal events that occur in those areas. Laughter, crying, moaning, and verbal automatisms have been described with lesions of the superior frontal gyrus and cingulate gyrus. In addition, complex gestures such as body rubbing, rearrangement of clothes, sexual automatism, mood changes, wandering, and agitation have all been reported with frontal lobe lesions. Finally, nonconvulsive frontal seizure states can produce prolonged behavioral disturbances (Riggio and Harner, 1992).

Lesions in the orbital prefrontal cortex are difficult to evaluate utilizing procedures such as EEG due to their proximity to the eye. Eye movements cause major artifacts that mask EEG abnormalities.

Miscellaneous conditions

Decreased metabolic activity has been reported in the OFC and particularly in the left hemisphere during protracted cocaine abstinence (Volkow et al., 1992). A decrease in cerebral blood flow in both the OFC and the DLPFC has been reported in patients with depression. Decreased blood flow has been seen in the orbital prefrontal cortex in phobic patients when presented with visual phobogenic stimuli (Figure 4.6).

Select bibliography

Fuster, J.M. *The Prefrontal Cortex* (4th ed.). (New York: Academic Press, 2008.)

Jasper, H.H., Riggio, S., and Goldman-Rakic, P.S. eds. *Epilepsy and the Functional Anatomy of the Frontal Lobe. Advances in Neurology* (vol. 66). (New York: Raven Press, 1995.)

Lunders, H.O. ed. *Supplementary Sensorimotor Area. Advances in Neurology* (vol. 70). (Philadelphia: Lippincott–Raven, 1996.)

Perecman, E. ed. *The Frontal Lobes Revisited.* (New York: IRBN Press, 1987.)

Roberts, A.C., Robbins, T.W., and Weiskrantz, L. *The Prefrontal Cortex. Executive and Cognitive Functions.* (New York: Oxford University Press, 2000.)

Stuss, D.T., and Benson, D.F. *The Frontal Lobes.* (New York: Raven Press, 1986.)

Uylings, H.B.M., Van Eden, C.G., DeBruin, J.P.C., Corner, M.A., and Feenstra, M.G.P. eds. *The Prefrontal Cortex. Its Structure, Function and Pathology. Progress in Brain Research* (vol. 85). (Amsterdam: Elsevier, 1990.)

References

Abell, F., Krams, M., Ashburner, J., Passingham, R., FristonK., Frackowiak, R.S.J., Happe, F., Frith, C.D., and Frith, U. 1999. The neuroanatomy of autism: A voxel-based whole brain analysis of structural scans. *Neuroreport* **10**:1647–1651.

Abi-Dargham, A., Mawlawi, O., Lombardo, I., Gil, R., Martinez, D., Huang, Y., Hwang, D.R., Keilp, J., Kochan, L., Van Heertum, R., Gorman, J.M., and Laruelle, M. 2002. Prefrontal dopamine D1 receptors and working memory in schizophrenia. *J. Neurosci.* **22**:3708–3719.

Adler, C.M., Holland, S.K., Schmithorst, V., Wilke, M., Weiss, K.L., Pan, H., and Strakowski, S.M. 2004. Abnormal frontal white matter tracts in bipolar disorder: A diffusion tensor imaging study. *Bipolar Disord.* **6**:197–203.

Aganova, E.Z., and Uranova, N.A. 1992. Morphometric analysis of synaptic contacts in the anterior limbic cortex in the endogenous psychoses. *Neurosci. Behav. Physiol.* **22**:59–65.

Akbarian, S., Kim, J.J., Potkin, S.G., Hetrick, W.P., Bunney, W.E., and Jones, E.G. 1996. Maldistribution of interstitial neurons in prefrontal white matter of the brains of schizophrenic patients. *Arch. Gen. Psychiatry* **53**:425–436.

Altshuler, L.L., Bookheimer, S.Y., Townsend, J., Proenza, M.A., Eisenberger, N., Sabb, F., Mintz, J., and Cohen, M.S. 2005a. Blunted activation in orbitofrontal cortex during mania: A functional magnetic resonance imaging study. *Biol. Psychiatry* **58**:763–769.

Altshuler, L., Bookheimer, S., Proenza, M.A., Townsend, J., Sabb, F., Firestine, A., Bartzokis, G., Mintz, J., Mazziotta, J., and Cohen, M.S. 2005b. Increased amygdala activation during mania: A functional magnetic resonance imaging study. *Am. J. Psychiatry* **162**:1211–1213.

Amuts, K., Weiss, P.H., Mohlberg, H., Pieperhoff, P., Eickhoff, S., Gurd, J.M., Marshall, J.C., Shah, N.J., Fink, G.R., and Zilles, K. 2004. Analysis of neural mechanisms underlying verbal fluency in cytoarchitectonically defined stereotaxic space –the roles of Brodmann's areas 44 and 45. *Neuroimage* **22**:42–56.

Anderson, M.C., Ochsner, K.N., Kuhl, B., Cooper, J., Robertson, E., Gabrieli, S.W., Glover, G.H., and Gabrieli, J.D.E. 2004. Neural systems underlying the suppression of unwanted memories. *Science* **303**:232–235.

Atmaca, M., Yildirim, G., Ozdmir, H., Yildirim, H., Ozdemir, H., Aydin, A., Tezcan, E., and Ozler, S. 2006. Volumetric MRI assessment of brain regions in patients with refractory obsessive-compulsive disorder. *Prog. Neuropsychopharmacol. Biol. Psychiatry* **30**:1051–1057.

Atmaca, M., Yildirim, H., Ozdemir, H., Tezcan, E., and Poyraz, K. 2007. Volumetric MRI study of key brain regions implicated in obsessive-compulsive disorder. *Prog. Neuropsychopharmacol. Biol. Psychiatry* **31**:46–52.

Bachevalier, J., and Loveland, K. 2006. The orbitofrontal-amygdala circuit and self-regulation of social-emotional behavior in autism. *Neurosci. Biobehav. Rev.* **30**:97–117.

Baddeley, A. 1992. Working memory. *Science* **255**:556–559.

Badre, D., and Wagner, A.D. 2007. Left ventrolateral prefrontal cortex and the cognitive control of memory. *Neuropsychologia* **45**:2883–2901.

Badre, D., Poldrack, R.A., Paré-Blagoev, E.J., Insler, R., and Wagner, A.D. 2006. Dissociable controlled retrieval and generalized selection mechanisms in ventrolateral prefrontal cortex. *Neuron* **47**:907–918.

Bagary, M.S., Hutton, S.B., Symms, M.R., Barker, G.J., Mutsatsa, S.H., and Barnes, T.R.E., 2004. Structural neural networks subserving oculomotor function in first-episode schizophrenia. *Biol. Psychiatry* **56**:620–627.

Barch, D.M. 2005. The cognitive neuroscience of schizophrenia. *Annu. Rev. Clin. Psychol.* **1**:321–353.

Baxter, L.R., Jr. 1992. Neuroimaging studies of obsessive compulsive disorder. *Psychiatr. Clin. North Am.* **15**:871–884.

Jr., Phelps, M.E., Mazziotta, J.C., Schwartz, J.M., Gerner, R.H., Selin, C.E., and Sumida, R.M. 1985. Cerebral metabolic rates for glucose in mood disorders –studies with positron emission tomography and fluorodeoxyglucose F18. *Arch. Gen. Psychiatry* **42**:441–447.

Baxter, L.R., Schwartz, J.M., Phelps, M.E., Mazziotta, J.E., Guze, B.H., Selin, C.E., Gerner, R.H., and Sumida,

R.M. 1989. Reduction of prefrontal cortex glucose metabolism common to three types of depression. *Arch. Gen. Psychiatry* **46**:243–250.

Baxter, L.R., Jr., Schwartz, J.M., Guze, B.H., Bergman, K., and Szuba, M.P. 1990. PET imaging in obsessive compulsive disorder with and without depression. *J. Clin. Psychiatry* **51**(Suppl.):61–69.

Bechara, A., Damasio, H., and Damasio, A.R. 2000. Emotion, decision making and the orbitofrontal cortex. *Cereb. Cortex* **10**:295–307.

Bench, C.J., Dolan, R.J., Friston, K.J., Brown, R., and Scott, L. 1992. The anatomy of melancholia: A positron emission tomography study of primary depression. *Psychol. Med.* **3**:602–615.

Benson, D.F., and Ardila, A. 1993. Depression in aphasia. In: S.E. Starkstein, and R.G.Robinson (eds.) *Depression in Neurologic Disease*. Baltimore: Johns Hopkins Press, pp.152–164.

Berthoz, S., Armony, J.L., Blair, R.J.R., and Dolan, R.J. 2002. An fMRI study of intentional and unintentional (embarrassing) violations of social norms. *Brain* **125**:1696–1708.

Bertolino, A., Breier, A., Callicott, J.H., Adler, C., Mattay, V.S., Shapiro, M., Frank, J.A., Pickar, D., and Weinberger, D.R. 2000. The relationship between dorsolateral prefrontal neuronal N-acetylasparate and evoked release of striatal dopamine in schizophrenia. *Neuropsycopharmacology* **22**:125–132.

Blair, R.J., Morris, J.S., Frith, C.D., Perrett, D.I., and Dolan, R.J. 1999. Dissociable neural responses to facial expressions of sadness and anger. *Brain* **122**:883–893.

Blakemore, S.-J. 2008. The social brain in adolescence. *Nat. Rev. Neurosci.* **9**:267–276.

Bleasel, A., Comair, Y., and Luders, H.O. 1996. Surgical ablations of the mesial frontal lobe in humans. In: H.O.Lunders (ed.) *Supplementary Sensorimotor Area*. Philadelphia: Lippincott–Raven, pp. 217–235.

Blumberg, H.P., Leung, H.C., Skudlarski, P., Lacadie, C.M., Fredericks, C.A., Harris, B.C., Charney, D.S., Gore, J.C., Krystal, J.H., and Peterson, B.S. 2003. A functional magnetic resonance imaging study of bipolar disorder: State- and trait-related dysfunction in ventral prefrontal cortices. *Arch. Gen. Psychiatry* **60**:601–609.

Boes, A.D., McCormick, L.M., Coryell, W.H., and Nopoulos, P. 2007. Rostral anterior cingulate cortex volume correlates with depressed mood in normal healthy children. *Biol. Psychiatry* **63**:391–397.

Bookheimer, S.Y., Zetiro, T.A., Blaxton, T.A., Gaillard, P.W., and Theodore, W.H. 2000. Activation of language cortex with automatic speech tasks. *Neurology* **55**:1151–1157.

Boone, K.B., Miller, B.L., Rosenberg, L., Durazo, A., McIntrye, M., and Weil, M. 1988. Neuro psychological

and behavioral abnormalities in an adolescent with frontal lobe seizure. *Neurology* **38**:583–586.

Botteron, K.N., Raichle, M.E., Drevets, W.C., Heath, A.C., and Todd, R.D. 2002. Volumetric reduction in left subgenual prefrontal cortex in early onset depression.*Biol. Psychiatry* **51**:342–344.

Breier, A. 1999. Cognitive deficit in schizophrenia and its neurochemical basis. *Br. J. Psychiatry* **174**(Suppl. 37):16–18.

Bremner, J.D. 2002. Neuroimaging of childhood trauma. *Semin. Clin. Neurospychiatry* **7**:104–112.

Brodal, A. 1981. *Neurological Anatomy*. New York: Oxford University Press.

Broffman, M. 1950. The lobotomized patient during the first year at home. In: M.Greenblatt, R.Arnot, and H.C.Solomon (eds.) *Studies in Lobotomy*. Orlando, FL: Grune and Stratton.

Brooks, J.O. III, Wang, P-W., Bonner, J.C., Rosen, A.C., Hoblyn, J.C., Hill, S.J., and Ketter, T.A. 2009. Dereased prefrontal, anterior cingulate, insula, and ventral striatal metabolism in medication-free depressed outpatients with bipolar disorder. *J. Psychiatric Res.* **43**:181–188.

Brunet, E., Sarfati, Y. Hardy-Bayle, M.C., and Decety, J. 2000. A PET investigation of the attibution of intentions with a nonverbal task.*Neuroimage* **11**:157–166.

Brunet, E., Sarfati, Y. Hardy-Bayle, M.C., and Decety, J. 2003. Abnormalities of brain function during a nonverbal theory of mind task in schizophrenia. *Neuropsychologia* **41**:1574–1582.

Buccino, G., Vogt, S., Ritzl, A., Fink, G.R., Zilles, K., Freund, H.J., and Rizzolatti, G. 2004. Neural circuits underlying imitation learning of hand actions: An event related fMRI study. *Neuron* **42**:323–334.

Buchanan, R.W., Vladar, K., Barta, P.E., and Pearlson, G.D. 1998. Structural evaluation of the prefrontal cortex in schizophrenia. *Am. J. Psychiatry* **155**:1049–1055.

Buckner, R.L., and Carroll, D.C. 2007. Self-projection and the brain. *Trends Cogn. Sci.* **11**:49–57.

Buckner, R.L., Andrews-Hanna, J.R., and Schacter, D.L. 2008. The brain's default network. *Ann. N. Y. Acad. Sci.* **1124**:1–38.

Burke, J.G., and Reveley, M.A., 2002. Improved antisaccade performance with risperidone in schizophrenia. *J. Neurol. Neurosurg. Psychiatry* **72**:449–454.

Butter, C.M., Mishkin, M., and Mirsky, A.F. 1968. Emotional response toward humans in monkeys with selective frontal lesions. *Psychol. Behav.* **4**:163–171.

Buttner-Ennever, J.A. (ed.) 1988. Neuroanatomy of the oculomotor system. *Reviews of Oculomotor Research* (vol. 2). New York: Elsevier.

Calvo-Merino, B., Glaser, D.E., Grezes, J., Passingham, R.E., and Haggard, P. 2005. Action observation and acquired motor skills: An fMRI study with expert dancers. *Cereb. Cortex* **15**:1243–1249.

Caplan, D., Alpert, N., Waters, G., and Olivieri, A. 2000. Activation of Broca's area by syntactic processing under conditions of concurrent articulation. *Hum. Brain Mapp.* **9**:65–71.

Carlsson, A., and Carlsson, M.L., 2006. A dopaminergic deficit hypothesis of schizophrenia: The path to discovery. *Dialogues Clin. Neurosci.* **8**:137–142.

Carper, R.A., and Courchesne, E. 2000. Inverse correlation between frontal lobe and cerebellum sizes in children with autism. *Brain* **123**:836–844.

Carr, L.A., Nigg, J.T., and Henderson, J.M. 2006. Attentional versus motor inhibition in adults with attention-deficit/hyperactivity disorder. *Neuropsychology* **20**:430–441.

Casanova, M.F., Buzhoeveden, D.P., Switala, A.E., and Roy, E. 2002. Minicolumnar pathology in autism. *Neurology* **58**:428–432.

Castelli, F., Frith, C., Happé, F., and Frith, U. 2002. Autism, Asperger syndrome and brain mechanisms for the attribution of mental states to animated shapes. *Brain* **125**:1839–1849.

Cavanna, A.E., and Trimble, M.R. 2006. The precuneus: a review of its functional anatomy and behavioural correlates. *Brain* **129**:564–583.

Charney, D.S. 2002. The Neurobiology of mood disorders. *Arch. Neurol.* **59**:326.

Chartrand, T.L., and Bargh, J.A. 1999. The chameleon effect: The perception-behavior link and social interaction. *J. Pers. Soc. Psychol.* **76**:893–910.

Choi, J.S., Kang, D.H., Kim, J.J., Ha, T.H., Lee, J.M., Youn, T., Kim, I.Y., Kim, S.I., and Kwon, J.S. 2004. Left anterior subregion of orbitofrontal cortex volume reduction and impaired organizational strategies in obsessive-compulsive disorder. *J. Psychiatr. Res.* **38**:193–199.

Clark, L., and Manes, F. 2004. Social and emotional decision-making following frontal lobe injury. *Neurocase* **10**:398–403.

Cohen, H., Kaplan, Z., Kotler, M., Kouperman, I., Moisa, R., and Grisaru, N. 2004. Repetitive transcranial magnetic stimulation of the right dorsolateral prefrontal cortex in posttraumatic stress disorder: a double-blind, placebo-controlled study. *Am. J. Psychiatry* **161**:515–524.

Cohen, R.M., Semple, W.E., Gross, M., Nordahl, T.E., King, A.C., Pickar, D., and Post, R.M. 1989. Evidence for common alterations in cerebral glucose metabolism in major affective disorders and schizophrenia. *Neuropsychopharmacology* **2**:241–254.

Coricelli, B., Critchley, H.D., Joffily, M., O'Doherty, J.P., Sirigu, A., and Dolan, R. 2005. Regret and its avoidance: A neuroimaging study of choice behavior. *Nat. Neurosci.* **8**:1255–1262.

Coryell, W., Nopoulos, P., Drevets, W., Wilson, T., and Andreasen, N.C., 2005. Subgenual prefrontal cortex volumes in major depressive disorder and schizophrenia: Diagnostic specificity and prognostic implications. *Am. J. Psychiatry* **162**:1706–1712.

Cotter, D.R., Mackay, D., Chana, G., Beasley, C., Landau, S., and Everall, I.P. 2002. Reduced neuronal size and glial cell density in area 9 of the dorsolateral prefrontal cortex in subjects with major depressive disorder. *Cereb. Cortex* **12**:386–394.

Cox, S.M., Andrade, A., and Johnsrude, I.S. 2005. Learning to like: A role for human orbitofrontal cortex in conditioned reward. *J. Neurosci.* **25**:2733–2740.

Croxson, P.L., Johansen-Berg, H., Behrens, T.E., Robson, M.D., Pinsk, M.A., Gross, C.G. Richter, W., Richter, M.C., Kastner, S., and Rushworth, M.F. 2005. Quantitative investigation of connections of the prefrontal cortex in the human and macaque using probabilistic diffusion tractography. *J. Neurosci.* **25**:8854–8866.

Cummings, J.L. 1993. The neuroanatomy of depression. *J. Clin. Psychiatry* **54**(Suppl.):14–20.

Cunningham, W.A., Raye, C.L., and Johnson, M.K. 2004. Implicit and explicit evaluation: fMRI correlates of valence, emotional intensity, and control in the processing of attitudes. *J. Cogn. Neurosci.* **16**:1717–1729.

Damasio, A.R. 1994. *Descartes' Error: Emotion, Reason, and the Human Brain*. New York: Grist/Putnam.

Damasio, A.R., and Anderson, S.W. 1993. The frontal lobes. In: K.M.Heilman and E.Valenstein (eds.) *Clinical Neuropsychology* (3rd ed.). New York: Oxford University Press.

Damasio, H., Tranel, D., Grabowski, T., Adolphs, R., and Damasio, A. 2004. Neural systems behind word and concept retrieval.*Cognition* **92**:179–229.

Dapretto, M., Davies, M.S., Pfeifer, J.H., Scott, A.A., Sigman, M., Bookheimer, S.Y., and Iacoboni, M. 2006. Understanding emotions in others: Mirror neuron dysfunction in children with autism spectrum disorders. *Nat. Neurosci.* **9**:28–30.

De La Fuente, J.M., Goldman, S., Stanus, E., Vizuete, C., Morlan, I., Bobes, J., and Mendlewicz, J. 1997. Brain glucose metabolism in borderline personality disorder. *J. Psychiatr. Res.* **31**:531–541.

Deiber, M-P., Honda, M., Ibañez, V., Sadato, N., and Hallett, M. 1999. Mesial motor areas in self-initiated versus externally triggered movements examined with fMRI: effect of movement type and rate. *J. Neurophysiol.* **81**:3065–3077.

Deiber, M-P., Ibanez, V., Caldara, R., Andrey, C., and Hauert, C-A., 2005. Programming effectors and coordination in bimanual in-phase mirror finger movements. *Cogn. Brain Res.* **23**:374–386.

Di Pellegrino, G., Fadiga, L., Fogassi, L., Gallese, V., and Rizzolatti, G. 1992. Understanding motor events: A neurophysiological study. *Exp. Brain Res.* **91**:176–180.

Diefendorf, A.R., and Dodge, R. 1908. An experimental study of ocular reaction of the insane from photographic records. *Brain* **31**:451–489.

Dimberg, U., and Petterson, M. 2000. Facial reactions to happy and angry facial expressions: evidence for right hemisphere dominance. *Psychophysiology* **37**:693–696.

Dolan, R.J., Bench, C.J., Brown, R.G., Scott, L.C., Friston, K.J., and Frackowiak, R.S.J. 1992. Regional cerebral blood flow abnormalities in depressed patients with cognitive impairment. *J. Neurol. Neurosurg. Psychiatry* **55**:768–773.

Donegan, N.H., Sanislow, C.A., Blumberg, H.P., Fulbright, R.K., Lacai, C., Skudlarski, P., Gore, J.C., Olson, I.R., McGlashan, T.H., and Wexler, B.E. 2003. Amygdala hyperreactivity in borderline personality disorder: Implications for emotional dysregulation. *Biol. Psychiatry* **54**:1284–1293.

Drevets, W.C., 2001. Neuroimaging and neuropathological studies of depression: Implications for the cognitive emotional manifestations of mood disorders. *Curr. Opin. Neurobiol.* **11**:240–249.

——— 2003. Neuroimaging abnormalities in the amygdala in mood disorders. *In: The Amygdala in Brain Function: Basic and Clinical Approaches. Ann. N. Y. Acad. Sci.* New York: New York Academy of Sciences.

Drevets, W.C., and Raichle, M.E. 1998. Reciprocal suppression of regional cerebral blood flow during emotional versus higher cognitive processes: Implications for interactions between emotion and cognition. *Cogn. Emot.* **12**:353–385.

Drevets, W.C., and Savitz, J. 2008. The subgenual anterior cingulate. *CNS Spectr.* **13**:663–678.

Drevets, W.C., Price, J.L., Simpson, J.R., Todd, R.D., Reich, T., Vannier, M., and Raichle, M.E. 1997. Subgenual prefrontal cortex abnormalities in mood disorders. *Nature* **386**:824–827.

Drevets, W.C., Bogers, W., and Raichle, M.E. 2002. Functional anatomical correlates of antidepressant drug treatment assessed using PET measures of regional glucose metabolism. *Eur. Neuropsychopharmacol.* **12**:527–544.

Drevets, W.C., Ryan, N., Bogers, W., Birmaher, B., Axelson, D., and Dahl, R. 2007. *Subgenual prefrontal cortex volume decreased in healthy humans at high familial risk for mood disorders.* Abstract present at: Annual Meeting of the Society for Neuroscience, Oct. 23, 2007, San Diego, CA.

Drevets, W.C., Price, J.L., and Furey, M.L. 2008. Brain structural and functional abnormalities in mood disorders: Implications for neurocircuitry models of depression. *Brain Struct. Funct.* **21**:93–118.

Drewe, E.A. 1974. The effect of type and area of brain lesion on Wisconsin Card Sorting Test performance. *Cortex* **10**:159–170.

Dum, R.P., and Strick, P.L. 1996. Spinal cord terminations of the medial wall motor areas in macaque monkeys. *J. Neurosci.* **16**:6513–6529.

Elliot, R., Dolan, R.J., and Frith, D.D. 2000. Dissociable functions in the medial and lateral orbitofrontal cortex: evidence from human neuroimaging studies. *Cereb. Cortex* **10**:308–317.

Elliot, R., Newman, J.L., Longe, O.A., and Deakin, J.F. 2003. Differential response patterns in the striatum and orbitofrontal cortex to financial reward in humans: A parametric functional magnetic resonance imaging study. *J. Neurosci.* **23**:303–307.

Elliot, R., Ogilvie, A., Rubinsztein, J.S., Calderon, G., Dolan, R.J., and Sahakian, B.J. 2004. Abnormal ventral frontal response during performance of an affective go/no go task in patients with mania. *Biol. Psychiatry* **55**:1163–1170.

Ernst, M., Liebenauer, L.L., King, C., Fitzgerald, G.A., Cohen, R.M., and Zametkin, A.J. 1994. Reduced brain metabolism in hyperactive girls. *J. Am. Acad. Child Adolesc. Psychiatry* **33**:858–868.

Ettinger, U., Kumari, V., Crawford, T.J., Flak, V., Sharma, T., Davis, R.E., and Corr, P.J. 2005. Saccadic eye movements, schizotypy, and role of neuroticism. *Biol. Psychol.* **68**:61–78.

Fabbri-Destro, M., and Rizzolatti, G., 2008. Mirror neurons and mirror systems in monkeys and humans. *Physiology* **23**:171–179.

Falconer, E.M., Felmingham, K.L., Allen, A., Clark, C.R., McFarlane, A.C., Williams, L.M., and Bryant, R.A. 2008. Developing an integrated brain, behavior and biological response profile in posttraumatic stress disorder (PTSD). *J. Integr. Neurosci.* **7**:439–456.

Farrow, T.F., Zheng, Y., Wilkinson, I.D., Spence, S.A., Deakin, J.F., Tarrier, N., Griffiths, P.D., and Woodruff, P.W. 2001. Investigating the functional anatomy of empathy and forgiveness. *Neuroreport* **12**:2433–2438.

Feinberg, T.E., Schindler, R.J., Flanagan, N.G., and Haber, L.D. 1992. Two alien hand syndromes. *Neurology* **42**:19–24.

Fogassi, L., Ferrari, P.F., Gesierich, B., Rozzi, S., Chersi, F., and Rizzolatti, G. 2005. Parietal lobe: From action organization to intention understanding. *Science* **308**:662–667.

Frank, M.J., Samanta, J., Moustafa, A.A., and Sherman, S.J. 2007. Hold your horses: Impulsivity, deep brain stimulation, and medication in parkinsonism. *Science* **318**:1309–1312.

Fransson, P. 2005. Spontaneous low-frequency BOLD signal fluctuations: An fMRI investigation of the resting-state default mode of brain function hypothesis. *Hum. Brain Mapp.* **26**:15–29.

111

Freund, H.-J., and Hummelsheim, H. 1984. Premotor cortex in man: Evidence for innervation of proximal limb muscles. *Exp. Brain Res.* **53**:479–482.

Frith, C.D. 2007. The social brain?*Phil. Trans. Roy. Lond. B Soc.* **362**:671–678.

Fuster, J.M. 1995. Memory and planning: Two temporal perspectives of frontal lobe function. In: H.H.Jasper, S.Riggio, and P.W.Goldman-Rakic (eds.) *Epilepsy and the Functional Anatomy of the Frontal Lobe. Advances in Neurology* (vol. 66). New York: Raven Press.

Fuster, J.M. 1996. Frontal lobe syndromes. In: B.Fogel, R.B.Schiffer, and S.M.Rao (eds) *Neuropsychiatry*. Baltimore: Williams & Wilkins, pp. 407–413.

Fuster, J.M. 2002. Frontal lobe and cognitive development. *J. Neurocytology* **31**:373–385.

Fuster, J.M. 2008. *The Prefrontal Cortex* (4th ed.). New York: Academic Press.

Gallagher, H.L., and Frith, C.D., 2003. Functional imaging of "theory of mind." *Trends Cogn. Sci.* **7**:77–83.

Gallagher, H.L., Jack, A.I., Roepstorff, A., and Frith, C.D. 2002. Imaging the intentional stance in a competitive game. *Neuroimage* **16**:814–821.

Gallese, V., Fadiga, L., Fogassi, L., and Rizzolatti, G. 1996. Action recognition in the premotor cortex. *Brain* **119**:593–609.

Galvan, A., Hare, T.A., Davidson, M., Spicer, J., Glover, G., and Casey, B.J. 2005. The role of ventral frontostriatal circuitry in reward-based learning in humans. *J. Neurosci.* **25**:2733–2740.

Galynker, I.I., Weiss, J., Ongseng, F., and Finestone, H. 1997. ECT treatment and cerebral perfusion in catatonia. *J. Nucl. Med.* **38**:251–254.

Garrity, A.G., Pearlson, G.D., McKiernan, K., Lloyd, D., Kiehl, K.A., and Calhoun, V.D. 2007. Aberrant "default mode" functional connectivity in schizophrenia. *Am. J. Psychiatry* **164**:450–457.

Giedd, J.N., Blumenthal, J., Jeffries, N.O., Castelleanos, F.X., Liu, H., Zijdenbos, A., Paus, T., Evans, A.C, and Rapaport, J.L. 1999. Brain development during childhood and adolescence: a longitudinal MRI study. *Nat. Neurosci.* **2**:861–863.

Glahn, D.C., Ragland, J.D., Abramoff, A., Barrett, J., Laird, A.R., Bearden, C.E., and Velligan, D.I. 2005. Beyond hypofrontality: A quantitative meta-analysis of functional neuroimaging studines of working memory in schizophrenia. *Hum. Brain Mapp.* **25**:60–69.

Glantz, L.A., and Lewis, D.A. 1993. Synaptophysin immunoreactivity is selectively decreased in the prefrontal cortex of schizophrenic subjects. *Soc. Neurosci. Abstr.* **19**:201.

Goel, V., Grafman, J., Tajik, J, Gana, S., and Danto, D. 1997. A study of the performance of patients with frontal lobe lesions in a financial planning task. *Brain* **120**:1805–1822.

Goldberg, M.E., and Bruce, C.J. 1986. The role of the arcuate frontal eye fields in the generation of saccadic eye movements. *Prog. Brain Res.* **64**:143–154.

Goldman-Rakic, P. 1997. Space and time in the mental universe. *Nature* **386**:559–560.

Goldman-Rakic, P.S. 1996. Dissolution of cerebral cortical mechanisms in subjects with schizophrenia. In: S.J.Watson (ed.) *Biology of Schizophrenia and Affective Disease*. Washington D.C.: American Psychiatric Press.

Goldman-Rakic, P.S., and Selemon, L.D. 1997. Functional and anatomical aspects of prefrontal pathology in schizophrenia. *Schizophr. Bull.* **23**:437–458.

Gooding, D.C., and Talent, K.A. 2001. The association between antisaccade task and working memory task performance in schizophrenia and bipolar disorder. *J. Nerv. Ment. Dis.* **189**:8–16.

Gooding, D.C., and Basso, M.A. 2008. The tell-tale tasks: A review of saccadic research in psychiatric patient populations. *Brain Cogn.* **68**:371–390.

Gooding, D.C., Mohapatra, L., and Shea, H.B. 2004. Temporal stability of saccadic task performance in schizophrenia and bipolar patients. *Psychol. Med.* **34**:921–932.

Gooding, D.C., Shea, H.B., and Matts, C.W. 2005. Saccadic performance in questionnaire-identified schizotypes over time. *Psychiatr. Res.* **133**:173–186.

Grafton, S.T., Mazziotta, J.C., Woods, R.P., and Phelps, M.E.1992a. Human functional anatomy of visually guided finger movements. *Brain* **115**:565–587.

Grafton, S.T., Mazziotta, J.C., Presty, S., Friston, K.J., Frackowiak, R.S.J., and Phelps, M.E.1992b. Functional anatomy of human procedural learning determined with regional cerebral blood flow and PET. *J. Neurosci.* **12**:2542–2548.

Gray, J.A. 1987. *The Psychology of Fear and Stress*. New York: Oxford University Press.

Grunwald, T., Bouteros, N.N., Pezer, N., von Oertzen, T., Fernandez, G., Schaller, C., and Elger, C.E. 2003. Neural substrates of sensory gating within the human brain. *Biol. Psychiatry* **53**:511–519.

Gurd, J.M., and Ward, C.D. 1989. Retrieval from semantic and letter-initial categories in patients with Parkinson's disease. *Neuropsychologia* **27**:743–746.

Gurd, J.M., Amunts, K., Weiss, P.H., Zafiris, O., Zilles, K., Marshall, J.C. and Fink, G.R. 2002. Posterior parietal cortex is implicated in continuous switching between verbal fluency tasks: an fMRI study with clinical implications. *Brain* **125**:1024–1038.

Gusnard, D.A., Akbudak, E., Shulman, G.L., and Raichle, M.E. 2001. Medial prefrontal cortex and self-referential mental activity: Relation to a default mode of brain function. *Proc. Natl. Acad. Sci. USA.* **98**:4259–4264.

Halsband, U., and Freund, H.J. 1990. Premotor cortex and conditional motor learning in man. *Brain* 113:207–222.

Halsband, U., Ito, N., Tanji, J., and Freund, H.J. 1993. The role of premotor cortex and the supplementary motor area in the temporal control of movement in man. *Brain* 116:243–266.

Happaney, K., Zelanzo, P.D., and Stuss, D.T., 2004. Development of orbitofrontal function: Current themes and future directions. *Brain Cogn.* 55:1–10.

Happé, F., Ehlers., S., Fletcher, P., Frith, U., Johansson, M., and Gillberg, C. 1996. Theory in the mind of the brain. Evidence from a PET scan study of Asperger syndrome. *Neuroreport* 8:197–201.

Hariri, A.R., Mattay, V.S., Tessitore, A., Fera, F., and Weinberger, D.R. 2003. Neocortical modulation of the amygdala response to fearful stimuli. *Biol. Psychiatry* 53:494–501.

Harris, M.S.H., Reilly, J.L., Keshavan, M.S., and Sweeney, J.A. 2006. Longitudinal studies of antisaccades in antipsychotic-naïve first-episode schizophrenia. *Psychol. Med.* 36:485–494.

Harrison, B.J., Yücel, M., Pujol, J., and Pantelis, C. 2007. Task-induced deactivation of midline cortical regions in schizophrenia assessed with fMRI. *Schizophr. Res.* 91:82–86.

Hazlett, E.A., Buchsbaum, J.S., Jeu, L.A., Nenadic, I., Fleischman, M.B., Shihabuddin, L., Haznedar, M.M., and Harvey, P.D. 2000. Hypofrontality in unmedicated schizophrenia patients studied with PET during performance of a serial verbal learning task. *Schizophr. Res.* 43:33–46.

Henderson, L.L, Yoder, P., Yale, M., and McDuffie, A. 2002. Getting the point: Electrophysiological correlates of protodeclarative pointing. *Int. J. Dev. Neurosci.* 20:449–458.

Herpertz, S.C., Dietrich, T.M., Wenning, B., Krings, T., Erberich, S.G., Willmes, K., Thron, A., and Sass, H. 2001. Evidence of abnormal amygdala functioning in borderline personality disorder: A functional MRI study. *Biol. Psychiatry* 50:292–298.

Hirayasu, Y., Shenton, M.E., Salisbury, D.F., Kwon, J.S., Wible, C.G., Fischer, I.A., Yurgelun-Todd, D., Zarate, C., Kikinis, R., Jolesz, F.A., and McCarley, R.W. 1999. Subgenual cingulate cortex volume in first episode psychosis. *Am. J. Psychiatry* 156:1091–1093.

Ho, A.P., Gillis, J.C., Buchsbaum, M.S., Wu, J.C., Abel, L., and Bunney, W.E. 1997. Brain glucose metabolism during non-rapid eye movement sleep in major depression: A positron emission tomography study. *Arch. Gen. Psychiatry* 53:645–652.

Hofer, A., Weiss, E.M., Golaszewski, S.M., Siedentopf, C.M., Brinkhoff, C., Kremser, Felber, C., and Fleischhacker, W.W. 2003. Neural correlates of episodic encoding and recognition of words in unmedicated patients during an acute episode of schizophrenia: A functional MRI study. *Am. J. Psychiatry* 160:1802–1808.

Hoffman, R.E., and McGlashan, T.H. 1997. Synaptic elimination, neurodevelopment, and the mechanism of hallucinated "voices" in schizophrenia. *Am. J. Psychiatry* 154:1683–1689.

Holahan, A.-L.V., and O' Driscoll, G.A. 2005. Antisaccade and smooth pursuit performance in positive- and negative-symptom schizotypy. *Schizophr. Res.* 76:43–54.

Hornak, J., Bramham, J., Rolls, E.T., Morris, R.G., O' Doherty, J., Bullock, P.R., and Polkey, C.E. 2003. Changes in emotion after circumscribed surgical lesions of the orbitofrontal and cingulate cortices. *Brain* 126:1691–1712.

Huttenlocher, P.R. 1979. Synaptic density in the human frontal cortex –developmental changes and effects of aging. *Brain Res.* 163:195–205.

Hutton, S.B. 2002. Improved antisaccade performance in schizophrenia with risperidone. Commentary. *J. Neurol. Neurosurg. Psychiatry* 72:429.

Hutton, S.B., Huddy, V., Barnes, T.R.E., Robbins, T.W., Crawford, T.J., Kennard, C., and Joyce, E.M. 2004. The relationship between antisaccades, smooth pursuit, and executive dysfunction in first-episode schizophrenia. *Biol. Psychiatry* 56:553–559.

Hynes, C.A., Baird, A.A., and Grafton, S.T. 2006. Differential role of the orbital frontal lobe in emotional versus cognitive perspective-taking. *Neuropsychologia* 44:374–383.

Iacoboni, M., and Dapretto, M. 2006. The mirror neuron system and the consequences of its dysfunction. *Nat. Rev. Neurosci.* 7:942–951.

Iacoboni, M., and Mazziotta, J.C. 2007. Mirror neuron system: basic findings and clinical applications. *Ann. Neurol.* 62:213–218.

Iacoboni, M., Woods, R.P., Brass, M. Bekkering, H., Mazziotta, J.C., and Rizzolati, G., 1999. Cortical mechanisms of human imitation. *Science* 286:2526–2528.

Ishai, A., 2007. Sex, beauty and the orbitofrontal cortex. *Int. J. Psychophysiol.* 63:181–185.

Jackson, P.L., Meltzoff, A.N., and Decety, J. 2005. How do we perceive the pain of others? A window into the neural processes involved in empathy. *Neuroimage* 24:771–779.

Jackson, P.L., Brunet, E., Meltzoff, A.N., and Decety, J. 2006. Empathy examined through the neural mechanisms involved in imagining how I feel versus how you feel pain. *Neuropsychologia* 44:752–761.

Jenkins, A.C., Macrae, C.N., and Mitchell, J.P. 2008. Repetition suppression of ventromedial prefrontal activity during judgments of self and others. *Pro. Nat. Acad. Sci. USA.* 105:4507–4512.

Johnson, D.L., Wiebe, J.S., Gold, S.M., Andreasen, N.C., Hichwa, R.D., Watkins, G.L., and BolesPonto, L.L. 1999. Cerebral blood flow and personality: A positron emission tomography study. *Am. J. Psychiatry* **156**: 252–257.

Johnson, K., and Everling, S. 2007. Primate prefrontal cortex sends cue, delay, saccade, and post-saccade activity to the superior colliculus. *Eur. J. Neurosci.* **26**:1381–1385.

Johnson, K., and Everling, S. 2008. Neurophysiology and neuroanatomy of reflexive and voluntary saccades in non-human primates. *Brain Cogn.* **68**:271–283.

Jonas, M., Sieber, H.R., Biermann-Ruben, K., Kessler, K., Bäumer, T., Büchel, C., Schnitzler, A., and Münchnau, A. 2007. Do simple intransitive finger movements consistently activate frontoparietal mirror neuron areas in humans? *Neuroimage* **36**:T44–T53.

Joseph, R. 1996. *Neuropsychology, Neuropsychiatry, and Behavioral Neurology* (2nd ed.). New York: Plenum Press.

Joseph, R. 1988. The right cerebral hemisphere: Emotion, music, visual-spatial skills, body-image, dreams and awareness. *J. Clin. Psychol.* **44**:630–673.

Kaneda, K. Phongphanphanee, P., Katoh, T., Isa, K. Yanagawa, Y., Obata, K., and Isa, T. 2008. Regulation of burst activity through presynaptic and postsynaptic GABA(B) receptors in mouse superior colliculus. *J. Neurosci.* **28**:816–827.

Kang, D.H., Kim, J.J., Choi, J.S., Kim, Y.I., Kim, C.W., Youn, T., Han, M.H., Chang, K.H., and Kwon, J.S. 2004. Volumetric investigation of the frontal-subcortical circuitry in patients with obsessive-compulsive disorder. *J. Neuropsychiatry Clin. Neurosci.* **16**:342–349.

Karama, S., Lecours, A.R., Leroux, J-M., Bourgouin, P., Beaudoin, G., Joubert, S., and Beauregard, M. 2002. Areas of brain activation in males and females during viewing of erotic film excerpts. *Hum. Brain Mapp.* **16**:1–13.

Kennedy, D.P., Redcay, E., and Courchesne, E. 2006. Failing to deactivate: Resting functional abnormalities in autism. *Proc. Natl. Acad. Sci. USA.* **103**:8275–7280.

Kéri, S., 2008. Interactive memory systems and category learning in schizophrenia. *Neurosci. Biobehav. Rev.* **32**:206–218.

Keshavan, M.S., Tandon, R., Boutros, N.N., and Nasrallah, H.A. 2008. Schizophrenia, "just the facts": What we know in 2008. Part III: Neurobiology. *Schizophr. Res.* **106**:89–107.

Kesler/West, M.L., Andersen, A.H., Smith, C.D., Avison, M.J., Davis, C.E., Kryscio, R.J., and Blonder, L.X. 2001. Neural substrates of facial emotion processing using fMRI. *Cog. Brain Res.* **11**:213–226.

Ketter, T., George, M., Ring, H., Pazzaglia, P., Marangel, L., Kimbrell, T., and Post, R. 1994. Primary mood disorders: Structural and resting functional studies. *Psychiatr. Ann.* **24**:642–647.

Ketter, T.A., and Drevets, W.C. 2002. Neuroimaging studies of bipolar depression: Functional neuropathology, treatment effects, and predictors of clinical response. *Clin. Neurosci. Res.* **2**:182–192.

Ketter, T.A., Kimbrell, T.A., George, M.S., Dunn, R.T., Speer, A.M., Benson, B.E., Willis, M.W., Danielson, A., Frye, M.A., Herscovitch, P., and Post, R.M. 2001. Effects of mood and subtype on cerebral glucose metabolism in treatment-resistant bipolar disorder. *Biol. Psychiatry* **49**:97–109.

Kieseppa, T., van Erp, T.G., Haukka, J., Partonen, T., Cannon, T.D., Poutanen, V.P., Kaprio, J., and Lonnqvist, J. 2003. Reduced left hemispheric white matter volume in twins with bipolar disorder. *Biol. Psychiatry* **54**: 896–905.

Kim, J-J., Lee, M.C., Kim, J., Kim, I.Y., Kim, S.I., Han, M.H., Chang, K-H., and Kwon, J.S. 2001. Grey matter abnormalities in obsessive –compulsive disorder: Statistical parametric mapping of segmented magnetic resonance images. *Br. J. Psychiatry* **179**:330–334.

Kim, H., Shimojo, S., and O ' Doherty, J.P. 2006. Is avoiding an aversive outcome rewarding? Neural substrates of avoidance learning in the human brain. *PLoS Biol.* **4**:e233.

Kimbrell, T.A., Ketter, T.A., George, M.S., Little, J.T., Benson, B.E., Willis, MW, Herscovitch, P., and Post, R.M. 2002. Regional cerebral glucose utilization in patients with a range of severities of unipolar depression. *Biol. Psychiatry* **51**:237–252.

Knight, R.T., Grabowecky, M.F., and Scabini, D. 1995. Role of human prefrontal cortex in attention control. In: H.H.Jasper, S.Riggio, and P.W.Goldman-Rakic (eds.) *Epilepsy and the Functional Anatomy of the Frontal Lobe. Advances in Neurology* (vol. 66). New York: Raven Press.

Knott, F., Lewis, C., and Williams, T. 1995. Sibling interaction of children with learning disabilities: A comparison of autism and Down's syndrome. *J. Child Psychol. Psychiatry* **36**:965–976.

Krainik, A., Lehericy, S., Duffau, H., Vlaicu, M., Poupon, F., Capelle, L., Cornu, P., Clemenceau, S., Sahel, M., Valery, C.A., Boch, A.L., Mangin, J.F., Bihan, D.L., and Marsault, C. 2001. Role of the supplementary motor area in motor deficit following medial frontal lobe surgery. *Neurology* **57**:871–878.

Krebs, M.-O., Gut-Fayand, A., Amado, I., Dabn, D., Bourdel, M.-C., Poirier, M.-F., and Berthoz, A. 2001. Impairment of predictive saccades in schizophrenia. *Neuroreport* **12**:465–469.

Lane, R.D., Reiman, E.M., Ahern, G.L., Schwartz, G.E., and Davidson, R.J. 1997. Neuroanatomical correlates of happiness, sadness, and disgust. *Am. J. Psychiatry* **154**:926–933.

Lanius, R.A., Williamson, P.C., Densmore, M.C., Boksman, K., Gupta, M.A., Neufeld, R.W., Gati, J.S., and Menon, R.S. 2001. Neural correlates of traumatic memories in posttraumatic stress disorder: A functional MRI investigation. *Am. J. Psychiatry* **158**:1920–1922.

Lanius, R.A., Williamson, P.C., Boksman, K., Densmore, M., Gupta, M., Gati, J.S., and Menon, R. 2002. Brain activation during script-driven imagery induced dissociative responses in PTSD: a functional MRI investigation. *Biol. Psychiatry* **52**:305–311.

Laplane, D., Talairach, J. Meininger, V., Bancaud, J., and Orgogozo, J.M. 1977. Clinical consequences of corticectomies involving the supplementary motor area in man. *J. Neurol. Sci.* **34**:301–314.

Larrison-Faucher, A.L., Matorin, A.A., and Sereno, A.B. 2004. Nicotine reduces antisaccade errors in task impaired schizophrenic subjects. *Prog. Neuropsychopharmacol. Biol. Psychiatry* **28**:505–516.

Lau, H.C., Rogers, R.D., Haggard, P., and Passingham, R.E. 2004. Attention to intention. *Science* **303**:1208–1210.

Lemogne, C., le Bastard, G., Mayberg, H., Volle, E., Bergouignan, L., Lehéricy, S., Allilaire, J-F., and Fossati, P. 2009. In search of the depressive self: extended medial prefrontal network during self-referential processing in major depression. *Soc. Cogn. Affect. Neurosci.* **4**: 305–312.

Leslie, K.R., Johnson-Frey, S.H., and Grafton, S.T. 2004. Functional imaging of face and hand imitation: towards a motor theory of empathy. *Neuroimage* **21**:601–607.

Levenson, R.W., Ekman, P., and Friesen, W.V. 1990. Voluntary facial action generates emotion-specific autonomic nervous system activity. *Psychophysiology* **27**:363–384.

Levin, H., and Kraus, M.F. 1994. The frontal lobes and traumatic brain injury. *J. Neuropsychiatry Clin. Neurosci.* **6**:443–454.

Leyton, M., Okazawa, H., Diksic, M., Paris, J., Rosa, P., Mzengeza, S., Young, S.N., Blier, P., and Benkelfat, C. 2001. Brain regional alpha-[11C]methyl-L-tryptophan trapping in impulsive subjects with borderline personality disorder. *Am. J. Psychiatry* **158**:775–782.

Lhermitte, F. 1986. Human autonomy and the frontal lobes. *Ann. Neurol.* **19**:335–343.

Liberzon, I., and Sripada, C.S. 2008. The functional neuroanatomy of PTSD: A critical review. *Prog. Brain Res.* **167**:151–169.

Liddle, P.R., Friston, K.J., Frith, C.D., Hirsch, S.R., Jones, T., and Frackowiak, R.S.J. 1992. Patterns of cerebral blood flow in schizophrenia. *Br. J. Psychiatry* **160**: 179–186.

Lidow, M.S., Goldman-Rakic, P.S., Gallager, D.W., and Rakic, P. 1991. Distribution of dopaminergic receptors in the primate cerebral cortex: Quantitative autoradiographic analysis using [3H]raclopride, [3H]spiperone and [3H]SCH23390. *Neuroscience* **40**:657–671.

Lindauer, R.J.L., Booij, J., Habraken, J.G.A., van Meijel, E.P.M., Uylings, H.B.M., Olff, M., Carlier, I.V.E., den Heeten, G.J., van Eck-Smit, B.L.F., and Gersons, B.P.R. 2008. Effects of psychotherapy on regional cerebral blood flow during trauma imagery in patients with post-traumatic stress disorder: A randomized clinical trial. *Psychol. Med.* **38**:543–554.

Lough, S., Kipps, C.M., Treise, C., Watson, P., Blair, J.R., and Hodges, J.R. 2006. Social reasoning, emotion and empathy in frontotemporal dementia. *Neuropsychologia* **44**:950–958.

Luna, B., Minshew, N.J., Garver, K.E., Lazar, N.A., Thulborn, K.R., Eddy, W.F., and Sweeney, J.A. 2002. Neocortical system abnormalities in autism: An fMRI study of spatial working memory. *Neurology* **59**:834–840.

Lyoo, I.K. 2005. Structural and functional imaging of patients with borderline personality disorder. In: M.C.Zanarini (ed.) *Borderline Personality Disorder*. New York: Taylor & Francis, pp. 305–333.

Lyoo, I.K., Han, M.H., and Cho, D.Y. 1998. A brain MRI study in subjects with borderline personality disorder: A functional MRI study. *Biol. Psychiatry* **50**:292–298.

MacDonald, A.W., III, and Carter, C.S. 2003. Event-related FMRI study of context processing in dorsolateral prefrontal cortex of patients with schizophrenia. *J. Abnorm. Psychol.* **112**:689–697.

Makuuchi, M. 2005. Is Broca's area crucial for imitation?*Cereb. Cortex* **15**:563–570.

Manoach, D.S., Gollub, R.L., Benson, E.S., Searl, M.M., Goff, D.C., Halpern, E., Saper, C.B., and Rauch, S.L. 2000. Schizophrenic subjects show aberrant fMRI activation of dorsolateral prefrontal cortex and basal ganglia during working memory performance. *Biol. Psychiatry* **48**:99–109.

Markowitsch, H.J., Vandekerckhove, M.M., Lanfermann, H., and Russ, M.O. 2003. Engagement of lateral and medial prefrontal areas in the ecphory of sad and happy autobiographical memories. *Cortex* **39**:643–665.

Martinot, J.L., Hardy, P., Feline, A., Huret, J.D., Mazoyer, B., Attar-Levy, D., Pappata, S., and Syrota, A. 1990. Left prefrontal glucose hypometabolism in the depressed state: A confirmation. *Am. J. Psychiatry* **147**:1313–1317.

Maruff, P., Purcell, R., Tyler, P., Pantelis, C., and Currie, J. 1999. Abnormalities of internally generated saccades in obsessive-compulsive disorder. *Psychol. Med.* **29**:1377–1385.

Marumo, K., Takizawa, R., Kawakubo, Y., Onitsuka, T., and Kasai, K. 2009. Gender difference in right lateral prefrontal hemodynamic response while viewing fearful faces: A multi-channel near-infrared spectroscopy study. *Neurosci. Res.* **63**:89–94.

Mason, M.F., Norton, M.I., VanHorn, J.D., Wegner, D.M., Grafton, S.T., and Macrae, N. 2007. Wandering minds: The default network and stimulus-independent thought. *Science* **315**:393–395.

Mayberg, H.S. 1997. Limbic-cortical dysregulation: A proposed model of depression. *J. Neuropsychiatry Clin. Neurosci.* **9**:471–481.

McAlonan, G.M., Cheung, V., Cheung, C., Suckling, J., Lam, G.Y., TaiK.S., Yip, L., Murphy, D.G.M., and Chua, S.E. 2005. Mapping the brain in autism: A voxel-based MRI study of volumetric differences and intercorrelations in autism. *Brain* **128**:268–276.

McCabe, K., Houser, D., Ryan, L., Smith, V., and Trouard, T. 2001. A functional imaging study of cooperation in two-person reciprocal exchange. *Proc. Natl. Acad. Sci. USA.* **98**:11832–11835.

McDowell, J.E., and Clementz, B.A. 2001. Behavioral and brain imaging studies of saccadic performance in schizophrenia. *Biol. Psychol.* **57**:5–22.

McGuire, P.K., Shah, G.M.S., and Murray, R.M. 1993. Increased blood flow in Broca's area during auditory hallucinations in schizophrenia. *Lancet* **342**:703–706.

McGuire, P.K., Silberswieg, D.A., Murray, R.M., David, A.S., Frackowiak, R.S.J., and Firth, C.D. 1996. Functional anatomy of inner speech and auditory verbal imagery. *Psychol. Med.* **26**:29–38.

Medendorp, W.P., Beurze, S.M., Van Pelt, S., and Van Der Werf, J. 2008. Behavioral and cortical mechanisms for spatial coding and action planning. *Cortex* **44**:587–597.

Mendez, M.F., and Zander, B.A. 1992. Reversible frontal lobe dysfunction from neurosarcoidosis. *Psychosomatics* **33**:215–217.

Mendez, M.F., and Clark, D.G. 2004. Aphemia-like syndrome from a right supplementary motor area lesion. *Clin. Neurol. Neurosurg.* **106**: 337–339.

Mendez, M.F., Bagart, B., and Edwards-Lee, T. 1997. Self-injurious behavior in frontotemporal dementia. *Neurocase* **3**:231–236.

Menzies, L., Chamberlain, S.R., Laird, A.R., Thelen, S.M., Sahakian, B.J., and Bullmore, E.T. 2008. Integrating evidence from neuroimaging and neuropsychological studies of obsessive-compulsive disorder: The orbitofronto-striatal model revisited. *Neurosci. Biobehav. Rev.* **32**:525–549.

Meyer-Lindenberg, A., Miletich, R.S., Kohn, P.D., Esposito, G., Carson, R.E., Quarantelli, M., Weinberger, D.R., and Berman, K.F. 2002. Reduced prefrontal activity predicts exaggerated striatal dopaminergic function in schizophrenia. *Nat. Neurosci.* **5**:267–271.

Miller, B.L., Cummings, J.L., McIntyre, H., Ebers, G., and Grode, M. 1986. Hypersexuality or altered sexual preference following brain injury. *J. Neurol. Neurosurg. Psychiatry* **49**:867–873.

Miller, E.K. 2000. The prefrontal cortex and cognitive control. *Nat. Rev. Neurosci.* **1**:59–65.

Milner, B. 1995. Aspects of human frontal lobe function. In: H.H.Jasper, S.Riggio, and P.W.Goldman-Rakic (eds.) *Epilepsy and the Functional Anatomy of the Frontal Lobe.* New York: Raven Press.

Mirzaei, S., Knoll, P., Keck, A., Preitler, B., Gurtierrez, E., Umek, H., Kohn, H., and Pechenstorfer, M. 2001. Regional cerebral blood flow in patients suffering from post-traumatic stress disorder. *Neuropsychobiology* **43**:260–264.

Mitchell, J.P., Macrae, C.N., and Banaji, M.R. 2006. Dissociable medial prefrontal contributions to judgments of similar and dissimilar others. *Neuron* **50**:655–663.

Monk, C.S., Nelson, E.E., McClure, E.B., Mogg, K., Bradley, B.P., Leibenluft, E., Blair, R.J.R., Chen, G., Charney, D.S., Ernst, M., and Pine, D.S. 2006. Ventrolateral prefrontal cortex activation and attentional bias in response to angry faces in adolescents with generalized anxiety disorder. *Am. J. Psychiatry* **163**:1091–1097.

Morris, P.L.P., Robinson, R.G., and Raphael, B. 1992. Lesion location and depression in hospitalized stroke patients. *Neuropsychiatry Neuropsychol. Behav. Neurol.* **5**:75–82.

Myers, R.E., Swett, C., and Miller, M. 1973. Loss of social group affinity following prefrontal lesions in free-ranging macaques. *Brain Res.* **64**:257–269.

Nachev, P. 2006. Cognition and medial frontal cortex in health and disease. *Curr. Opin. Neurol.* **19**:586–592.

Nachev, P., Kennard, C., and Husain, M. 2008. Functional role of the supplementary and pre-supplementary motor areas. *Nat. Rev. Neurosci.* **9**:856–869.

Nagaratnam, N., Nagaratnam, K., Ng, K., and Diu, P. 2004. *J. Clin. Neurosci.* **11**:25–30.

Nakamura, K., Sakai, K., and Hikosaka, O. 1999. Effects of local inactivation of monkey medial frontal cortex in learning of sequential procedures. *J. Neurophysiol.* **82**:1063–1068.

Nestler, E.J. 1997. Schizophrenia: An emerging pathophysiology. *Nature* **385**: 578–579.

Nitschke, J.B., Nelson, E.E., Rusch, B.D., Fox, A.S., Oakes, T.R., and Davidson, R.J. 2004. Orbitofrontal cortex tracks positive mood in mothers viewing pictures of their newborn infants. *Neuroimage* **21**: 583–592.

Nitschke, J.B., Sarinopoulos, I., Mackiewicz, K.L., Schaefer, H.S., and Davidson, R.J. 2006. Functional neuroanatomy of aversion and its anticipation. *Neuroimage* **29**:109–116.

Oberman, L.M., and Ramachandran, V.S. 2007. The simulating social mind: The role of the mirror neuron system and simulation in the social and communicative deficits of autism spectrum disorders. *Psychol. Bull.* **133**:310–327.

Oberman, L.M., Ramachandran, V.S., and Pineda, J.A. 2008. Modulation of mu suppression in children with autism spectrum disorders in response to familiar or unfamiliar stimuli: The mirror neuron hypothesis. *Neuropsychologia* **46**:1558–1565.

Ochsner, K.N., and Gross, J.J. 2007. The neural architecture of emotion regulation. In: J.J. Gross (ed.) *Handbook of Emotion Regulation.* New York: Guilford Press, pp. 87–109.

Ochsner, K.N., Bunge, S.A., Gross, J.J., and Gabrieli, J.D.E. 2002. Rethinking feelings: an fMRI study of the cognitive regulation of emotion. *J. Cogn. Sci.* **14**:1215–1229.

Ochsner, K.N., Beer, J.S., Robertson, E.R., Cooper, J.C., Gavrieli, J.D., Kihsltrom, J.F., and D'Esposito, M. 2005a. The neural correlates of direct and reflected self-knowledge. *Neuroimage* **28**:757–762.

O'Doherty, J., Winston, J., Critchley, H., Perrett, D., Burt, D.M., and Dolan, R.J. 2003. Beauty in a smile: the role of medial orbitofrontal cortex in facial attractiveness. *Neuropsychologia* **41**:147–155.

Olsson, A., and Ochsner, K.N. 2008. The role of social cognition in emotion. *Trends Cogn. Sci.* **12**:65–71.

Ongür, D., Ferry, A.T., and Price, J.L., 1998. Glial reduction in the subgenual prefrontal cortex in mood disorders. *Proc. Natl. Acad. Sci. USA.* **95**:13290–13295.

Osuch, E.A., Benson, B., Geraci, M., Podell, D., Hersocovitch, P., McCann, U.D., and Post, R.M. 2001. Regional cerebral blood flow correlated with flashback intensity in patients with posttraumatic stress disorder. *Biol. Psychiatry* **50**:246–253.

Owen, A.M. 2000. The role of the lateral frontal cortex in mnemonic processing: the contribution of functional neuroimaging. *Exp. Brain Res.* **133**:33–43.

Quintana, J., and Fuster, J.M. 1992. Mnemonic and predictive functions of cortical neurons in a memory task. *Neuroreport* **3**:721–724.

Parsons, L.M., Sergent, J., Hodges, D.A., and Fox, P.T. 2005. The brain basis of piano performance. *Neuropsychologia* **43**:199–215.

Parton, A., Nachev, P., Hodgson, T., Mort, D., Thomas, D., Ordidge, R., Morgan, P., Jackson, S., Rees, G., and Husain, M., 2007. Role of the human supplementary eye field in the control of saccadic eye movements. *Neuropsychologia* **45**:897–1008.

Pelphrey, K.A., Morris, J.P., and McCarthy. 2004. Grasping the intentions of others: The perceived intentionality of an action influences activity in the superior temporal sulcus during social perception. *J. Cogn. Neurosci.* **16**:1706–1716.

Penn, H.E. 2006. Neurobiological correlates of autism: A review of recent research. *Child Neuropsychol.* **12**:57–79.

Petrides, M., Cadoret, G., and Mackey, S. 2005. Orofacial somatomotor responses in the macaque monkey homologue of Broca's area. *Nature* **435**:1235–1238.

Pfefferbaum, A., Desmond, J.E., Galloway, C., Menon, V., Glover, G.H., and Sullivan, E.V. 2001. Reorganization of frontal systems used by alcoholics for spatial working memory: an fMRI study. *Neuroimage* **14**:7–20.

Phillips, M.L., Drevets, W.C., Rauch, S.L., and Lane, R. 2003. Neurobiology of emotion perception I: The neural basis of normal emotion perception. *Biol. Psychiatry* **54**:504–514.

Phillips, M.L., Ladouceur, C.D., and Drevets, W.C. 2008. A neural model of voluntary and automatic emotion regulation: Implications for understanding the pathophysiology and neurodevelopment of bipolar disorder. *Mol. Psychiatry* **13**:833–857.

Picard, N., and Strick, P.L. 1996. Motor areas of the medial wall: a review of their location and functional activation. *Cereb. Cortex* **6**:342–353.

Pissiota, A., Frans, O., Fernandez, M., Von Knorring, L., Fischer, H., and Fredrikson, M. 2003. Neurofunctional correlates of posttraumatic stress disorder: A PET symptom provocation study. *Eur. Arch. Psychiatry Clin. Neurosci.* **252**:68–75.

Polli, F.E., Barton, J.J.S., Thakkar, K.N., Greve, D.N., Goff, D.S., Rauch, S.L., and Manoach, D.S. 2008. Reduced error-related activation in two anterior cingulated circuits is related to impaired performance in schizophrenia. *Brain* **131**:971–986.

Price, J.L. 2007. Definition of the orbital cortex in relation to specific connections with limbic and visceral structures and other cortical regions. *Ann. N. Y. Acad. Sci.* **1121**:54–71.

Price, J.L., Carmichael, S.T., Carnes, K.M., Clugnet, M-C., Kuroda, K., and Ray, J.P. 1991. Olfactory input to the prefrontal cortex. In: J.L.Davis and H.Eichenbaum (eds.) *Olfaction: A Model System for Computational Neuroscience.* Cambridge, MA: MIT Press, pp. 101–120.

Price, C.J., Howard, D., Patterson, K., Warburton, E.A., Friston, K., and Frackowiak, R.S.J. 1998. A functional neuroimaging description of two deep dyslexi patients. *J. Cogn. Neurosci.* **10**:305–315.

Radant, A.D., Dobie, D.J., Calkins, M.E., Olincy, A., Braff, D.L. Cadenhead, K.S., Freedman, R., Green, M.F., Greenwood, T.A., Gur, R.E., Light, G.A., Meichle, S.P., Mintz, J. Nuechterlein, K.H., Schork, N.J., Seidman, L.J., Siever, L.J., Silverman, J.M. Stone, W.S., Swerdlow, N.R., Tsuang, M.T., Turetsky, B.I., and Tsuang, D.W. 2007. Successful multi-site measurement of antisaccade performance deficits in schizophrenia. *Schizophr. Res.* **89**:320–329.

Ragland, J.D., Yoon, J., Minzenberg, M.J., and Carter, C.S. 2007. Neuroimaging of cognitive disability in schizophrenia: Search for a pathophysiological mechanism. *Int. Rev. Psychiatry* **19**:417–427.

Rajkowska, G., Miguel-Hidalgo, J.J., Wei, J., Dilley, G., Pitman, S.D., Meltzer, H.Y., Overholser, J.C., Roth, B.L., and Stockmeier, C.A. 1999. Morphometric evidence for neuronal and glial prefrontal cell pathology in major depression. *Biol. Psychiatry* **45**:1085–1098.

Rajkowska, G., Halaris, A., and Selemon, L.D. 2001. Reductions in neuronal and glial density characterize the dorsolateral prefrontal cortex in bipolar disorder. *Biol. Psychiatry* **49**:741–752.

Rangaswamy, M., Porjesz, B., Ardekani, B.A., Choi, S.J., Tanabe, J.L., Lim, K.O., and Begleiter, H. 2004. A functional MRI study of visual oddball: evidence for frontoparietal dysfunction in subjects at risk for alcoholism. *Neuroimage* **21**:329–339.

Rauch, S.L., Jenike, M.A., Alpert, N.M., Baer, L., Breiter, H.C., Savage, C.R., and Fischman, A.J. 1994. Regional cerebral blood flow measured during symptom provocation in obsessive-compulsive disorder using oxygen 15-labeled carbon dioxide and positron emission tomography. *Arch. Gen. Psychiatry* **51**: 62–70.

Rauch, S.L., Savage, C.R., Alpert, N.M., Miguel, E.C., Baer, L., Breiter, H.C., Fischman, A.J., Manzo, P.A., Moretti, C., and Jenike, M.A. 1995. A positron emission tomographic study of simple phobic symptom provocation. *Arch. Gen. Psychiatry*, **52**:20–28.

Rauch, S.L., van der Kolk, B.A., Fisler, R.E., Alpert, N.M., Orr, S.P., Savage, C.R., Fischman, A.J., Jenike, M.A., and Pitman, R.K. 1996. A symptom provocation study of posttraumatic stress disorder using positron emission tomography and script-driven imagery. *Arch. Gen. Psychiatry* **53**:380–387.

Redoute, J., Stoleru, S., Gregoire, M.C., Costes, N., Cinotti, L., Lavenne, F., Le Bars, D., Forest, M.G., and Pujol, J.F. 2000. Brain processing of visual sexual stimuli in human males. *Hum. Brain Mapp.* **11**:162–177.

Reichenberg, A., and Harvey, P.E. 2007. Neuropsychological impairments in schizophrenia: Integration of performance-based and brain imaging findings. *Psychol. Bull.* **133**:833–858.

Reiman, E.M., Lane, R.D., Ahern, G.L., Schwartz, G.E., Davidson, R.J., Friston, K.J., Yun, L.-S., and Chen, K. 1997. Neuroanatomical correlates of externally and internally generated human emotion. *Am. J. Psychiatry* **154**:918–925.

Reuter, B., Rakusan, L., and Kathmann, N. 2005. Poor antisaccade performance in schizophrenia: An inhibition deficit? *Psychiatry Res.* **135**:1–10.

Reynolds, J.R., Donaldson, D.I., Wagner, A.D., and Braver, T.S. 2004. Item- and task-level processes in the left inferior prefrontal cortex: positive and negative correlates of encoding. *Neuroimage* **21**:1472–1483.

Riggio, S., and Harner, R.N. 1992. Frontal lobe epilepsy. *Neuropsychiatry Neuropsychol. Behav. Neurol.* **5**:283–293.

Rizzolatti, G., and Craighero, L. 2004. The mirror-neuron system. *Annu. Rev. Neurosci.* **27**:169–192.

Rizzolatti, G., Fadiga, L., Matelli, M., Bettinardi, V., Paulesu, E., Perani, D., and Fazio, F. 1996a. Localization of grasp representation in humans by PET: 1. Observation versus execution. *Exp. Brain Res.* **111**: 246–252.

Rizzolatti, G., Luppino, G., and Matelli, M. 1996b. The classic supplementary motor area is formed by two independent areas. In: H.O.Lunders (ed.) *Supplementary Sensorimotor Area.* Philadelphia: Lippincott–Raven, pp. 45–56.

Rizzolatti, G., Fogassi, L., and Gallese, V. 2001. Neurophysiological mechanisms underlying the understanding and imitation of action. *Nat. Rev. Neurosci.* **2**:661–670.

Rogers, R.D., Owen, A.M., Middleton, H.C., Williams, E.J., Pickard, J.D., Sahakian, B.J., and Robbins, T.W. 1999. Choosing between small, likely rewards and large, unlikely rewards activates inferior and orbital prefrontal cortex. *J. Neurosci.* **19**:9029–9038.

Rolls, E.T. 1990. A theory of emotion, and its applications to understanding the neural basis of emotions. *Cogn. Emot.* **4**:161–1990.

Rolls, E.T. 1997. Taste and olfactory processing in the brain and its relation to the control of eating. *Crit. Rev. Neurobiol.* **11**:263–287.

Rolls, E.T. 2000. The orbitofrontal cortex and reward. *Cereb. Cortex* **10**:284–294.

Rolls, E.T., and Grabenhorst, F. 2008. The orbitofrontal cortex and beyond: From affect to decision-making. *Prog. Neurobiol.* **86**:216–244.

Rolls, E.T., Kringelbach, M.L., and de Araujo, I.E. 2003a. Different representations of pleasant and unpleasant odours in the human brain. *Eur. J. Neurosci.* **18**:695–703.

Rolls, E.T., Verhagen, J.V., and Kadohisa, M. 2003b. Representations of the texture of food in the primate orbitofrontal cortex: Neurons responding to viscosity, grittiness, and capsaicin. *J. Neurophysiol.* **90**: 3711–3724.

Rolls, E.T., Browning, A.S., Inoue, K., and Hernandi, I. 2005. Novel visual stimuli activate a population of neurons in the primate orbitofrontal cortex. *Neurobiol. Learn. Mem.* **84**:111–123.

Rosano, C., Sweeney, J.A., Melchitzky, D.S., and Lewis, D.A. 2003. The human precentral sulcus: chemoarchitecture of a region corresponding to the frontal eye fields. *Brain Res.* **972**:16–30.

Rubinsztein, J.S., Fletcher, P.C., Rogers, R.D., Ho., L.W., Aigbirhio, F., Paykel, E.S., Robbins, T.W., and Sahakian,

B.J. 2001. Decision-making in mania: A PET study. *Brain* 124:2550–2563.

Rusch, N., val Elst, L.T., Ludaescher, P., Wilke, M., Huppertz, H.J., Thiel, T., Schmahl, C., Bohus, M., Lieb, K., Hesslinger, B., Hennig, J., and Ebert, D. 2003. A voxel-based morphometric MRI study in female patients with borderline personality disorder. *Neuroimage* 20:385–392.

Sackeim, H.A., Prohovnik, I., Moeller, J.R., Brown, R.P., Apter, S., Prudic, J., Devanand, D.P., and Mukherjee, S. 1990. Regional cerebral blood flow in mood disorders. I. Comparison of major depressives and normal controls at rest. *Arch. Gen. Psychiatry* 47:60–70.

Sahyoun, C., Floyer-Lea, A., Johansen-Berg., H., and Matthews, P.M. 2003. Towards an understanding of gait control: brain activation during the anticipation, preparation and execution of foot movements. *Neuroimage* 21:568–575.

Saleem, K.S., Kondo, H., and Price, J.L. 2008. Complementary circuits connecting the orbital and medial prefrontal networks with the temporal, insular, and opercular cortex in the macaque monkey. *J. Como. Neurol.* 506:659–693.

Sandson, J., and Albert, M.L. 1987. Perseveration in behavioral neurology. *Neurology* 37:1736–1741.

Saxe, R. 2006. Uniquely human social cognition. *Curr. Opin. Neurobiol.* 16:235–239.

Schall, J.E., and Boucher, L. 2007. Executive control of gaze by the frontal lobes. *Cogn. Affect. Behav. Neurosci.* 7:396–421.

Schmahl, C.G., Vermetten, E., Elzinga, B.M., and Bremner, J.D. 2003. Magnetic resonance imaging of hippocampal and amygdala volume in women with childhood abuse and borderline personality disorder. *Psychiatry Res.* 122:109–115.

Schmitz, T.W., and Johnson, S.C. 2007. Relevance to self: a brief review and framework of neural systems underlying appraisal. *Neurosci. Biobehav. Rev.* 31:585–596.

Schultz, W. 2006. Behavioral theories and the neurophysiology of reward. *Annu. Rev. Psychol.* 57: 87–115.

Seeman, M.V. 1997. Psychopathology in women and men: Focus on female hormones. *Am. J. Psychiatry* 154:1641–1647.

Selemon, L.D., Rajkowska, G., and Goldman-Rakic, P.S. 1995. Abnormally high neuronal density in the schizophrenic cortex. A morphometric analysis of prefrontal area 9 and occipital area 17. *Arch. Gen. Psychiatry* 52:805–818.

Semple, W.E., Goyer, P.F., and McCormick, R. 2000. Higher brain flood flow at amygdala and lower frontal cortex blood flow in PTSD patients with comorbid cocaine and alcohol abuse compared with normals. *Psychiatry* 63:65–74.

Shamay-Tsoory, S.G., and Aharon-Peretz, J. 2007. Dissociable prefrontal networks for cognitive and affective theory of the mind: A lesion study. *Neuropsychologia* 45:3054–3067.

Shaw, P., Bramham, J., Lawrence, E. J., Morris, R., Baron-Cohen, S., and David, A.S. 2005. Differential effects of lesions of the amygdala and prefrontal cortex on recognizing facial expressions of complex emotions. *J. Cogn. Neurosci.* 17:1410–1419.

Shin, L.M., Whalen, P.J., Pitman, R.K., Bush, G., Macklin, M.L., Lasko, N.B., Orr, S.P., McInerney, S.G., and Rauch, S.L. 2001. An fMRI study of anterior cingulate function in posttraumatic stress disorder. *Biol. Psychiatry* 50:932–942.

Siever, L.J., Buchsbaum, M.S., New, A.S., Spiegel-Cohen, J. Wei, T., Hazlett, E.A., Sevin, E., Nunn, M., and Mitropoulou, V. 1999. d,l-fenfluramine response in impulsivie personality disorder assessed with [18F]fluorodeoxyglucose positron emission tomography. *Neuropsychopharmacol* 20:431–432.

Sirigu, A., Cohen, L., Zalla, T., Pradat-Diehl, P., Van Eeckhout, P., Grafman, J., and Agid, Y. 1998. Distinct frontal regions for processing sentence syntax and story grammar. *Cortex* 34:771–778.

Small, D.M., Gregory, M.D., Mak, Y.E., Gitelman, D., Mesulam, M.M., and Parrish, T. 2003. Dissociation of neural representation of intensity and affective valuation in human gustation. *Neuron* 14(39): 581–583.

Smith, E.E., and Jonides, J. 1999. Storage and executive processes in the frontal lobes. *Science* 283:1657–1661.

Smith, J.D., Reisberg, D., and Wilson, M. 1992. Subvocalization and auditory imagery: Interactions between the inner ear and inner voice. In: D.Reisberg (ed.) *Auditory Imagery*. New Jersey: Lawrence Erlbaum, pp. 95–119.

Soloff, P.H., Meltzer, C.C., Grer, P.J., Constantine, D., and Kelly, T.M. 2000. A fenfluramine-activated FDG-PET study of borderline personality disorder. *Biol. Psychiatry* 47:540–547.

Soloff, P.H., Meltzer, C.C., Becker, C., Greer, P.J., Kelly, T.M., and Constantine, D. 2003. Impulsivity and prefrontal hypometabolism in borderline personality disorder. *Psychiatry Res.* 123:153–163.

Sonnby-Borgström, M. 2002. Automatic mimicry reactions as related to differences in emotional empathy. *Scand. J. Psychol.* 43:433–443.

Sowell, E.R., Thompson., P.M., Tessner, K.D., and Toga, A.W. 2001. Mapping continued brain growth and gray matter density reduction in dorsal frontal cortex: inverse relationhships during post adolescent brain maturation. *J. Neurosci.* 21:8819–8829.

Starkstein, S.E., and Robinson, R.G. 1993. Depression in cerebrovascular disease. In: S.E.Starkstein, and

R.G.Robinson (eds.) *Depression in Neurologic Disease*. Baltimore: Johns Hopkins Press, pp. 28–49.

Starkstein, S.E., Robinson, R.G., and Price, T.R. 1987. Comparison of cortical and subcortical lesions in the production of post-stroke mood disorders. *Brain* **110**:1045–1059.

Strakowski, S.M. 2002. Differential brain mechanisms in bipolar and unipolar disorders: Considerations from brain imaging. In: J.E. Soares (ed.) *Brain Imaging in Affective Disorders*. New York: Marcel Dekker, Inc.

Sukhwinder, S.S., Bullmore, E., Simmons, A., Murray, R., and McGuire, P. 2000. Functional anatomy of auditory verbal imagery in schizophrenic patients with auditory hallucinations. *Am. J. Psychiatry* **157**:1691–1693.

Swedo, S.E., Pietrini, P., Leonard, H.L., Schapiro, M.B., Rettew, D.C., Goldberger, E.L., Rapoport, S.I., Rapoport, J.L., and Grady, C.L. 1992. Cerebral glucose metabolism in childhood-onset obsessive-compulsive disorder. Revisualization during pharmacotherapy. *Arch. Gen. Psychiatry* **49**:690–694.

Tamminga, C.A. 1999. Pruning during development. *Am. J. Psychiatry* **156**:168.

Tamminga, C.A., Thaker, G.K., Buchanan, R., Kirkpatrick, B., Alphs, L.D., Chase, T.N., and Carpenter, W.T. 1992. Limbic system abnormalities identified in schizophrenia using positron emission tomography with flurodeoxyglucose and neocortical alterations with deficit syndrome. *Arch. Gen. Psychiatry* **49**: 522–530.

Tanji, J., Kurata, K., and Okano, K. 1985. The effect of cooling of the supplementary motor cortex and adjacent cortical areas. *Exp. Brain Res.* **60**:423–426.

Teasdale, J.D., Howard, R.J., Cox, S.F., Ha, Y., Brammer, M.J., Williams, S.C.R., and Checkley, S.A. 1999. Functional MRI study of the cognitive generation of affect. *Am. J. Psychiatry* **156**:209–215.

Tebartz, van Elst, L., Hesslinger, B., Thierl, T., Geiger, E., Haegele, K., Lemieux, L., Lieb, K., Bohus, M., Hennig, J., and Ebert, D. 2003. Frontolimbic brain abnormalities in patients with borderline personality disorder: A volumetric magnetic resonance imaging study. *Biol. Psychiatry* **54**:163–171.

Thaler, D., Chen, Y.C., Nixon, P.D., Stern, C.E., and Passingham, R.E. 1995. The functions of the medial premotor cortex. I. Simple learned movements. *Exp. Brain Res.* **102**:445–450.

Thampi, A., Campbell, C., Clarke, M., Barrett, S., and King, D.J. 2003. Eye movements and neurocognitive function in treatment resistant schizophrenia: A pilot study. *Ir. J. Psychol. Med.* **20**:6–10.

Todorov, A., Harris, L.T., and Fiske, S.T. 2006. Toward socially inspired social neuroscience. *Brain Res.* **1079**:76–85.

Torrey, E.F., Webster, M., Knable, M., Johnston, N., and Yolken, R.H. 2000. The Stanley Foundation brain collection and Neuropathology Consortium. *Schizophr. Res.* **44**:151–155.

Tsunoda, M., Kawaski, Y., Matsui, M., Tonoya, Y., Hagion, H., Suzuki, M., Seta, H., and Kurachi, M. 2005. Relationship between exploratory eye movements and brain morphomology in schizophrenia spectrum patients. *Eur. Arch. Psychiatry Clin. Neurosci.* **255**: 104–110.

Turella, L., Pierno, A.C., Tubaldi, F., and Castiello, U. 2009. Mirron neurons in humans: Consisting or confounding evidence? *Brain Lang.* **108**:10–21.

Uddin, L.Q., Iacoboni, M., Lang, C., and Keenan, J.P. 2007. The self and social cognition: The role of cortical midline structures and mirror neurons. *Trends Cogn. Sci.* **11**:153–157.

Uranova, N.A., Vostrikov, V.M., Orlovskaya, D.D., and Rachmanova, V.I., 2004. Oligodendroglial density in the prefrontal cortex in schizophrenia and mood disorders: A study from the Stanley Neuropathology Consortium. *Schizophr. Res.* **67**:269–275.

Ursu, S., and Carter, C.S. 2005. Outcome representations, counterfactual comparisons and the human orbitofrontal cortex; Implications for neuroimaging studies of decision-making. *Brain Res. Cogn. Brain Res.* **23**:51–60.

van den Heuvel, O.A., Veltman, D.J., Groenewegen, J.J., Witter, M.P., Merkelbach, J., Cath, D.C., Van Balkom, A.J., Van Oppen, P., and van Dyck, R. 2005. Disorder-specific neuroanatomical correlates of attentional bias in obsessive-compulsive disorder, panic disorder, and hypochondriasis. *Arch. Gen. Psychiatry*. **62**:922–933.

Volkow, N.D., Hitzemann, R., Wang, G.-J., Fowler, J.S., Wolf, A.P., Dewey, S.L., and Handlessman, L. 1992. Long-term frontal brain metabolic changes in cocaine abusers. *Synapse* **11**:184–190.

Vollm, B., Richardson, P., Stirling, J., Elliott, R., Dolan, M., Chaudhry, I., Del Ben, C., McKie, S., Anderson, I., and Deakin, B. 2004. Neurobiological substrates of antisocial and borderline personality disorder: Preliminary results of functional fMRI study. *Crim. Behav. Ment. Health* **14**:39–54.

Wager, T.D., and Smith, E.E. 2003. Neuroimaging studies of working memory: a meta-analysis. *Cogn. Affect. Behav. Neurosci.* **3**:255–274.

Wagner, A.D., Shannon, B.J., Kahn, I., and Buckner, R.L. 2005. Parietal lobe contributions to episodic memory retrieval. *Trends Cogn. Sci.* **9**:445–453.

Weinberger, D.R., Berman, K.F., and Chase, T.N. 1986. Prefrontal cortex physiological activation in Parkinson disease: effect of L-dopa. *Neurology* **36**(Suppl.):170.

Whalen, C., and Schreibman, L. 2003. Joint attention training for children with autism using behavior modification procedures. *J. Child Psychol. Psychiatry* **44**:456–468.

Wicker, B., Keyseres, C., Plailly, J., Royet, J.P., Gallese, V., and Rizzolatti, G. 2003. Both of us disgusted in my insula: the common neural basis of seeing and feeling disgust. *Neuron* **40**:655–664.

Williams, J.H.G., Waiter, G.D., Gilchrist, A., Perrettr, D.I., Murray, A.D., and Whiten, A. 2006. Neural mechanisms of imitation and mirror neuron functioning in autistic spectrum disorder. *Neuropsychologia* **44**:610–621.

Winograd-Gurvich, C., Georgiou-Karistianis, N. Fitzgerald, P.B., Millist, L., and White, O.B., 2006. Self-paced and reprogrammed saccades: Differences between melancholic and non-melancholic depression. *Neurosci. Res.* **56**:253–260.

Winston, J.S., Strange, B.A., O'Doherty, J., and Dolan, R.J. 2002. Automatic and intentional brain responses during evaluation of trustworthiness of faces. *Nat. Neurosci.* **5**:277–283.

Winston, J.S., O'Doherty, J., Kilner, J.M., Perrett, D.I., and Dolan, R.J. 2007. Brain systems for assessing facial attractiveness. *Neuropsychologia* **45**:195–206.

Winterer, G., Musso, F., Beckmann, C., Mattay, V., Egan, M.F., Jones, D.W., Callicott, J.H., Coppola, R., and Weinberger, D.R. 2006. Instability of prefrontal signal processing in schizophrenia. *Am. J. Psychiatry* **163**:1960–1968.

Wise, S.P., Fried, I., Olivier, A., Paus, T., Rizzolatti, G., and Zilles, K.J. 1996. Workshop on the anatomic definition and boundaries of the supplementary sensorimotor area. In: H.O.Lunders (ed.) *Supplementary Sensorimotor Area*. Philadelphia: Lippincott–Raven, pp. 489–496.

Wise, S.P., Boussaloud, D., Johnson, P.B., and Caminiti, R. 1997. Premotor and parietal cortex: Corticocortical connectivity and combinatorial computations. *Annu. Rev. Neurosci.* **20**:25–42.

Woo, T.U., Whitehead, R.E., Melchitzky, D.S., and Lewis, D.A. 1998. A subclass of prefrontal gamma-aminobutyric acid axon terminals are selectively altered schizophrenia. *Proc. Natl. Acad. Sci. USA.* **95**:5341–5346.

Yingling, C.D., and Skinner, J.E. 1977. Gating of thalamic input to cerebral cortex by nucleus reticularis thalami. In: J.Desmedt (ed.) *Attention, Voluntary Contraction and Event Related Cerebral Potential*. Basel: Karger, pp. 70–96.

Zald, D.H., and Kim, S.W. 1996. Anatomy and function of the orbital frontal cortex: II function and relevance to obsessive-compulsive disorder. *J. Neuropsychiatry Clin. Neurosci.* **8**:249–261.

Zametkin, A.J., Nordahl, T.E., Gross, M., King, A.L., Semple, W.E., Rumsey, J., Hamberger, S., and Cohen, R.M. 1990. Cerebral glucose metabolism in adults with hyperactivity of childhood onset. *N. Engl. J. Med.* **323**:1361–1366.

Zhang, J.X., Zhuang, J., Ma., L., Yu, W., Peng, D., Ding, G., Zhang, Z., and Weng, X. 2004. Semantic processing of Chinese in left inferior prefrontal cortex studied with reversible words. *Neuroimage* **23**:975–982.

Zhou, Y., Liang, M., Tian, L., Wang, K., Hao, Y., Liu, H., Liu, Z., and Jiang, T. 2007. Functional disintegration in paranoid schizophrenia using resting-state fMRI. *Schizophr. Res.* **97**:194–205.

Introduction

The basal ganglia (basal nuclei) have been regarded traditionally as a motor control system. Lesions in the basal ganglia almost always result in movement disorders. Recently, these structures have been found to influence other emotionally related behaviors. Research on the behavioral influence of the basal ganglia was prompted by the repeated observation that emotional and cognitive dysfunctions frequently accompany movement disorders of basal ganglia origin. In some cases, psychiatric manifestations precede the onset of motor symptoms. With the advent of neuroimaging techniques, investigation into the anatomy and metabolic physiology of these structures in the awake human has revealed intriguing behavioral relationships.

Motor activity is controlled by the intricate interaction of three major systems: the cerebral cortex, the cerebellum, and the basal ganglia. The few milliseconds that intervene between thought and action are crucial for our adjustment in modern society. Increased understanding of structures such as the basal ganglia that influence those few milliseconds is helping unravel some of the mysteries of human behavior. It is interesting that the main input to the basal ganglia comes from the cerebral cortex and that its output returns (via the thalamus) to the frontal cortex (motor, premotor, and prefrontal cortex). The frontal cortex, including the prefrontal areas, thus mediates and plays a significant role in the various functions of the basal ganglia.

Originally the basal ganglia were described as a group of cerebral (telencephalic) nuclei. These classical basal ganglia included the caudate nucleus, putamen, globus pallidus, claustrum, and amygdala. Since the time the classical basal ganglia were described, the amygdala has been reassigned to the limbic system. Little is known of the function of the claustrum, and it is not considered here. A diencephalic nucleus, the subthalamic nucleus, has been added to the group since it is closely tied to the caudate/putamen–globus pallidus. The substantia nigra and ventral tegmental

area (mesencephalic nuclei) and the pedunculopontine tegmental nucleus (a midbrain–pontine nucleus; Chapter 10) have been added for the same reason (Figure 7.1). Some authors describe the nigral complex as consisting of the substantia nigra proper and the ventral tegmental area, which lies just medial to it.

The basal ganglia are divided into dorsal and ventral divisions [Figure 7.2; see Haber and Fudge (1997a) for a detailed review]. In a general sense the dorsal division is concerned with motor function whereas the ventral division functions in support of behavior in the emotional realm. Included as part of the substantia innominata is the basal nucleus (of Meynert).

The basal ganglia receive signals from the cerebral cortex and route integrated responses to these

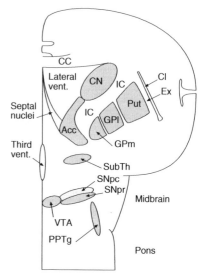

Figure 7.1. A schematic representation of the basal ganglia and nearby structures. Clinically significant basal ganglia are shaded. Acc, nucleus accumbens; CC, corpus callosum; Cl, claustrum; CN, caudate nucleus (head); IC, internal capsule; Ex, external capsule; GPl, lateral segment of globus pallidus; GPm, medial segment of globus pallidus; PPTg, pedunculopontine tegmental nucleus; Put, putamen; SNpc, substantia nigra pars compacta; SNpr, substantia nigra pars reticulata; SubTh, subthalamic nucleus; VTA, ventral tegmental nucleus.

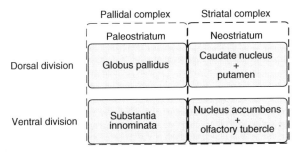

	Pallidal complex	Striatal complex
	Paleostriatum	Neostriatum
Dorsal division	Globus pallidus	Caudate nucleus + putamen
Ventral division	Substantia innominata	Nucleus accumbens + olfactory tubercle

Figure 7.2. The basal ganglia consist of a dorsal division and a ventral division. The dorsal division contains the globus pallidus (paleostriatum) and the caudate nucleus and putamen (neostriatum). The paleostriatum is continuous ventrally with the substantia innominata. The neostriatum is continuous ventrally with the nucleus accumbens and the olfactory tubercle.

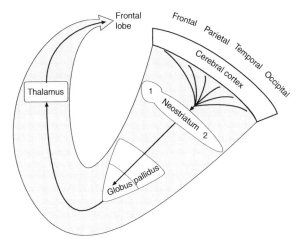

Figure 7.3. The generalized pattern of connections involving the basal ganglia form a loop from the cortex to the basal ganglia and back to the cortex by way of the thalamus. 1, caudate nucleus; 2, putamen. Compare with Figure 7.1 and the direct pathway of Figure 7.4.

signals back to the cerebral cortex (Figure 7.3). The cortical information is processed through a series of multiple parallel channels as the signals pass through the basal ganglia. The basic mechanism of operation of the basal ganglia is through a process of disinhibition. Consequently, damage to the basal ganglia often results in the release of behavior, usually in the form of uncontrollable motor activity (e.g., the tremor seen in Parkinson disease).

The basal ganglia are viewed as part of a planning mechanism that drives motor pattern generators. They work closely with executive levels of the frontal lobe to help select the motor response appropriate to the current situation. The basal ganglia also operate in close harmony with the frontal lobes in the acquisition, retention, and expression of cognitive behavior (Graybiel, 1997). Regions of the caudate nucleus (dorsal striatum) as well as the ventral striatum seem to be important in cognitive function.

Dorsal striatopallidum and associated nuclei

Neostriatum (dorsal striatum)

The neostriatum is made up of the putamen and the caudate nucleus (Figure 7.2). The putamen and caudate are separated anatomically by fibers of the internal capsule (Figure 7.1). The caudate nucleus occupies a position in the floor of the lateral ventricle dorsolateral to the thalamus. It consists of a head, body, and tail. The body continues caudally, lateral to the thalamus, and tapers gradually to form the tail, which curves ventrally into the temporal lobe to end near the amygdala. The putamen lies behind the anterior limb of the internal capsule and medial to the external capsule (Figure 9.1).

The neostriatum is the gateway to the basal ganglia (Figure 7.3). It receives fibers from all portions of the cerebral cortex and from the intralaminar nuclei of the thalamus. The neurotransmitter from the cortex is glutamate. Afferent fibers from regions of the frontal and parietal lobes may have preferential targets within the neostriatum. Fibers from the motor area of the frontal lobe [Brodmann's area (BA) BA 6] and from the primary somesthetic cortex (BA 1, BA 2, and BA 3) end predominantly on cells in the putamen. Fibers from

123

the dorsolateral prefrontal cortex and from the somesthetic association cortex (BA 5 and BA 7) terminate on cells in the caudate nucleus. These differences in cortical projection fibers support the concept of differences in function between the caudate nucleus and putamen. Neurons located within the neostriatum (interneurons) use acetylcholine as a neurotransmitter. Efferent fibers from both components of the neostriatum are γ-aminobutyric acid (GABA)ergic. GABA is one of the major inhibitory neurotransmitters of the central nervous system. Efferent fibers from the neostriatum terminate in the substantia nigra and in both the lateral and the medial segments of the globus pallidus (Figure 7.3).

It has been theorized that the neostriatum is a repository of common motor programs and acts as a comparator that serves gating and screening functions. It can act in response to external sensory signals or to commands from various regions of the cortex. Normally the neostriatum works in conjunction with the frontal cortex to inhibit motor and thought impulses that are inappropriate to the task at hand. For example, it is normal to generate a waving action of the arm in response to the sight of a person leaving the house. However, it is inappropriate to generate the same arm-waving motor response to the sight of a spouse leaving the house to put the trash out on the kerb. It is suggested that the putamen deals with motor behaviors whereas portions of the caudate nucleus deal with thoughts and sensations (Baxter *et al.*, 1990).

The caudate nucleus plays a key role in the serial order of movements and behavior (Aldridge and Berridge, 1998). Dopaminergic input from the substantia nigra correlates with learning-related activation of the left dorsolateral prefrontal cortex and anterior

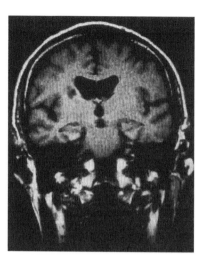

Figure 7.4. A magnetic resonance image (T1-weighted), coronal view, taken two months after the patient's acute event showed predominant dorsolateral involvement of the right caudate nucleus. (Reprinted with permission from Mendez *et al.*, 1989.)

cingulate area. This correlation is lost in early stage Parkinson patients (Carbon *et al.*, 2004), however, these patients show an increase in cortical activation, suggesting cortical compensation for loss in striatal function in sequential learning (Nakamura *et al.*, 2001).

Continuous administration of D-amphetamine over three days produces degeneration of axons in the neostriatum as well as in the motor frontal cortex of rats. The damage to dopamine axon terminals appears much like that seen in the neostriatum after administration of 1-methyl-4-phenyl-1,2,3,6-tetrahydro pyridine (MPTP) (Ryan *et al.*, 1990).

In the motor sphere, lesions in the rostroventral caudate nucleus can produce choreoathetosis on the contralateral side. In the behavioral sphere, abulia is the most common disturbance reported with lesions of the caudate nucleus. Abulia includes apathy, loss of initiative, and loss of spontaneous thoughts and emotional responses (Bhatia and Marsden, 1994).

A suggestion of reduced caudate nucleus volume in schizophrenic patients has been reported by DeLisi and associates (1991). More recently a marked (14%) reduction was seen in the volume of the caudate nucleus in neuroleptic-naïve schizophrenic patients (Keshavan *et al.*, 1998). This reduction does not appear to be diagnostically specific, since reductions in caudate nucleus volume have been reported in nonschizophrenic psychotic patients and in patients with depression (Krishnan *et al.*, 1992). These reductions were not accompanied by volume reductions of the putamen.

Clinical vignette

A 52-year-old hypertensive man developed delirium, which slowly cleared leaving a profoundly apathetic state. He remained detached and disinterested and would not initiate any activity. When spoken to he would reply in a few words, and he would never initiate a conversation. A computed tomography (CT) scan showed a recent infarct in the head of the right caudate, which was clearly delineated on magnetic resonance imaging (MRI) two months later (Figure 7.4). One year following the event he was distractible, irritable, and easily frustrated. There was decreased initiative, disengagement from prior activities, and decreased attention to his appearance and weight. He eventually lost his job as school principal.

Striatal binding sites have been reported to be significantly more abundant in cocaine users. The severity of cocaine use is correlated with the number of binding sites (Little *et al.*, 1999).

Dorsal pallidum (paleostriatum)

The globus pallidus is the dorsal division of the paleostriatum (Figure 7.2) and lies medial to the putamen (Figures 7.1, 7.3, and 9.1). It consists of a lateral segment and a medial segment separated by a band of fibers. Cell bodies in the lateral segment project fibers that terminate in the medial segment. The medial segment is a major output nucleus of the basal ganglia. The putamen and the globus pallidus lie directly adjacent to one another and collectively are called the lentiform nucleus.

Depression is a common finding in diseases that affect the globus pallidus. A neuroanatomical model of depression after pallidal lesions focuses on enhanced inhibition of the prefrontal cortex (Lauterbach *et al.*, 1997; Lauterbach, 1999).

Ames *et al.* (1994) found that of 46 patients with frontal lobe degeneration, 78% demonstrated repetitive behaviors ranging from motor stereotypies to complex obsessive-compulsive behavior. These patients had additional damage in the basal ganglia, caudate, and pallidal regions. It is postulated that the combined damage to the frontal lobe, caudate nucleus, and globus pallidus may account for the repetitive behavior seen in the frontal lobe degeneration and possibly in idiopathic obsessive-compulsive disorder (OCD). Anoxic injury, such as that produced by carbon monoxide poisoning, can result in bilateral infarctions of the globus pallidus and can cause obsessions, compulsions, and a Tourette-like syndrome (Salloway and Cummings, 1994).

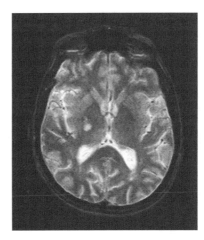

Figure 7.5. A magnetic resonance image (T2-weighted) demonstrated increased signal intensity in the ventrolateral globus pallidus on the right. (Reprinted with permission from Mendez *et al.*, 2004.)

Subthalamic nucleus (subthalamus)

The subthalamic nucleus lies below the thalamus and is contiguous with the substantia nigra at its caudal end. Cell bodies located in the lateral segment of the globus pallidus project to the subthalamus (Figure 7.6). Efferent fibers from the subthalamus project to the medial segment of the globus pallidus and to the substantia nigra pars reticulata. The subthalamus is a key component of the indirect pathway through the basal ganglia. Strokes or tumors that affect the subthalamus produce contralateral hemiballismus. The affected extremities often exhibit a decrease in muscle tone.

Substantia nigra

The substantia nigra is one of the basal ganglia and is located in the midbrain (Figure 7.1). Neuromelanin found in the substantia nigra pars compacta is a by-product of dopamine metabolism and gives the "nigra" its dark appearance as seen at autopsy. The substantia nigra consists of two distinct divisions, the pars reticulata and pars compacta.

The substantia nigra pars compacta contains cells that produce dopamine and give rise to fibers that project to the caudate nucleus and to the putamen. These fibers make up the nigrostriatal (mesostriatal) tract. The axons that make up the nigrostriatal projection are believed to interact with dopamine receptor sites, where neuroleptics cause movement disorders. The substantia nigra pars compacta sends dopaminergic fibers to the neostriatum, involving both the direct pathway and the indirect pathway.

Dopaminergic fibers that act on D_1 dopamine receptors activate the direct pathway and increase motor activity. In contrast, dopaminergic fibers that act on D_2 receptors activate the indirect pathway and

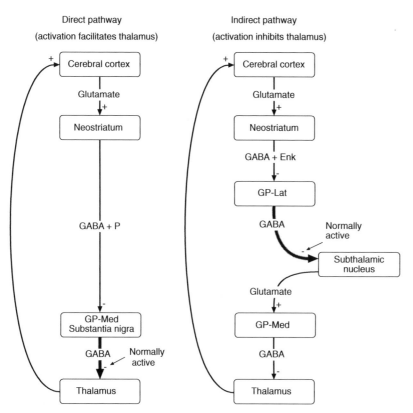

Direct pathway
(activation facilitates thalamus)

Indirect pathway
(activation inhibits thalamus)

Figure 7.6. There are two pathways through the basal ganglia: the direct pathway and the indirect pathway. When the body is at rest, the thalamus is inhibited. When muscular activity is called for, the thalamus is disinhibited. When activated by the cerebral cortex, the direct pathway increases the output of the thalamus. The indirect pathway decreases the output of the thalamus. Substantia nigra identified in this illustration represents only substantia pars reticulata. γ-Aminobutyric acid (GABA) in the neostriatal direct pathway is accompanied by the cotransmitter substance P (P). GABA in the neostriatal indirect pathway is accompanied by the cotransmitter enkephalin (Enk). GP, globus pallidus; Med, medial; Lat, lateral.

decrease motor activity. D_2 receptors tend to be concentrated in the lateral segment of the globus pallidus. Overall it appears that an increase in the level of dopamine in the neostriatum shifts the balance toward the direct pathway and an increase in activity (Figure 7.6).

Dopamine is a relatively slow-acting neurotransmitter, and because of this slow action, some authors describe it as a neuromodulator. Release of dopamine precedes motor activity. Dopamine is inhibitory on neurons of the striatum; when released, it decreases the spontaneous firing rate of these neurons. The suppression of spontaneous firing makes individual striatal neurons more sensitive to excitatory signals from the cerebral cortex. In this manner, the release of dopamine primes the striatum for motor activity under the direction of the cerebral cortex.

Dopamine neurons from pars compacta project mainly to the dorsal and ventral striatum, where they are crucial for reward-based motor control. Their signals provide a reward prediction error (difference between actual reward value and expected reward value) for motor behavior to maximize reward (Schultz, 1998). Their signals also encode novel environmental events that can produce an immediate change in motor behavior (Redgrave and Gurney, 2006). Overall they modulate the anticipated reward value of an impending action (Hikosaka et al., 2006; Nakamura and Hikosaka, 2006).

Evidence from mouse studies supports the hypothesis that midbrain stem cells result in neurogenesis in the substantia nigra. The rate of turnover is less than that of the dentate gyrus (Chapter 11). Lesions result in an increase in neuronal replacement (Zhao et al., 2003).

The substantia nigra pars reticulata is an output nucleus of the basal ganglia much like the medial segment of the globus pallidus. This division of the substantia nigra gives rise to the nigrothalamic fibers. The substantia nigra pars reticulata and the medial segment of the globus pallidus are the two major output nuclei of the basal ganglia. Both project to the thalamus.

Extrapyramidal side effects of antipsychotic drugs are due to their ability to block D_2 receptor sites. These side effects include dystonia, akathisia, pseudoparkinsonism, and tardive dyskinesia. Akathisia is motor restlessness and may be mistaken for psychotic restlessness and agitation. Tardive dyskinesia is the worst of the side effects and is associated with long-term therapy. It is seen in up to 50% of patients who are receiving long-term treatment and may not disappear even when the drug is discontinued. Although dopamine or dopamine receptors or both may be involved in schizophrenia, Okubo et al. (1997) found no difference in the density of D_2 receptors in the neostriatum of drug-free schizophrenic patients and control subjects.

Atrophy of neuron cell bodies in the substantia nigra pars compacta leads to dopamine loss and Parkinson disease. Side effects of dopamine replacement therapy (levodopa, L-dopa) include dyskinesias and hallucinations. Intracerebral transplantation of dopaminergic fetal mesencephalic tissue has few reported psychiatric sequelae; however, transplantation of adrenal medullary tissue often causes psychosis or delirium (Price et al., 1995). Patients with Parkinson disease have been shown to exhibit cognitive impairment. Impairments in visuospatial function, executive function, and memory have been described (Savage, 1997).

Neuroimaging studies have revealed that metabolism in the caudate nuclei and orbitofrontal cortex of depressed patients with Parkinson disease is lower than that of nondepressed patients with Parkinson disease (Mayberg et al., 1990). Left anterior lesions involving the caudate nucleus have the greatest risk of depression regardless of the level of disability caused by the stroke (Starkstein et al., 1987). These and other results (George et al., 1993) indicate that depression associated with Parkinson disease may involve the caudate nucleus (Lafer et al., 1997).

Patients with Parkinson disease are diagnosed with depression significantly more frequently than are patients with other disabilities (Ehmann et al., 1990; Menza and Mark, 1994). The mean frequency of depression in Parkinsonian patients is 40%, and the depression is accompanied by a high rate of anxiety symptoms (Cummings, 1992; Starkstein and Mayberg, 1993). Parkinson patients with depression show significant cell loss in the ventral tegmental area (Torack and Morris, 1988). This area lies just medial to the substantia nigra and supplies dopamine to the limbic system and cortex (see later in text). It has been suggested that depression in Parkinson disease is seen more commonly in patients with more prominent dopamine-responsive signs such as gait disturbance and rigidity. Parkinson patients with left brain dysfunction have a higher incidence of depression than do patients with right brain dysfunction (Cummings,

1992; Starkstein and Mayberg, 1993). Depression correlates with lowered metabolism in the head of the caudate and the orbitofrontal cortex (Mayberg et al., 1990).

> A 79-year-old man presented to medical attention with an acute personality change. He had suddenly begun to act strangely, telling strange stories, and doing unusual things such as serving his wife tuna in milk. His neighbors complained that he had stopped caring for his house and allowed his dogs to urinate and defecate throughout the interior. On examination, the patient was found to be distractible, disinhibited, and unconcerned, particularly about his unkempt appearance. He was friendly, loquacious, and winked and made sexual innuendoes toward the female hospital staff. There were no other neurological findings, and computed tomography showed a recent left caudate lacunar stroke.

Connections of the dorsal striatopallidal system (skeletomotor circuit)

Parallel circuits

Four distinct circuits are recognized involving the basal ganglia. These circuits run parallel to each other, but each serves a separate behavior. The best known circuit is associated with the movement disorders of basal ganglia disease. It is called the skeletomotor circuit and consists of both a direct and an indirect circuit (Figure 7.6). The oculomotor circuit controls the action of the extraocular muscles. Two additional circuits are recognized but are less well known. These are the association circuit, which is believed to serve cognition, and the limbic circuit, which is thought to serve emotions. All four circuits have certain elements in common. First, each receives input from many areas of the cortex. Second, each sends signals through the basal ganglia, but the specific regions used by each of the circuits may differ. Third, all four circuits relay in the thalamus before sending signals back to the cortex. Fourth, all four circuits send signals back to the frontal lobe, but the exact portion of the frontal lobe targeted by each circuit differs. Although each of the circuits is separate, it is thought that each of their actions is influenced by actions of the others by way of interneurons located within the basal ganglia. Three of the circuits are associated with the dorsal striatopallidal system. The fourth, the limbic circuit, is associated with the ventral striatopallidal system.

Skeletomotor circuit

Direct pathway

The connections of the classical basal ganglia are relatively well known even though their exact mode of operation remains unclear (Graybiel, 1995). The direct pathway is a loop that has its origin in the cerebral cortex (Figures 7.3 and 7.6). The pathway loops down into the basal ganglia and then returns to the cortex by way of the thalamus. Fibers from many areas of the cortex project into the neostriatum (caudate nucleus and putamen), effectively funneling many fibers onto relatively few cells. Fibers from the neostriatum course to the medial segment of the globus pallidus. Efferents from the globus pallidus terminate in the anterior division of the ventrolateral nucleus of the thalamus, which projects back to the frontal lobe. Cortical neurons that receive input from the basal ganglia seem to have common properties. They receive significant sensory input, they are commonly involved in premovement activities, and they respond to stimuli that have motivational significance. Lesions in these cortical areas result in attentional deficits and defective movements.

The direct (basic) pathway functions on the principle of disinhibition. The cells of the ventrolateral thalamus project to the supplementary motor cortex and facilitate motor activity. These cells would fire constantly if it were not for the fact that the output cells of the medial segment of the globus pallidus are tonically active. These tonically active cells contain GABA, which inhibits activity in the ventrolateral nucleus of the thalamus. Efferent fibers from the cortex contain glutamate, an excitatory neurotransmitter. When a signal arrives in the neostriatum from the cortex requesting a particular motor response, glutamate causes selected cells in the neostriatum to fire. The cells of the neostriatum contain GABA, which inhibits the tonically active GABA cells of the medial segment of the globus pallidus. The action of the neostriatal GABA inhibits the action of the GABAergic cells of the globus pallidus, which normally inhibit the action of the thalamus. By inhibiting the action of inhibitory globus pallidus neurons, the neurons of the ventrolateral nucleus of the thalamus are released (disinhibited); the thalamus fires and activates motor regions of the frontal lobe.

Indirect pathway

The components of the indirect pathway are similar to those of the direct pathway but with the addition of a detour through the lateral segment of the globus pallidus and the subthalamic nucleus (Figure 7.6). In the case of the indirect pathway, the ventrolateral nucleus of the thalamus is inhibited by the activity of GABAergic neurons of the medial segment of the globus pallidus –just the same as with the direct pathway. However, these GABAergic neurons are encouraged to fire more rapidly only when the normally active GABAergic neurons of the lateral segment of the globus pallidus are inhibited.

The overall effect of activation of the direct pathway is to increase cortical activity. The overall effect of activation of the indirect pathway is to decrease cortical activity. During a normal resting state the two pathways are in balance with a slight edge given to the indirect pathway. Note that the neostriatal GABAergic neurons serving the two pathways each carry a different cotransmitter (Figure 7.6).

A number of parallel circuits, probably thousands, run from the prefrontal cortex to the basal ganglia and then to the thalamus and back to the cortex. Each of these circuits contains a direct and an indirect pathway. The striatum plays a role in supporting movement and thought and is active in procedural learning.

Oculomotor circuit

The oculomotor circuit is involved with the control of eye movements and arises from more restricted areas of the cortex than the other circuits. The input to the oculomotor circuit arises from cell bodies located in the frontal eye field (see "Frontal eye field," Chapter 6, page 89) and the posterior parietal cortex. The oculomotor circuit targets oculomotor control areas in the frontal cortex.

Association circuit

The association circuit receives input from many areas of the cortex. It is hypothesized that this circuit is responsible for relating motor activity to targets in the extrapersonal space and may play a special role in eye–hand coordination. The association circuit projects to the frontal association area. This area, especially the dorsolateral prefrontal cortex, is important in organizing behavior in space and in time (see "Dorsolateral prefrontal cortex," Chapter 6, page 94).

Ventral striatopallidum and associated nuclei

Ventral striatum (limbic striatum)

The ventral striatum is also known as the limbic striatum and includes a number of structures found in the basal forebrain, including the nucleus accumbens, the olfactory tubercle, and the ventral extensions of the caudate nucleus and putamen. Much of the ventral pallidum appears to be a ventral extension of the globus pallidus and includes the substantia innominata and basal nucleus (of Meynert).

Nucleus accumbens

The nucleus accumbens is a small nucleus near the midline just rostral to the diencephalon. It lies at the base of the septum pellucidum. The nucleus accumbens is continuous above with the caudate/putamen and extends ventrally as the olfactory tubercle (Figure 7.1). Two major subdivisions of the nucleus are recognized: the core and the shell. The core represents a ventromedial extension of the caudate/putamen. There is no distinguishable border between the caudate/putamen and the core. The shell of the nucleus accumbens surrounds the core on its medial and ventral borders. The shell extends caudomedially to blend with the central division of the extended amygdala, providing evidence of the close relationship between the nucleus accumbens and the limbic system. The bed nucleus of the stria terminalis is part of the extended amygdala and is anatomically similar to the shell of nucleus accumbens (Carboni et al., 2000). Distinctive cell clusters throughout the nucleus accumbens suggest that different regions of the nucleus may operate selectively under different functional conditions (deOlmos and Heimer, 1999).

Projections from the prefrontal cortex, from the midline nuclei of the thalamus, and from the hippocampus and basal amygdala terminate in both the core and the shell of the nucleus accumbens. Projections from the shell terminate in the nucleus basalis (of Meynert), which is the source of cholinergic fibers to the cortex. These connections through the nucleus basalis may allow the shell of the nucleus accumbens to influence arousal, attention, and cognitive function (Heimer et al., 1997). The shell is different from the core in that it has fibers that project directly to the central nucleus of the extended amygdala and to the lateral hypothalamus. The connections of the shell to the amygdala suggest that the nucleus accumbens

may facilitate autonomic and goal-directed behavior (Alheid and Heimer, 1996).

The nucleus accumbens has been described as a limbic–motor interface. It is in a position to bring together input from limbic "motivational" structures, and its output goes to structures associated with motor processes, including the globus pallidus, substantia nigra, and pedunculopontine tegmental nucleus (Winn et al., 1997).

The nucleus accumbens and dopamine have been closely associated with the rewarding effects of carbohydrates as well as abusive drugs including alcohol, cocaine, amphetamine, and morphine (Blum et al., 1996a). The nucleus accumbens is also involved with both withdrawal effects related to these drugs and effects of antipsychotic drugs (Alheid and Heimer, 1996). One model of schizophrenia proposes that an increase in the quantity of dopamine released in the nucleus accumbens by the mesolimbic pathway from the ventral tegmental area is responsible for positive psychotic symptoms (Gray et al., 1991; Gray, 1998). Another model of the pathophysiology of schizophrenia suggests that abnormalities in the projection from the hippocampus to the nucleus accumbens are responsible for the psychosis and thought disorganization of schizophrenia (Csernansky and Bardgett, 1998).

Ventral pallidum

Several nuclei within the substantia innominata along with the lateral preoptic area make up the ventral pallidum. The ventral pallidum is continuous with the globus pallidus (dorsal pallidum), which lies above it.

Basal nucleus (of Meynert)

The basal nucleus makes up a large portion of the substantia innominata. The majority of acetylcholine found in the brain arises from the neurons of the basal nucleus. It projects fibers to the neocortex, hippocampus, amygdala, thalamus, and brainstem. It receives fibers from the amygdala, hypothalamus (Chapter 8), pedunculopontine nucleus, and midbrain (Chapter 10).

The basal nucleus is believed to be important in integrating subcortical functions. Drugs such as scopolamine that block acetylcholine can cause confusion and memory disorders. Loss of the acetylcholinergic neurons of the basal nucleus has been described in Alzheimer disease (Price et al., 1982). However, acetylcholine disappears from the axon terminals before it is reduced in the cell bodies in the basal nucleus. This suggests that nerve cell loss in the basal nucleus is secondary to dying back of the axons (Sofroniew *et al.*, 1983; Herholz *et al.*, 2004).

Ventral tegmental area

The ventral tegmental area has recently been included as one of the basal ganglia (Figures 7.1, 10.3 and 10.4). It is located in the midbrain and appears as a ventromedial extension of the substantia nigra pars compacta. In addition to their close proximity, the ventral tegmental area and substantia nigra pars compacta serve similar functions and they have a similar histochemical makeup. For this reason they have been identified as the two components of the "nigral complex" (Ma, 1997). Like substantia nigra pars compacta, the ventral tegmental area contains a large population of dopaminergic neurons.

Similarity between cells found in the substantia nigra and the ventral tegmental area has suggested the existence of a dorsal tier and a ventral tier of dopaminergic neurons. The dorsal tier includes a band of neurons stretching across the dorsal substantia nigra pars compacta and contiguous ventral tegmental area. The ventral tier consists of cells of the ventral substantia nigra pars compacta and a corresponding ventral group of ventral tegmental area neurons. Evidence suggests that the dorsal tier neurons are tightly linked with the limbic system. The ventral tier dopaminergic neurons are influenced by limbic regions but are more closely linked with areas of the striatum that are important in sensorimotor control (Haber and Fudge, 1997b).

Descending projections to the ventral tegmental area include indirect connections from the hippocampus by way of septal nuclei and the hypothalamus. These close connections with limbic system structures led Nauta (1958) to include the ventral tegmental area as part of the "midbrain limbic area." The ventral tegmental area projects through the medial forebrain bundle to limbic areas (mesolimbic system) and to cortical areas (mesocortical system). Targets of the dopaminergic fibers from the ventral tegmental area include the dorsolateral and medial prefrontal cortex, the anterior cingulate gyrus (mesocortical system) and nucleus accumbens, the hippocampus, and the amygdala (mesolimbic system). The midline and medial thalamic nuclei are considered part of the limbic thalamus and are also targets of ascending dopaminergic fibers (Chapter 9).

There is evidence that many of the fibers that make up the mesocortical projection arise from neurons both from the ventral tegmental area and from adjacent areas of the midbrain. The adjacent areas include widespread regions of the substantia nigra and the retrorubral field. A few fibers even originate from within the parabrachial nucleus. Although this is described as a dopaminergic system, a surprising number of the fibers are not from dopamine-producing neurons. It appears that the mesocortical projections to the dorsal prefrontal cortex, to the ventromedial prefrontal cortex, and to the anterior cingulate cortex are served by midbrain neurons from three different regions of the midbrain (Williams and Goldman-Rakic, 1998).

The ventral tegmental area dopaminergic system is postulated to be involved in reward associated with newly learned behaviors in contrast to the maintenance of previously learned behaviors (Schultz *et al.*, 1995). This system responds to the novelty of an unexpected stimulus, to primary rewards, and to the conditioned stimulus associated with that reward (Haber and Fudge, 1997a). Systemic injection of cocaine in rats has been shown to produce an increase in extracellular glutamate in the ventral tegmental area, and this may underlie behavioral sensitization to cocaine (Kalivas and Duffy, 1998).

Bogerts *et al.* (1983) found that the size of neuromelanin-containing neurons in the ventral tegmental area was decreased and the volume of the substantia nigra area was reduced in the brains of six schizophrenic patients. There was no change in the number of neurons or glia cells. An increase in activity in the mesolimbic system has been reported in schizophrenia (Kapur *et al.*, 2005). This is accompanied by a decrease in activity in the prefrontal area. It has been suggested that the positive symptoms of schizophrenia may reflect mesolimbic hyperactivity, and the negative symptoms may reflect mesocortical hypoactivity (Weinberger, 1987).

Pedunculopontine tegmental nucleus

The pedunculopontine tegmental nucleus extends caudally from the substantia nigra just medial to the lateral lemniscus (Figures 7.1 and 10.3). It is usually considered as one of the reticular formation nuclei (Chapter 10); however, its connections with the basal ganglia and importance in motor control have motivated some authors to include it among the basal ganglia (Winn *et al.*, 1997). Like the nucleus basalis, the pedunculopontine tegmental nucleus is an important source of acetylcholine; however, it also contains noncholinergic neurons, much the same as the substantia nigra contains dopaminergic and nondopaminergic neurons. Fibers from the pedunculopontine nucleus project to the frontal cortex, septum, amygdala, globus pallidus, substantia nigra, hypothalamus, and thalamus. The largest and most studied are those projections to the thalamus. The pedunculopontine tegmental nucleus receives fibers from the dorsal striatum (putamen, globus pallidus, substantia nigra pars reticulata, subthalamic nucleus), the ventral striatum (nucleus accumbens), amygdala, and brainstem reticular formation (raphe nuclei and locus ceruleus) (Jones, 1990; Wainer and Mesulam, 1990).

Limbic connections of the pedunculopontine nucleus (septum, amygdala, ventral pallidum, prefrontal cortex), along with behavioral studies, underscore its importance in working memory and cognition. The pedunculopontine nucleus plays a role in the regulation of the basal nucleus (Decker and McGaugh, 1991). Connections with other basal ganglia nuclei suggest its importance in motor activity. It is known to be important in locomotion and possibly may be involved in the pill-rolling tremor of Parkinson disease. It appears to be critical in the reward effects of opiates and other stimulants and plays a role in attention and arousal (Steckler et al., 1994). The pedunculopontine tegmental nucleus like nucleus accumbens is considered a limbic–motor interface and may be involved with response switching and perseveration. It is speculated to be in a position to respond to signals from the ventral striatum in order to inhibit an ongoing response maintained by the dorsal striatum (Winn et al., 1997).

Neuron cell loss in the pedunculopontine tegmental nucleus has been reported in Parkinson disease (Jellinger, 1991), Alzheimer disease (Mufson et al., 1988), and progressive supranuclear palsy (Jellinger, 1988). Impairment of attentional processes is a common denominator of all of these disorders.

Connections of the ventral striatopallidal system (limbic circuit)

In addition to the other circuits of the basal ganglia, the ventral striatopallidal system forms yet another circuit called the limbic circuit (Figure 7.7). It is the least known of the circuits. It is believed to provide an interface between the limbic system and the motor systems. From what is known of the connections of the ventral striatopallidal system, there appear to be many similarities between the general pattern of connectivity of this system and the dorsal striatopallidal system (Figures

7.3 and 7.8). Limbic fibers to the ventral striatopallidal system arise from the hippocampus and the amygdala (Burns et al., 1996). Fibers from many cortical areas and from several brainstem nuclei, including the raphe nuclei and locus ceruleus, funnel together and converge on the ventral striatum. A large contingent of fibers is from the ventral tegmental area. The bulk of the efferent fibers from the nucleus accumbens project to the ventral pallidum. The ventral pallidum projects back to both cortical and brainstem targets. The primary cortical target is the prefrontal cortex directly and via the mediodorsal nucleus of the thalamus indirectly. Brainstem targets include the pedunculopontine tegmental nucleus. Evidence indicates that the ventral striatal system is involved in emotional behavior and with motivational aspects of motor behavior (Graybiel, 1995).

Serotonin is much less studied than dopamine but also plays a role in the function of the basal ganglia

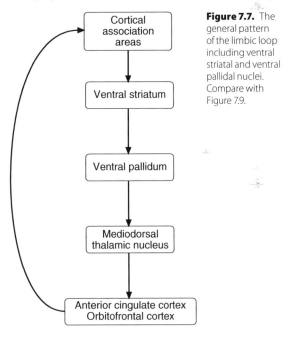

Figure 7.7. The general pattern of the limbic loop including ventral striatal and ventral pallidal nuclei. Compare with Figure 7.9.

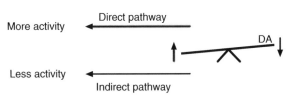

Figure 7.8. The indirect system is the normally active pathway. The action of an increase in the level of dopamine is to facilitate motor activity. DA, dopamine.

and is found throughout the caudate nucleus and putamen (Pazos and Palacios, 1985; Pazos *et al.*, 1985). Clomipramine, which acts on the serotonergic system, has been useful in treating symptoms of OCD. It has been questioned whether serotonin may play a role in this disorder (Insel and Winslow, 1992).

Deep brain stimulation

Deep brain stimulation (DBS) involves the placement of an electrode array in a specific part of the brain. The electrode array is connected to an implanted pulse generator (IPG) located subcutaneously usually just inferior to the clavicle. The array is placed in the ventral intermediate (ventrointermedial) nucleus of the thalamus for essential familial tremor. For dystonia and the rigidity, bradykinesia/akinesia and tremor associated with Parkinson disease, the globus pallidus or subthalamic nucleus is targeted. The ventral posterior medial and ventral posterior lateral thalamic nuclei have been stimulated for the control of pain. Stimulation of the subgenual region of the anterior cingulate gyrus (BA 25) has been effective in some cases of depression (Lozano *et al.*, 2008; Mayberg *et al.*, 2005). (See also lateral habenular nucleus in Chapter 8). A major advantage of DBS is that it changes brain activity in a controlled manner and its effects are reversible (Krauss, 2002).

The mechanism of action of DBS is unclear and the cellular pathway(s) are not fully understood. DBS has been shown to be associated with a marked increase in the release of adenosine triphosphate (ATP) by nearby astrocytes. ATP release results in accumulation of its catabolic product adenosine. Activation of the adenosine A1 receptor in mice depresses excitatory transmission in the thalamus and reduces both tremor- and DBS-induced side effects. In addition intrathalamic infusion of A1 receptor agonists in mice directly reduces tremor. These findings implicate adenosine mechanisms in the production of tremor (Latini and Pedata, 2001; Bekar *et al.*, 2008).

Neuropsychiatric side effects have been reported, including cognitive dysfunction, apathy, depression, hallucinations, compulsive gambling, and hypersexuality (Burn and Troster, 2004; Smeding *et al.*, 2006).

Behavioral considerations

Obsessive-compulsive disorder (OCD)

Obsessive-compulsive disorder is a multidimensional disorder that includes obsessions, checking, symmetry and ordering, cleanliness and washing, and hoarding (Leckman *et al.*, 1997). A response bias exists toward stimuli related to socioterritorial concerns about danger, violence, hygiene, order, and sex. These behaviors are mediated by orbitofrontal-subcortical circuits. In healthy individuals socioterritorial concerns and responses to stimuli perceived as dangerous are processed through the orbitofrontal-caudate circuit and inhibited when appropriate by the indirect pathway. Patients with OCD are particularly sensitive to socioterritorial stimuli and related concerns of danger, violence, hygiene, order, etc., and have an imbalance in the direct/indirect pathway that prevents them from inhibiting behaviors related to these stimuli and switching to alternative behaviors (Saxena *et al.*, 1998). Luxenberg and associates (1988) and Robinson and colleagues (1995) reported atrophy of the caudate in patients with OCD. An increase in metabolism over control subjects has been reported in the whole cerebral hemispheres, the orbital gyri, and the heads of the caudate nuclei in patients with OCD (Figure 12.7; Baxter, 1992; Saxena *et al.*, 1998). It is theorized that small, restricted caudate lesions may be responsible for OCD, whereas larger lesions of the caudate nuclei result in more global symptoms such as those seen in Huntington disease (Baxter *et al.*, 1990). Baxter and coworkers (1990) have proposed that chronic motor tics are due to small lesions in the putamen. Baxter (1992) theorized that a deficit in caudate function leads to inadequate repression (i.e., filtering) of input from the orbital cortex ("worry"). This deficit allows input from other cortical areas to continue on to the globus pallidus, where it frees the thalamus to drive the cortex to carry out a behavior (Figure 7.9). For example, sensations that signal dirty hands may normally match with an appropriate response: hand washing. However, in the case of OCD, the screening capability of the neostriatum is decreased, and the slightest sensory input from the hands may trigger hand washing. In this scenario even sensory input unrelated to the hands may cross over and produce hand washing. Motivation and the initiation of the activity may originate in the anterior cingulate gyrus (Chapter 12). According to Houck and Wise (1995) the basal ganglia make use of old rules when presented with familiar environmental and contextual stimuli. It is up to the frontal cortex to alter a learned response pattern when old rules need to be rejected and new rules applied (Rapoport and Fiske, 1998). The presence of dopamine in the frontal cortex may be important both in activating old rules and in learning new rules (Houck and Wise, 1995).

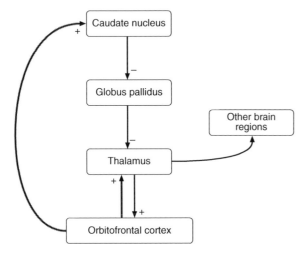

Figure 7.9. It is proposed that overactivity in the orbital prefrontal cortex ("worry") drives the caudate nucleus. The resulting increase in the output of the caudate nucleus reduces inhibition on the thalamus. The thalamus becomes overactive and further drives the orbital prefrontal cortex. In the model, the orbital prefrontal cortex also drives the thalamus directly. Successful treatment may reduce the input to the caudate nucleus and/or it may reduce the facilitation of the thalamus by direct input from the prefrontal orbital cortex. (After Baxter, 1992.)

Effective therapy allows the patient to enhance the filtering effect of the caudate to limit behavioral responses from signals from the orbital cortex. Positron emission tomography (PET) scans of OCD patients revealed that the metabolic rates in the basal ganglia and in the orbital cortex are higher in OCD patients than in controls (Baxter *et al.*, 1990). The increase in metabolism may reflect attempts by the patient to control the disorder. Similar changes seen in caudate metabolism following successful therapy reflect the role played by the caudate in learning new habits and skills (Schwartz *et al.*, 1996).

Stereotaxic lesions of the bifrontal pathways located beneath and in front of the head of the caudate nucleus (subcaudate tractotomy or capsulotomy; Chapter 12) have been used as a surgical treatment of intractable affective disorder (Kartsounis *et al.*, 1991). Capsulotomy has been found to benefit intractable cases of obsessive-compulsive disorder. The effect is believed to result from interrupting the connections between the caudate and frontal and anterior cingulate cortex (Rapoport, 1991).

Tourette syndrome

Neuroimaging studies provide evidence that the head of the caudate is involved in Tourette syndrome (Hyde *et al.*, 1995). The caudate nucleus is smaller in

volume in both children and adults with Tourette, but there is no correlation between size and severity of symptoms (Peterson *et al.*, 2003). It is speculated that the dysfunction of the caudate seen in patients with Tourette syndrome is responsible for the compulsive component of tics (Wolf *et al.*, 1996). It is suggested that patients with Tourette syndrome exhibit super-sensitivity of the D_2 dopamine receptor or have an excess of dopamine in the caudate nucleus (Singer, 1997). The similarity in caudate nucleus abnormalities seen both in patients with OCD and in those with Tourette, along with the fact that OCD is frequently a comorbid condition with Tourette syndrome, suggests that the caudate may be involved in both conditions. These two disorders may represent overlapping neurobehavioral conditions, although OCD involves, in addition, the orbitofrontal and cingulate areas (Wolf *et al.*, 1996).

The right putamen is larger than the left in control subjects. Singer *et al.* (1993) reported that 13 of 37 Tourette syndrome patients demonstrated reverse asymmetry, with the right larger than the left putamen. The abnormal anatomical asymmetry is paralleled by abnormal asymmetry in behavioral tests performed by these patients (Yank *et al.*, 1994).

Hyperkinetic movement disorders

Chorea and athetosis are common hyperkinetic movement disorders. Choreoathetoid movements are typical of Huntington disease. These movement disorders correlate with loss of striatal neurons. Ballism is seen rarely but is usually as a result of an infarction of the subthalamic nucleus. The violent movements of ballism may represent extreme choreoathetoid movements. Tics are also a form of hyperkinetic movement disorder. The forced vocalizations of Tourette syndrome may represent a form of complex tic. Hyperkinetic movements may be suppressed with D_2 receptor antagonists. Cholinergic agonists are sometimes used for control of chorea in Huntington disease.

Hypokinetic movement disorders

Akinesia, bradykinesia, and rigidity are examples of hypokinesis, which are seen in Parkinson disease. A loss of dopamine-producing cells in the substantia nigra pars compacta occurs in Parkinson disease. Tardive dyskinesia may appear after long-term treatment with antipsychotic agents (phenothiazines and the butyrophenones). These drugs appear to block dopaminergic transmission and may eventually cause dopaminergic receptors in the basal ganglia to become hypersensitive to dopamine.

Pallidotomy and subthalamic DBS for Parkinson disease have demonstrated positive effects for motor function. Decreased semantic verbal fluency has been reported but unaccompanied by cognitive defects (Gironell et al., 2003). Hypersexuality (Roane et al., 2002; Mendez et al., 2004), transient manic behavior (Okun et al., 2003), and confusion have also been reported (Higuchi and Iacono, 2003; Hua et al., 2003).

Huntington disease

Atrophy of the caudate has been reported in patients with Huntington disease (Luxenberg et al., 1988). Cell loss is seen first in the dorsomedial caudate nucleus. The greatest neuron loss is in the caudate, then the putamen, with more subtle cell loss in the ventral tegmental area (Peyser and Folstein, 1993). Both motor disturbances and mood disorder seen in Huntington disease correlate with cell loss in the caudate nucleus. Depression, seen in 41% of 186 Huntington patients in the study by Folstein et al. (1990), preceded other symptoms by an average of five years. In many cases patients experience episodes of depression before they are even aware that they are at risk for Huntington disease (Folstein et al., 1990).

Other behavioral considerations

Trichotillomania (repetitive hair-pulling) has been referred to as compulsive and contains elements similar to the compulsions of OCD (Swedo and Leonard, 1992). In studies, patients with trichotillomania exhibit significantly smaller left putamen volume (13.2%) than control subjects. These differences more closely parallel those seen in Tourette syndrome than those seen in OCD (O'Sullivan et al., 1997).

Pearlson et al. (1995) reported that the density of D_2-like dopamine receptors is increased in the caudate nucleus of patients with bipolar disorder and psychotic symptoms compared with normal control subjects and with nonpsychotic patients with bipolar disorder. It has been suggested that changes in the dopamine system are secondary to primary abnormalities in the serotonergic and norepinephrinergic systems.

Peyser and Folstein (1993) propose that when the caudate is damaged or caudate function is disrupted by lesions elsewhere in the brain, depression is often produced. This fits with the "subcortical triad" of depression, movement disorder, and dementia that often result from damage to the caudate and nearby structures

(Folstein et al., 1990; McHugh, 1990; Folstein et al., 1991). Mayberg (1993) found that stroke patients identified as having mood disorders and unilateral lesions restricted to the head of the caudate, with or without extension into the internal capsule, exhibited depression if the lesion was on the left and mania if it was on the right.

There is some evidence that the basal ganglia may be involved in schizophrenia (Buchsbaum, 1990; Liddle et al., 1992). Catatonia in schizophrenia may be related to cell loss and gliosis found in the globus pallidus (Falkai and Bogerts, 1993). In contrast other investigators have found an increase in size in the striatum and pallidum (Heckers et al., 1991), although more recent findings suggest that the increased size is due to the use of neuroleptics (Heckers, 1998).

Wilson disease is a neurodegenerative disorder that results from an abnormality in copper metabolism and manifests mainly through a movement disorder, psychiatric symptoms, and liver disease. The abnormal movements include rigidity, coarse proximal tremor, and choreoathetosis. Patients may have a facial expression of silliness or indifference, but their emotions are usually not affected. The disorder may start at an early age (7–15 years) or at a late age (after 30 years). Psychiatric symptoms include impulsiveness, irritability, and affective changes. The late form has been more closely associated with psychosis, usually of a paranoid type. In approximately 20% of patients, psychiatric symptoms precede other signs or symptoms of the disease (Lohr and Wisniewski, 1987).

The A1 allele of the D_2 dopamine receptor gene is dysfunctional in some cases of alcoholism. Variants of the D_2 dopamine receptor gene have been correlated with crack/cocaine dependency, obesity, carbohydrate binge eating, attention-deficit hyperactivity disorder, Tourette syndrome, pathological gambling, and smoking. The association of these various behavioral disorders with a single genetic anomaly supports the concept of a "reward deficiency syndrome" (Blum et al., 1996a, b).

Lesions in the striatum on the dominant side can cause atypical aphasias. This indicates a possible role of the basal ganglia in language. Neurological conditions that commonly accompany psychotic episodes suggest basal ganglia involvement.

In summary, evidence from several different sources indicates that the basal ganglia may be partially involved in the regulation of attentional and cognitive functions by correlating and integrating motor and sensory information. Both operate by way of a simple loop from the cortex down into the basal ganglia and back to the cortex (Figure 7.3). The motor loops are concerned with motor functions, whereas the limbic circuit is concerned with emotions. The filtering and gating functions of the basal ganglia appear to be used by both the motor and the limbic circuits.

Select bibliography

Bolam, J.P., Ingham, C.A., and Magill, P.J. (eds.) *The Basal Ganglia VIII. Advances in Behavioral Biology* (vol. 56). (New York: Springer Science and Business Media, 2005.)

Kandel, E.R., Schwartz, J.H., and Jessell, T.M. *Principles of Neural Science* (3rd ed.). (Norwalk CT: Appleton & Lange, 1991.)

Kultas-Ilinsky, K., and Llinsky, I.A. eds. *Basal Ganglia and Thalamus in Health and Movement Disorders*. (New York: Kluwer Academic/Plenum Publishers, 2001.)

Ma, T.P. The basal ganglia. In: D.E. Haines (ed.) *Fundamental Neuroscience*. (New York: Churchill Livingstone, 1997, pp. 363–378.)

Miguel, E.C., Rauch, S.L., and Leckman, J.F. *Psychiatric Clinics of North America: Neuropsychiatry of the Basal Ganglia* (vol. 20). (Philadelphia: Saunders, 1997.)

Moretti, R. ed. *Basal Ganglia and Thalamus: Their Role in Cognition and Behavior*. (New York: Nova Science, 2009.)

Nolte, J. *The Human Brain: An Introduction to Its Functional Anatomy*; Chapter 19, Basal Ganglia. (Philadelphia: Mosby/Elsevier, 2009.)

Weiner, W.J., and Lang, A.E. eds. *Behavioral Neurology of Movement Disorders. Advances in Neurology* (vol. 65). (New York: Raven Press, 1995.)

References

Alheid, G.F., and Heimer, L. 1996. Theories of basal forebrain organization and the "emotional motor system." In: G.Holstege, R.Bandler, and C.B.Saper (eds.) *The Emotional Motor System, Progress in Brain Research*, volume 107. New York: Elsevier, pp. 461–484.

Aldridge, J.W., and Berridge, K.C. 1998. Coding of serial order by neostriatal neurons: a "natural action" approach to movement sequence. *J. Neurosci.* **18**: 2777–2787.

Ames, D., Cummings, J.L., Wirshing, W.C., Quinn, B., and Mahler, M. 1994. Repetitive and compulsive behavior in frontal lobe degenerations. *J. Neuropsychiatry Clin. Neurosci.* **6**:100–113.

Baxter, L.R. Jr. 1992. Neuroimaging studies of obsessive compulsive disorder. *Psychiatr. Clin. North Am.* **15**: 871–884.

Baxter, L.R., Schwartz, J.M., Guze, B.H., Bergman, K., and Szuba, M.P. 1990. Neuroimaging in obsessive-compulsive disorder: Seeking the mediating neuroanatomy. In: M.A.Jenike, L.Baer, and W.E. Minichiello (eds.) *Obsessive-Compulsive Disorders: Theory and Management*. Littleton MA: Year Book Medical Publishers.

Bekar, L., Libionka, W., Tian, G., Xu, Q., Torres, A., Wang, X., Lovatt, D., Williams, E., Takano, T., Schnermann, J., Bakos, R., and Nedergaard, M. 2008. Adenosine is crucial for deep brain stimulation–mediated attenuation of tremor. *Nat. Med.* **14**:75–80.

Bhatia, K.P., and Marsden, C.D. 1994. The behavioural and motor consequences of local lesions of the basal ganglia in man. *Brain* **117**:859–876.

Blum, K., Cull, J.G., Braverman, E.R., and Comings, D.E.1996a. Reward deficiency syndrome. *Am. Sci.* **84**:132–145.

Blum, K., Sheridan, P.J., Wood, R.C., Braverman, E.R., Chen, T.J.H., Cull, J.G., and Comings, D.E.1996b. The D2 dopamine receptor gene as a determinant of reward deficiency syndrome. *J. R. Soc. Med.* **89**: 396–400.

Bogerts, B., Hantsch, J., and Herzer, M. 1983. A morphometric study of the dopamine-containing cell groups in the mesencephalon of normals, Parkinson patients, and schizophrenics. *Biol. Psychiatry* **18**: 951–969.

Buchsbaum, M.S. 1990. The frontal lobes, basal ganglia, and temporal lobes as sites for schizophrenia. *Schizophr. Bull.* **16**:379–389.

Burn, D., and Troster, A. 2004. Neuropsychiatric complications of medical and surgical therapies for Parkinson's disease. *J. Geriatr. Psychiatr. Neurol.* **17**: 172–180.

Burns, L.H., Annett, L., Kelley, A.E., Everitt, B.J., and Robbins, T.W. 1996. Effects of lesions to amygdala, ventral subiculum, medial prefrontal cortex, and nucleus accumbens on the reaction to novelty: Implication for limbic-striatal interactions. *Behav. Neurosci.* **110**:60–73.

Carbon, M., Ma, Y., Barnes, A., Dhawan, V., Chaly, T., Ghilardi, M.F., and Eidelberg, D. 2004. Caudate Nucleus: influence of dopaminergic input on sequence learning and brain activation in Parkinsonism. *Neuroimage* **21**:1497–1507.

Carboni, E., Silvagni, A., Rolando, M.T., and Di Chiara, G. 2000. Stimulation of in vivo dopamine transmission in the bed nucleus of stria terminalis by reinforcing drugs. *J. Neurosci.* **20**:RC102.

Casanova, M.F., Crapanzano, K.A., Mannheim, G., and Kruesi, M. 1995. Sydenham's chorea and schizophrenia: A case report. *Schizophr. Res.* **16**: 73–76.

Csernansky, J.G., and Bardgett, M.E. 1998. Limbic-cortical neuronal damage and the pathophysiology of schizophrenia. *Schizophr. Bull.* **24**:231–248.

Cummings, J.L. 1992. Depression and Parkinson's disease: A review. *Am. J. Psychiatry* **149**:443–454.

Decker, M.W., and McGaugh, J.L. 1991. The role of interactions between the cholinergic system and other neuromodulatory systems in learning and memory. *Synapse* 7:151–168.

DeLisi, L.E., Hoff, A.L., Schwartz, J.E., Shields, G.W., Halthore, S.N., Gupta, S.M., Henn, F.A., and Anand, A.K. 1991. Brain morphology in first-episode schizophrenic-like psychotic patients: A quantitative magnetic resonance imaging study. *Biol. Psychiatry* **29**:159–175.

deOlmos, J.S., and Heimer, L. 1999. The concepts of the ventral striatopallidal system and the extended amygdala. *Ann. N. Y. Acad. Sci.* **877**:1–32.

Ehmann, T.S., Beninger, R.J., Gawel, M.J., and Riopelle, R.J. 1990. Depressive symptoms in Parkinson's disease: A comparison with disabled control subjects. *J. Geriatr. Psychiatr. Neurol.* 1:3–9.

Falkai, P., and Bogerts, B., 1993. Cytoarchitectonic and developmental studies in schizophrenia. In: R.W.Kerwin (ed.) *Cambridge Medical Reviews: Neurobiology and Psychiatry*, vol. 2. Cambridge, England: Cambridge University Press, pp. 43–52.

Folstein, S.E., Folstein, M.F., and Starkstein, S.E. 1990. Diseases of the caudate as a model for a manic depressive disorder. In: A.J.Franks (ed.) *Function and Dysfunction in the Basal Ganglia*. Manchester: Manchester University Press, pp. 239–246.

Folstein, S.E., Peyser, C.E., Starkstein, S.E., and Folstein, M.F. 1991. The subcortical triad of Huntington's disease: A model for a neuropathology of depression, dementia and dyskinesia. In: B.J.Carroll and J.E.Barrett (eds.) *Psychopathology and the Brain*. New York: Raven Press, pp. 65–75.

George, M.S., Ketter, T.A., and Post, R.M. 1993. SPECT and PET imaging in mood disorders. *J. Clin. Psychiatry* **54**(Suppl. 11):6–13.

Gironell, A., Kulisevsky, J., Rami, L., Fortuny, N., Garcia-Sanchez, C., and Pascual-Sedano, B. 2003. Effects of pallidotomy and bilateral subthalamic stimulation on cognitive function in Parkinson disease. A controlled comparative study. *J. Neurol.* **250**:917–923.

Gray, J.A. 1998. Integrating schizophrenia. *Schizophr. Bull.* **24**:249–266.

Gray, J.A., Feldon, J., Rawlins, J.N.R., Hemsley, D.R., and Smith, A.D. 1991. The neuropsychology of schizophrenia. *Behav. Brain Res.* 14:1–20.

Graybiel, A.M. 1995. The basal ganglia. *Trends Neurosci.* **18**:60–62.

Graybiel, A.M. 1997. The basal ganglia and cognitive pattern generators. *Schizophr. Bull.* **23**:459–469.

Haber, S.N., and Fudge, J.L.1997a. The primate substantia nigra and VTA: Integrative circuitry and function. *Crit. Rev. Neurobiol.* **11**:323–342.

Haber, S.N., and Fudge, J.L.1997b. The interface between dopamine neurons and the amygdala: Implications for schizophrenia. *Schizophr. Bull.* **23**:471–482.

Heckers, S. 1998. Neuropathology of schizophrenia: Cortex, thalamus, basal ganglia, and neurotransmitter-specific projection systems. *Schizophr. Bull.* **23**:403–421.

Heckers, S., Heinsen, H., Heinsen, Y.C., and Beckmann, H. 1991. Cortex, white matter, and basal ganglia in schizophrenia: A volumetric postmortem study. *Biol. Psychiatry* **29**:556–566.

Heimer, L., Alheid, G.F., de Olmos, J.S., Groenewegen, H.J., Haber, S.N., Harlan, R.E., and Zahm, D.S. 1997. The accumbens: Beyond the core-shell dichotomy. *J. Neuropsychiatry Clin. Neurosci.* 9:354–381.

Herholz, K., Weisenbach, S., Zündorf, G., Lenz, O., Schröder, H., Bauer, B., Kalbe, E., and Heiss, W.-D. 2004. In vivo study of acetylcholine esterase in basal forebrain, amygdala, and cortex in mild to moderate Alzheimer disease. *Neuroimage* **21**:136–143.

Higuchi, Y., and Iacono, R.P. 2003. Surgical complications in patients with Parkinson's disease after posterioventral pallidotomy. *Neurosurgery* **52**:568–571.

Hikosaka, O., Nakamura, K., and Nakahara, H. 2006. Basal ganglia orient eyes to reward. *J. Neurophysiol.* **95**:567–584.

Houck, J., and Wise, S.P. 1995. Distributed modular architectures linking basal ganglia, cerebellum, and cerebral cortex: Their role in planning and controlling action. *Cereb. Cortex* **5**:95–110.

Hua, Z., Guodong, G., Qinchuan, L., Yaqun, A., Qinfen, W., and Xuelian, W. 2003. Analysis of complications of radiofrequency pallidotomy. *Neurosurgery* **52**:99–101.

Hyde, T.M., Stacey, M.E., Coppola, R.C., Handel, S.F., Rickler, K.C., and Weinberger, D.R. 1995. Cerebral morphometric abnormalities in Tourette's syndrome: A quantitative MRI study in monozygotic twins. *Neurology* **45**:1176–1182.

Insel, T.R., and Winslow, J.T. 1992. Neurobiology of obsessive compulsive disorder. *Psychiatr. Clin. North Am.* **15**:813–824.

Jellinger, K. 1988. The pedunculopontine nucleus in Parkinson's disease, progressive supranuclear palsy and Alzheimer's disease. *J. Neurol. Neurosurg. Psychiatry* **51**:540–543.

Jellinger, K. 1991. Pathology of Parkinson's disease: Changes other than the nigrostriatal pathway. *Mol. Chem. Neurpathol.* **14**:153–197.

Jones, B.E. 1990. Immunohistochemical study of choline acetyltrasferase-immunoreactive processes and cells innervating the pontomedullary reticular formation in the rat. *J. Comp. Neurol.* **295**:485–491.

Kalivas, P.W., and Duffy, P. 1998. Repeated cocaine administration alters extracellular glutamate in the ventral tegmental area. *J. Neurochem.* **70**:1497–1502.

Kapur, S., Mizrahi, R., and Li, M. 2005. From dopamine to salience to psychosis: Linking biology, pharmacology and phenomenology of psychosis. *Schizophr. Res.* **79**:59–68.

Kartsounis, L.D., Poynton, A., Bridges, P.K., and Bartlett, J.R. 1991. Neuro-psychological correlates of stereotactic subcaudate tractotomy. *Brain* **114**:2657–2673.

Keshavan, M.S., Rosenberg, D., Sweeney, J.A., and Pettegrew, J.W. 1998. Decreased caudate volume in neuroleptic-naive psychotic patients. *Am. J. Psychiatry* **155**:774–778.

Krauss, J.K. 2002. Deep brain stimulation for dystonia in adults. Overview and developments. *Stereotact. Funct. Neurosurg.* **78**:168–182.

Krishnan, K.R.R., McDonald, W.M., Escalona, P.R., Doraiswamy, P.M., Na, C., Husain, M.M., Figiel, G.S., Boyko, O.B., Ellinwood, E.H., and Nemeroff, C.B. 1992. Magnetic resonance imaging of the caudate nuclei in depression: Preliminary observations. *Arch. Gen. Psychiatry* **49**:553–557.

Lafer, B., Renshaw, P.F., and Sachs, G.S. 1997. Major depression and the basal ganglia. *Psychiatr. Clin. North Am.* **20**:885–896.

Latini, S., and Pedata, F. 2001. Adenosine in the central nervous system: release mechanisms and extracellular concentrations. *J. Neurochem.* **79**:463–484.

Lauterbach, E.C. 1999. The external globus pallidus in depression. *J. Neuropsychiatry Clin. Neurosci.* **11**:515–516.

Lauterbach, E.C., Jackson, J.G., Price, S.T., Wilson, A.N., Kirsh, A.D., and Dever, G.E.A. 1997. Clinical, motor, and biological correlates of depressive disorders after focal subcortical lesions. *J. Neuropsychiatry Clin. Neurosci.* **9**:259–266.

Leckman, J.F., Grice, D.E., Boardman, J., Zhang, H., Vitale, A., Bondi, C., Alsobrook, J., Peterson, B.S., Cohen, D.J., Rasmussen, S.A., Goodman, W.K., McDougle, C.J., and Pauls, D.L. 1997. Symptoms of obsessive-compulsive disorder. *Am. J. Psychiatry* **154**:911–917.

Liddle, P.F., Friston, K.J., Frith, C.D., Hirsch, S.R., Jones, T., and Frackowiak, R.S. 1992. Patterns of cerebral blood flow in schizophrenia. *Br. J. Psychiatry* **160**:179–186.

Little, K.Y., Zhang, L., Desmond, T., Frey, K.A., Dalach, G.W., and Cassin, B.J. 1999. Striatal dopaminergic abnormalities in human cocaine users. *Am. J. Psychiatry* **156**:238–245.

Lohr, J.B., and Wisniewski, A.A. 1987. *Movement Disorders; A Neuropsychiatric Approach*. New York: Guilford.

Lozano, A.M., Mayberg, H.S., Giacobbe, P., Hamani, C., Craddock, R.C., and Kennedy, S.H. 2008. Subcallosal cingulate gyrus deep brain stimulation for treatment-resistant depression. *Biol. Psychiatry* **64**:461–467.

Luxenberg, J.S., Swedo, S.E., Flament, M.F., Friedland, R.P., Rapoport, J., and Rapoport, S.I. 1988. Neuroanatomical abnormalities in obsessive-compulsive disorder determined with quantitative x-ray computed tomography. *Am. J. Psychiatry* **145**:1089–1093.

Ma, T.P. 1997. The basal ganglia. In: D.E.Haines (ed.) *Fundamental Neuroscience*. New York: Churchill Livingstone, pp. 363–378.

Mayberg, H.S. 1993. Neuroimaging studies of depression in neurologic disease. In: S.E.Starkstein, and R.G.Robinson (eds.) *Depression in Neurologic Disease*. Baltimore: Johns Hopkins Press, pp. 186–216.

Mayberg, H.S., Starkstein, S.E., Sadzot, B., Preziosi, T., Andrezejewski, P.L., Dannals, R.F., Wagner, H.N., Jr., and Robinson, R.G. 1990. Selective hypometabolism in the inferior frontal lobe in depressed patients with Parkinson's disease. *Ann. Neurol.* **28**:57–64.

Mayberg, H.S., Lozano, A.M., Voon, V., McNeely, H.E., Seminowicz, D., Hamani, C., Schwalb, J.M., and Kennedy, S.H. 2005. Deep brain stimulation for treatment-resistant depression. *Neuron* **45**:651–660.

McHugh, P.R. 1990. The basal ganglia: The region, the integration of its systems and implications for psychiatry and neurology. In: A.J.Franks (ed.) *Function and Dysfunction in the Basal Ganglia*. Manchester, England: Manchester University Press, pp. 259–269.

Mendez, M.F., Adams, N.L., and Skoog, K.M. 1989. Neurobehavioral changes associated with caudate lesions. *Neurology* **39**:349–354.

Mendez, M.F., O'Connor, S.M., and Gerald, T.H. 2004. Hypersexuality after right pallidotomy for Parkinson's disease. *J. Neuropsychiatry Clin. Neurosci.* **16**:37–40.

Menza, M.A., and Mark, M.H. 1994. Parkinson's disease and depression: The relationship to disability and personality. *J. Neuropsychiatry Clin. Neurosci.* **6**:165–169.

Mufson, E.J., Mash, D.C., and Hersh, L.B. 1988. Neurofibrillary tangles in cholinergic pedunculopontine neurons in Alzheimer's disease. *Ann. Neurol.* **24**:623–629.

Nakamura, K., and Hikosaka, O. 2006. Role of dopamine in the primate caudate nucleus in reward modulation of saccades. *J. Neurosci.* **26**:5360–5369.

Nakamura, T., Ghilardi, M.F., Mentis, M., Dhawan, V., Fukuda, M., Hacking, A., Moeller, J.R., Ghez, C., and Eidelberg, D. 2001. Functional networks in motor sequence learning: abnormal topographies in Parkinson's disease. *Hum. Brain Mapp.* **12**:42–60.

Nauta, W.J.H. 1958. Hippocampal projections and related neural pathways to the midbrain in the cat. *Brain* **81**:319–340.

Okubo, Y., Suhara, T., Suzuki, K., Kobayashi, K., Inoue, O., Terasaki, O., Someya, Y., Sassa, T., Sudo, Y., Matsushima, E., Iyo, M., Tateno, Y., and Toru, M. 1997. Decreased prefrontal dopamine D1 receptors in schizophrenia revealed by PET. *Nature* **385**:634–636.

Okun, M.S., Bakay, R.A.E., DeLong, M.R., and Vitek, J.L. 2003. Transient manic behavior after pallidotomy. *Brain Cogn.* **52**:281–283.

O'Sullivan, R.L., Rauch, S.L., Breitr, H.C., Grachev, I.D., Baer, L., Kennedy, D.N., Keuthen, N.J., Savage, C.R., Manzo, P.W., Caviness, V.S., and Jenike, M.A. 1997. Reduced basal ganglia volumes in trichotillomania measured via morphometric magnetic resonance imaging. *Biol. Psychiatry* **42**:39–45.

Pazos, A., and Palacios, J.M. 1985. Quantitative autoradiographic mapping of serotonin receptors in the rat brain, I: Serotonin-1 receptors. *Brain Res.* **346**:205–230.

Pazos, A., Cortes, R., and Palacios, J.M. 1985. Quantitative autoradiographic mapping of serotonin receptors in the rat brain, II: Serotonin-2 receptors. *Brain Res.* **346**:231–249.

Pearlson, G.D., Wong, D.F., Tune, L.E., Ross, C.A., Chase, G.A., Links, J.M., Dannals, R.F., Wilson, A.A., Ravert, H.T., Wagner, H.N., and DePaulo, J.R. 1995. In vivo D2 dopamine receptor density in psychotic and nonpsychotic patients with bipolar disorder. *Arch. Gen. Psychiatry* **52**:471–477.

Peterson, B.S., Thomas, P., Kane, M.J., Scahill, L., Zhang, H., Bronen, R., King, R.A., Leckman, J.F., and Staib, L. 2003. Basal ganglia volumes in patients with Gilles de las tournette syndrome. *Arch. Gen. Psychiatry* **60**:415–424.

Peyser, C.E., and Folstein, S.E. 1993. Depression in Huntington disease. In: S.E.Starkstein and R.G.Robinson (eds.) *Depression in Neurologic Disease.* Baltimore: Johns Hopkins Press, pp. 117–138.

Price, D.L., Whitehouse, P.J., Struble, R.G., Clark, A.W., Coyle, J.T., DeLong, M.R., and Hedreen, J.C. 1982. Basal forebrain cholinergic systems in Alzheimer's disease and related dementia. *Neurosciences* **1**:84–92.

Price, L.H., Spencer, D.D., Marek, K.L., Robbins, R.J., Leranth, C., Farhi, A., Naftolin, F., Roth, R.H., Bunney, B.S., Hoffer, P.B., Makuch, R., and Redmond, D.E. Jr. 1995. Psychiatric status after human fetal mesencephalic tissue transplantation in Parkinson's disease. *Biol. Psychiatry* **38**:498–505.

Rapoport, J.L. 1991. Basal ganglia dysfunction as a proposed cause of obsessive-compulsive disorder. In: B.J.Carroll and J.E.Barrett (eds.) *Psychopathology and the Brain.* New York: Raven Press, pp. 77–95.

Rapoport, J.L., and Fiske, A. 1998. The new biology of obsessive-compulsive disorder: Implications for evolutionary psychology. *Perspec. Biol. Med.* **41**:159–175.

Redgrave, P., and Gurney, K. 2006. The short-latency dopamine signal: A role in discovering novel actions? *Nat. Rev. Neurosci.* **7**:967–975.

Roane, D.M., Yu, M. Feinberg, T.E., and Rogers, J.D. 2002. Hypersexuality after pallidal surgery in Parkinson disease. *Neuropsychiatry Neuropsychol. Behav. Neurol.* **15**:247–251.

Robinson, D., Wu, H., Munne, R.A., Ashtari, M., Alvir, J., Ma, J., Lerner, G., Koreen, A., Cole, K., and Bogerts, B. 1995. Reduced caudate nucleus volume in obsessive-compulsive disorder. *Arch. Gen. Psychiatry* **52**:393–398.

Ryan, L., Martone, M., Linder, J., and Groves, P. 1990. Histological and ultrastructural evidence that d-amphetamine causes degeneration in neostriatum and frontal cortex of man. *Brain Res.* **518**:67–77.

Salloway, S., and Cummings, J. 1994. Subcortical disease and neuro-psychiatric illness. *J. Neuropsychiatry* **6**:93–97.

Savage, C. 1997. Neuropsychology of subcortical dementias. *Psychiatr. Clin. North Am.* **20**:911–933.

Saxena, S., Brody, A.L., Schwartz, J.M., and Baxter, L.R. 1998. Neuroimaging and frontal-subcortical circuitry in obsessive-compulsive disorder. *Br. J. Psychiatry* **173**(Suppl. 35):26–37.

Schultz, S.K., Miller, D.D., Arndt, S., Ziebell, S., Gupta, S., and Andreasen, N.C. 1995. Withdrawal-emergent dyskinesia in patients with schizophrenia during antipsychotic discontinuation. *Biol. Psychiatry* **38**:713–719.

Schultz, W. 1998. Predictive reward signal of dopamine neurons. *J. Neurophysiol.* **80**:1–27.

Schwartz, J.M., Stoessel, P.W., Baxter, L.R., Jr., Martin, K.M., and Phelps, M.E. 1996. Systematic changes in cerebral glucose metabolic rate after successful behavior modification treatment of obsessive-compulsive disorder. *Arch. Gen. Psychiatry* **53**:109–113.

Singer, H.S. 1997. Neurobiology of Tourette syndrome. *Neurol. Clin. North Am.* **15**:357–379.

Singer, H.S., Reiss, A.L., Brown, J.E., Aylwar, E.H., Shih, B., Chee, B., Harris, E.L., Reader, M.J., Chase, G.A., and Bryan, R.N. 1993. Volumetric MRI changes in basal ganglia of children with Tourette's syndrome. *Neurology* **43**:950–956.

Smeding, H., Speelman, J., Koning-Haanstra, M., Esselink, R.A.J., de Bie, R.M.A., de Haan, Lenders, W.P.M., Nijssen, C.G., Staal, J., Smeding, H.M.M., Schuurman, P.R. Bosch, D.A., and Speelman, J.D. 2006. Neuropsychological effects of bilateral STN stimulation in Parkinson disease: A controlled study. *Neurology* **66**:1830–1836.

Sofroniew, M.V., Pearson, R.C., Eckenstein, F., Cuello, A.C., and Powell, T.P. 1983. Retrograde changes in cholinergic neurons in the basal forebrain of the rat following cortical damage. *Brain Res.* **289**:370–374.

Starkstein, S.E., and Mayberg, H.S. 1993. Depression in Parkinson disease. In: S.E.Starkstein and R.G.Robinson (eds.) *Depression in Neurologic Disease*. Baltimore: Johns Hopkins Press, pp. 97–116.

Starkstein, S.E., Robinson, R.G., and Price, T.R. 1987. Comparison of cortical and subcortical lesions in the production of post-stroke mood disorders. *Brain* **110**:1045–1059.

Steckler, T., Inglis, W., Winn, P., and Sahgal, A. 1994. The pedunculopontine tegmental nucleus: A role in cognitive processes?*Brain Res. Rev.* **19**:298–318.

Swedo, S.E., and Leonard, H.L. 1992. Trichotillomania: An obsessive compulsive spectrum disorder? *Psychiatr. Clin. North Am.* **151**:777–790.

Torack, R.M., and Morris, J.C. 1988. The association of ventral tegmental area histopathology with adult dementia. *Arch. Neurol.* **45**:497–501.

Wainer, B.H., and Mesulam, M.M. 1990. Ascending cholinergic pathways in the rat brain. In: M.Steriade and D.Biesold (eds.) *Brain Cholinergic Systems*. Oxford, England: Oxford University Press, pp. 65–199.

Weinberger, D.R. 1987. Implications of normal brain development for the pathogenesis of schizophrenia. *Arch. Gen. Psychiatry* **44**:660–669.

Williams, S.M., and Goldman-Rakic, P.S. 1998. Widespread origin of primate mesofrontal dopamine system. *Cerebr. Cortex* **8**:321–345.

Winn, P., Brown, V.J., and Inglis, W.L. 1997. On the relationships between the striatum and the pedunculopontine nucleus. *Crit. Rev. Neurobiol.* **11**:241–261.

Wolf, S.S., Jones, D.W., Knable, M.B., Gorey, J.G., Lee, K.S., Hyde, T.M., Coppola, R., and Weinberger, D.R. 1996. Tourette syndrome: Prediction of phenotypic variation in monozygotic twins by caudate nucleus D2 receptor binding. *Science* **273**:1225–1227.

Yank, M., Yazgan, B.P., Wexler, B.E., and Leckman, J.F. 1994. Behavioral laterality in individual with Gilles de la Tourette's syndrome and basal ganglia alterations: A preliminary report. *Biol. Psychiatry* **38**:386–390.

Zhao, M., Momma, S., Delfani, K., Carlén, M., Cassidy, R.M., Johansson, C.B., Brismar, H., Shupliakov, O., Frisén, J., and Janson, A.M. 2003. Evidence for neurogenesis in the adult mammalian substantia nigra. *Proc. Natl. Acad. Sci. USA.* **100**:7925–7930.

Diencephalon: Hypothalamus and epithalamus

Hypothalamus

The hypothalamus is the region of the mammalian brain that is most important in the coordination of behaviors essential for the maintenance and continuation of the species. Although the hypothalamus occupies only about 0.15% of the volume of the human brain, it plays a major role in the regulation and release of hormones from the pituitary gland, maintenance of body temperature, and organization of goal-seeking behaviors such as feeding, drinking, mating, and aggression. It is the primary center for the control of autonomic function. It also is the region of the brain that is essential for behavioral adjustments to changes in the internal or external environment (Figure 8.1). The hypothalamus is a very old structure with striking similarity between humans and lower animals. It is made up of a number of nuclei and scattered cell groups. Some hypothalamic cell groups control specific functions (e.g., blood pressure, heart rate, etc.) through the coordinated action of short intrahypothalamic connections. Other nuclei operate by projections to structures outside the confines of the hypothalamus.

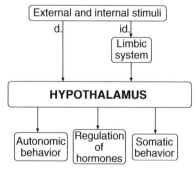

Figure 8.1. The hypothalamus is positioned between incoming sensory signals and the body's response to those signals. Some sensory signals arrive directly (d.) from the sensory receptor. Other sensory signals are processed through higher centers and are considered indirect (id.). Output may involve only internal controls (e.g., change in heart rate) or may be more complex (e.g., eating behavior).

Anatomy and behavioral considerations

The hypothalamus lies on either side of the walls of the third ventricle below the level of the hypothalamic sulcus (Figures 8.2, 9.2, 9.3, and 14.6). It is bounded in front (anteriorly) by the lamina terminalis and optic chiasm, laterally by the optic tracts, and behind by the mammillary bodies. Some hypothalamic nuclei are continuous across the floor of the third ventricle. On the bottom (ventral surface) of the hypothalamus is the infundibulum, to which the pituitary (hypophysis) is attached. The median eminence forms the floor of the third ventricle and is the staging area from which the hypothalamic releasing factors leave to enter the hypothalamohypophyseal portal system (Figure 8.2). The borders of the individual hypothalamic nuclei are often indistinct and the location of some borders varies from author to author. Some hypothalamic subdivisions are referred to as areas or zones because of the difficulty in establishing distinct borders.

Hamann et al. (2004) found that the hypothalamus and amygdala showed greater activity bilaterally in men than women when viewing identical sexual stimuli even when the females reported greater arousal.

The organization of the hypothalamus can be simplified by viewing it as made up of one area and three zones (Figure 8.3). The preoptic area makes up the anterior (rostral) portion of the hypothalamus. Its major components are the medial and lateral preoptic nuclei (Figure 8.4). The thin periventricular zone lies just inside the walls of the third ventricle and makes up the most medial of the three zones. The medial zone contains the majority of the hypothalamic nuclei (Figure 8.5). The separation between the medial and lateral zones is formed by the fibers of the fornix. The lateral zone contains incoming axons from limbic and other structures. The lateral zone also contains the nerve cell bodies that give rise to many of the axons that leave the hypothalamus. The medial forebrain bundle is a diffuse fiber system that passes through the lateral

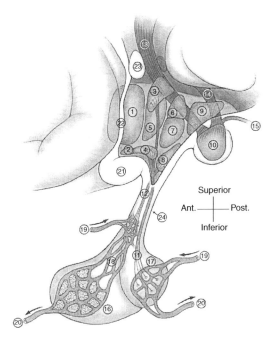

Hypothalamic nuclei:
1. Preoptic
2. Suprachiasmatic
3. Paraventricular
4. Supraoptic
5. Anterior
6. Dorsomedial
7. Ventromedial
8. Arcuate
9. Posterior
10. Mamillary

Tracts:
11. Hypothalamohypophyseal
12. Tuberohypophyseal
13. Column of fornix
14. Mammillothalamic

Other structures:
15. Mammillotegmental tr.
16. Anterior pituitary
17. Posterior pituitary
18. Hypophyseal portal system
19. Hypophyseal arteries
20. Hypophyseal veins
21. Optic chiasm
22. Lamina terminalis
23. Anterior commissure
24. Infundibulum

Figure 8.2. A three-dimensional view of the medial zone of the hypothalamus showing the principal nuclei and surrounding structures. (Reproduced by permission from Young, P.A., and Young, P.H. 1997. Basic Clinical Anatomy. Baltimore: Williams & Wilkins.)

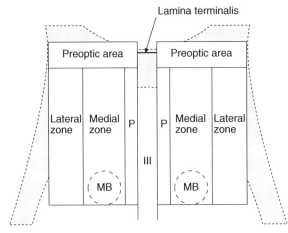

Figure 8.3. The hypothalamus viewed from above consists of the preoptic area in front and three parallel zones behind. From the cavity of the third ventricle (III) moving laterally are the periventricular zone (P), the medial zone, and the lateral zone. The medial zone is further subdivided and includes the mammillary bodies (MB). The optic nerve, chiasm, and optic tract are shown by the dotted lines.

zone interconnecting structures above and below with the hypothalamus.

The pituitary is made up of the posterior lobe and the anterior lobe (nos. 17 and 16, respectively, Figure 8.2). The posterior lobe of the pituitary is innervated directly by neurons whose cell bodies lie in the hypothalamus. The axons from these neurons make up the hypothalamohypophyseal tract (no. 11,

Figure 8.2). Neurotransmitters (vasopressin and oxytocin) from these neurons are released directly into capillaries located in the posterior lobe of the pituitary. The anterior lobe is controlled indirectly via "releasing substances." Neurotransmitters (releasing substances) from many of the hypothalamic nuclei enter into the hypophyseal portal system to be passed downstream to the anterior lobe of the pituitary, where they control the release of many anterior pituitary lobe hormones (Table 8.1).

There are both monosynaptic (direct) and polysynaptic (indirect) inputs to the hypothalamus (Figure 8.1). Both inputs reflect sensory signals from internal (visceral) and external (somatosensory) domains (Figure 8.6). Several monosynaptic pathways arise from within the dorsal horn of the spinal cord and from within the trigeminal spinal nucleus. These fibers project directly to many areas of the hypothalamus. The monosynaptic pathways provide a route for reflex autonomic and endocrine behaviors (Katter *et al.*, 1991). These behaviors include heart rate change in response to pain, shivering in response to cold, milk letdown in response to suckling, and so forth.

Polysynaptic pathways receive sensory signals that are relayed from spinal cord and brainstem autonomic nuclei (e.g., solitary and parabrachial nuclei). These afferent signals are processed through structures such as the amygdala, nucleus accumbens, and

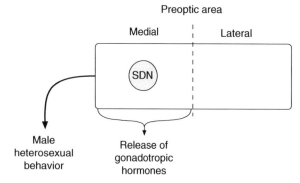

Figure 8.4. The medial preoptic nucleus produces luteinizing hormone-releasing hormone and influences motor behaviors. SDN, sexually dimorphic nucleus.

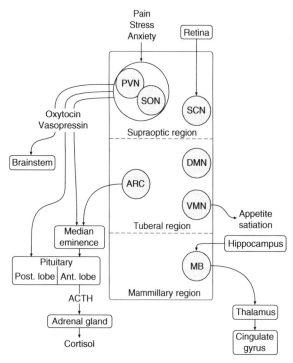

Figure 8.5. The medial hypothalamic zone is rich in nuclei. Efferents link the medial zone of the hypothalamus with the pituitary and with other brain centers. Oxytocin/vasopressin from the PVN/SON follow three separate pathways. ACTH, adrenocorticotropic hormone; ARC, arcuate nucleus; MB, mammillary body; PVN, paraventricular nucleus; SON, supraoptic nucleus; SCN, suprachiasmatic nucleus; DMN, dorsomedial nucleus; VMN, ventromedial nucleus.

limbic association cortex before being relayed to the hypothalamus. Polysynaptic pathways are responsible for behaviors such as sleep, food intake, freezing and flight, and affects such as depression, rage, and fear (Burstein, 1996).

Preoptic hypothalamic area

The preoptic area (no. 1, Figure 8.2) includes the medial and lateral preoptic nuclei (Figure 8.4). Many neurons in the preoptic area and nearby anterior hypothalamus contain both androgen and estrogen receptors. Stimulation of these areas has been shown to initiate sexual behavior in animals. Lesions of the preoptic area reduce or abolish copulatory behavior in many species (Van de Poll and Van Goozen, 1992).

Fibers that project to the medial preoptic area arise in the cingulate cortex, hippocampus, septum, and lateral habenular nucleus. These are all limbic structures (Corodimas *et al.*, 1993). The medial preoptic area receives input from the olfactory system by way of the amygdala and the stria terminalis and projects heavily to the periaqueductal gray of the midbrain and to the anterior ventral medulla. Both of these brainstem areas have been implicated in the control of incoming pain signals, in sexual behavior, and in the initiation of maternal and defensive/aggressive behaviors (Shipley *et al.*, 1996). It is hypothesized that this pathway is important in the olfactory cues related to these behaviors.

One or more nuclei found within the medial preoptic area are sexually dimorphic in animals; however, the concept remains controversial in the human (Martin, 1996). One cluster of neurons is called the sexually dimorphic nucleus (SDN). It is also known as INAH1 (interstitial nucleus of the anterior hypothalamus, number 1). It contains at birth only about 20% of the number of neurons that are seen at 2–4 years of age. After 4 years, the cell number decreases in girls but remains constant in boys. No difference in cell number in the SDN is seen between homosexual and heterosexual men (Swaab *et al.*, 1995). The anterior nucleus (Figure 8.2), sometimes described as INAH3, is also sexually dimorphic (LeVay, 1991; LeVay and Hamer, 1994). It is larger in the male and contains approximately twice the number of neurons in adult male than in adult female humans. However, Friedman and Downey (1993) reported the size to be similar on average when comparing the brains of male homosexuals and female heterosexuals. Before birth the anterior nucleus is similar in size in both male and female rats. It is smaller in male offspring of rats that are stressed while pregnant. It is larger in sexually active male rats. Many of the cells of INAH3 die in the female shortly after birth. However, testosterone present from 4 days before until 10 days following birth protects these neurons from cell death in the male rat. Differential

Table 8.1. Hypothalamic releasing hormones and their actions on the anterior pituitary.

Releasing hormone	Action on anterior pituitary
Corticotropin-releasing hormone (CRH)	Stimulates secretion of adrenocorticotropic hormone (ACTH)
Thyrotropin-releasing hormone (TRH)	Stimulates secretion of thyroid-stimulating hormone (TSH)
Gonadotropin-releasing hormone (GnRH), Luteinizing hormone-releasing hormone (LHRH)	Stimulate secretion of follicle-stimulating hormone (FSH) and luteinizing hormone (LH)
Growth hormone-releasing hormone (GHRH)	Stimulates secretion of growth hormone (GH)
Somatostatin, somatotropin release-inhibiting hormone (SRIH)	Inhibits secretion of growth hormone (GH)
Dopamine	Inhibits biosynthesis and secretion of prolactin (PRL)

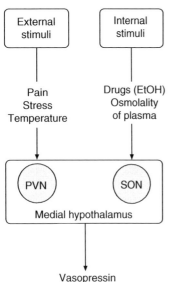

Figure 8.6. Both external and internal stimuli can affect the release of hormones controlled by the hypothalamus. In this example the output of vasopressin (antidiuretic hormone) is increased by heat and dehydration and decreased by pain, stress, and alcohol. PVN, paraventricular nucleus; SON, supraoptic nucleus; EtOH, ethyl alcohol.

Activity in the medial preoptic area increases in the male monkey during sexual arousal but decreases during copulation and ceases after ejaculation. A lesion of the medial preoptic area produces a major reduction in female-directed sexual behavior, although the capacity for masturbation continues. Electrical stimulation of the medial preoptic area initiates sexual behavior only if a receptive female is available. The medial preoptic area shows the greatest testosterone uptake of any region of the brain. Efferent connections from the medial preoptic area include projections to the dorsomedial hypothalamic nucleus and to brainstem areas linked with penile erection. Stimulation of the medial preoptic area in the female rat inhibits lordosis. In contrast, stimulation in the male rat induces copulation (Marson and McKenna, 1994).

Periventricular hypothalamic zone

The periventricular zone is a thin layer that lies just lateral to the ependymal cells that form the lining of the third ventricle. This zone is important in regulating the release of hormones from the anterior pituitary.

Medial hypothalamic zone

The medial hypothalamic zone includes the majority of the well-defined nuclei of the hypothalamus (Figures 8.2 and 8.5). Several important regions in this zone include, from front to back, the supraoptic, the tuberal, and the mammillary regions. In addition to containing important nuclei, the tuberal region is continuous below with the infundibular stalk of the pituitary gland.

Supraoptic region

The supraoptic region is located directly above the optic chiasm and includes the supraoptic, the paraventricular, and the suprachiasmatic nuclei (Figures 8.2

cell death accounts for the sexual dimorphism of this nucleus. These same neurons in human females begin to undergo programmed death at about 4 years of age.

The medial preoptic area contains neurons that produce luteinizing hormone-releasing hormone. In the pituitary, this releasing hormone regulates the level of gonadotropins. The medial preoptic area plays an important role in maternal behavior (Numan and Sheenan, 1997). Surgical or chemical lesions of the medial preoptic area severely disrupt the induction as well as the maintenance of maternal behavior (DeVries and Villalba, 1997). The ventral tegmental area (Chapter 7) may be the target of fibers that arise from the medial preoptic area (Numan and Smith, 1984; Hansen and Ferreira, 1986).

The medial preoptic area is also critical in the expression of male-typical heterosexual behavior.

and 8.5). Clusters of magnocellular neurons within the supraoptic and paraventricular nuclei produce oxytocin and vasopressin. The paraventricular nucleus consists of one subdivision that projects to the median eminence and a second subdivision that projects to the posterior pituitary. A third subdivision, which also produces oxytocin and vasopressin, projects to brainstem and to spinal cord autonomic nuclei. The axons from the third subdivision enter the medial forebrain bundle and descend in the dorsolateral brainstem. Axons of some neurons pass through the infundibular stalk to terminate on capillaries in the posterior lobe of the pituitary. When these neurons depolarize, their neurotransmitter (oxytocin or vasopressin) is released directly into the bloodstream. These neurons receive input from brainstem autonomic nuclei (solitary nucleus) and from circumventricular organs. The latter are vascular neural structures that lack the blood–brain barrier. One of these, the subfornical region located in the wall of the third ventricle, sends axons that terminate in the hypothalamus. It is presumed that the circumventricular organs sense osmolality and bloodborne chemicals. Many areas of the hypothalamus are sensitive to hormones. Some hormones cross the blood–brain barrier, and others bind to intracellular receptors.

Other neurons in the paraventricular nucleus that also produce oxytocin and vasopressin project to limbic structures, including the amygdala and hippocampus. Descending fibers project to the brainstem to terminate in the locus ceruleus and in the raphe nuclei (Chapter 10). Some oxytocin axons extend to the spinal cord where they terminate on presynaptic neurons of the sympathetic nervous system (Sofroniew, 1983).

Oxytocin release causes contraction of the smooth muscles of the uterus during childbirth as well as contraction of the myoepithelial cells of the mammary gland during nursing. Surprisingly, the number of oxytocin-producing cells is about the same in the female and male. Intraventricular injection of oxytocin in the female rat rapidly stimulates maternal behavior (Pedersen and Prange, 1979). In contrast, oxytocin infusion in males results in an increase in nonsexual social interaction (Witt, 1997). Receptors for oxytocin in both the medial preoptic area of the hypothalamus and the ventral tegmental area of the midbrain are critical for the postpartum onset of maternal behavior in the rat. The oxytocin-producing neurons are located in the lateral preoptic area and in the paraventricular nucleus. Proximal separation of rat pups from their mothers (i.e., the pups remain in olfactory and auditory contact) markedly depletes oxytocin levels in the mothers. It is speculated that stimuli that reactivate the mechanisms of attachment between mother and offspring contribute to the sense of longing and other strong emotions that accompany the loss of a close relationship in humans (Pedersen, 1997). These emotions may be related to a reduction in the level of oxytocin. Oxytocin released by the paraventricular nucleus may play a role in the sedation, relaxation, and decreased sympathoadrenal activity at the hypothalamic level that occurs during friendly social interaction (Uvnas-Moberg, 1997).

There appears to be a central dysregulation of vasopressin secretion in patients with anorexia nervosa (Demitrack and Gold, 1988). The number of vasopressin- and oxytocin-expressing neurons in the paraventricular nucleus of patients with mood disorder is significantly increased (Purba et al., 1996). An increase in both vasopressin and oxytocin was reported in bulimic patients (Demitrack et al., 1990). The levels of vasopressin and oxytocin are altered in the cerebrospinal fluid of depressed patients (Legros et al., 1993). No correlation has been found between the extent of the depressive symptomatology and the level of reduction of vasopressin (Gjerris, 1990).

The suprachiasmatic nucleus (Figures 8.2 and 8.5) is found in the supraoptic region of the medial zone. It lies just above the optic chiasm and just below and lateral to the supraoptic nucleus. The suprachiasmatic nucleus is critical in controlling the day–night circadian rhythm of the body and functions as the "master clock." It receives primary visual afferents from the retina and secondary afferents from the lateral geniculate body of the visual system. The suprachiasmatic nucleus has intimate connections with the pineal gland and plays a key role in circadian functions as well as in seasonal function (Pevet et al., 1996; Reuss, 1996).

The suprachiasmatic nucleus may be related to seasonal fluctuations in mood (seasonal affective disorder or SAD), and the number of vasopressin-expressing neurons is greatest in October and November, when the incidence of depression is greatest (Hofman et al., 1993). Exposure to prolonged periods of light following transportation to a distant time zone can facilitate recovery from jet lag. More specifically, exposure to bright light in the morning delays the light–dark cycle (phase advance), whereas exposure to bright light in the evening advances this cycle (phase delay). Most SAD patients with winter depression experience abnormal phase delays and therefore respond positively to bright morning light. The bright light itself is not an antidepressant, but the reversal of the abnormal phase delay acts as an antidepressant (Lewy and Sack, 1996).

Tuberal region

The arcuate nucleus (Figures 8.2 and 8.5) as well as other hypothalamic nuclei contain neurons that produce various release and release-inhibiting hormones. These include gonadotropin-releasing hormone, luteinizing hormone-releasing hormone, and corticotropin-releasing hormone (CRH). The close connections between the hypothalamus, the pituitary, and the adrenal gland are recognized as the hypothalamic–pituitary–adrenal (HPA) axis. CRH is responsible for triggering the release of adrenocorticotropic hormone (ACTH) from the anterior lobe of the pituitary gland. Abnormalities in the HPA axis have been linked to several disorders.

The neurons of the paraventricular nucleus that control the HPA are strongly activated in depression (Raadsheer et al., 1994). Excessive ACTH secretion and a concomitant increase in cortisol by the adrenal cortex are seen in 40%–60% of depressed patients, primarily during afternoon and evening hours. The hypersecretion of cortisol is not dependent on stress. The synthetic corticosteroid dexamethasone, when administered to normal individuals, suppresses CRH. HPA activity can be assessed by measures of cortisol in the blood, urine, saliva, and in cerebrospinal fluid (DeMoranville and Jackson, 1996). When synthetic corticosteroid dexamethasone is administered to depressed patients during the evening, approximately 40% show no decline in cortisol levels. Improvement in the dexamethasone suppression test is seen in successful antidepressant treatment (Holsboer-Trachsler et al., 1991).

Subtle alterations in HPA function have been observed in patients with panic disorder (Abelson and Curtis, 1996). Weinstock (1997) hypothesized that prenatal stress impairs the ability of the child's HPA to cope in novel situations.

The periventricular hypothalamus, the arcuate nucleus, and other hypothalamic regions that produce CRH represent the origin of the HPA axis. The regulation of the HPA axis depends on three major factors. First, the pulsatile release of CRH is under the control of the suprachiasmatic nucleus. Second, psychological and physical stresses are mediated by way of pathways from the brainstem and limbic system to the hypothalamus. Third, circulating levels of glucocorticoids are sensed by the hypothalamus in a negative feedback mechanism that regulates the output of CRH. The hippocampus also has many glucocorticoid receptors and appears to play an important role in monitoring stress and regulating the production and release of CRH by the hypothalamus. Exposure to stress downregulates glucocorticoid receptors in both the hippocampus and hypothalamus. Therefore, the feedback receptors are less sensitive to circulating glucocorticoids and the hypothalamus secretes inordinately high levels of CRH (Herman et al., 1995). The separation of partners which show signs of emotional attachment, activates the HPA axis, whereas separation of partners which show little emotional attachment has little or no effect on the HPA (Hennessy, 1997). Significantly decreased bone density in women with depression is consistent with dysfunction of the HPA axis (Michelson et al., 1996).

Many neurons in the arcuate nucleus produce β-endorphin. This peptide is known to play an important role in the control of pain. In addition, some of these same neurons project to the periaqueductal gray, which is a midbrain region known to function in the suppression of incoming pain signals (Chapter 10). The arcuate nucleus and its connections with the paraventricular nucleus also are a hypothalamic pathway involved in the control of body weight. This pathway may be the target of the hormone leptin, which is secreted by fat cells (Horvath, 2005; Schwartz and Seeley, 1997). A nucleus adjacent to the arcuate nucleus (the periventricular nucleus) produces dopamine, which inhibits prolactin release.

Abnormal levels of endorphins have been reported in the hypothalamic tissue of schizophrenia patients. Both "endorphin excess" and "endorphin deficiency" hypotheses of schizophrenia have been proposed (Wiegant et al., 1992). Goldstein et al. (2007) found that the total hypothalamic volume was increased in patients with schizophrenia and in nonpsychotic relatives. The increase was greater in the region of the paraventricular nuclei and mammillary body and correlated positively with anxiety. These findings suggest a relationship between schizophrenia and the high rate of endocrine disorders.

Neurons located in the arcuate (infundibular) nucleus of the medial zone are hypertrophied in postmenopausal women. Some cells of the arcuate nucleus are sensitive to circulating levels of estrogen and regulate the activity of substance P-producing neurons found there. Substance P production in neurons in the arcuate nucleus varies with the sexual cycle and may regulate the release of gonadotropin-releasing hormone from the hypothalamus into the hypophyseal portal system. It has been hypothesized that an increase in the pulsatile release of substance P may coincide with menopausal flushes (Rance, 1992).

The dorsomedial nucleus (Figures 8.2 and 8.5) lies immediately above the ventromedial nucleus. Stimulation of the dorsomedial nucleus in laboratory animals produces unusually aggressive behavior that lasts only as long as the stimulus is present. This aggressive behavior is known as sham rage and can be produced by stimulation in other regions of the hypothalamus.

The ventromedial nucleus (Figures 8.2 and 8.5) lies near the midline just anterior to the mammillary bodies. It receives input from the amygdala. It projects heavily to the magnocellular nuclei of the basal forebrain including the basal nucleus (of Meynert). These nuclei in turn project to all areas of the cerebral cortex. The ventromedial nucleus has been described in the past as the satiety center. It regulates the amount of food consumed in order to maintain a normal body weight. It is interconnected with the lateral hypothalamic zone (see the following section), which has been described in the past as the hunger center. The concept of hunger and satiety centers is a convenient concept. Feeding control is probably more complex than this comparison would imply, however, and involves a number of additional structures (Kupfermann, 1991).

Clinical vignette

A 36-year-old man was found to have an anterior hypothalamic tumor when he was evaluated for a 65-lb weight gain, hallucinations, paranoid delusions, and confusion. After surgical removal of the tumor, he became apathetic and akinetic mutism developed. He responded well to treatment with dopamine agonists (bromocriptine) (Ross and Stewart, 1981). The case suggests that akinesia may be related to loss of dopaminergic input to anterior cingulate or other frontal lobe regions. The postsurgical clinical picture may have been produced by damage to the mesolimbic/mesocortical dopamine fibers. These fibers are found within the medial forebrain bundle, which courses from the ventral tegmental area to the cingulate cortex and passes through the lateral hypothalamic zone.

A lesion of the ventromedial nucleus results in appetite disorders and marked increase in body weight. Stereotactic lesions of the ventromedial nucleus have been used in an attempt to treat alcoholism, drug addiction, and hypersexuality. Increase in body weight is a common side effect of these lesions (Nadvornik et al., 1975).

The ventrolateral portion of the ventromedial nucleus is responsible for typical female sexual behavior. Stimulation of this area produces lordosis in rats. The ventromedial nucleus is a site of action of estrogen and progesterone hormones. Projections from the ventromedial nucleus to the periaqueductal gray may be the route by which this region of the hypothalamus induces sexual behavior (Pfaff et al., 1994).

A number of nuclei in the hypothalamus have receptor sites for estrogen. Under experimental conditions food intake is increased when estrogen levels decrease. There is evidence that during the second half of the menstrual cycle when estrogen levels drop there is also an increase in food intake and preference for carbohydrates (Bray, 1992).

The mammillary bodies and the cells of the posterior hypothalamic nucleus that lie dorsal to the mammillary bodies mark the posterior (caudal) extent of the medial hypothalamus. The largest number of afferents to the mammillary bodies come from the hippocampus by way of the fornix (nos. 20 and 2, respectively, Figure 13.5). This connection with the hippocampus suggests that the mammillary bodies are also involved in emotion as well as memory. For example, the mammillary bodies have been implicated in penile erection (Segraves, 1996). Fibers from the mammillary bodies ascend to the anterior nucleus of the thalamus and make up the mammillothalamic tract (no. 8, Figure 13.5). The anterior nucleus of the thalamus is a major component of the limbic thalamus (Figure 9.2). Cell loss is seen in the mammillary bodies as well as in the mediodorsal nucleus of the thalamus in alcoholic Wernicke–Korsakoff syndrome (Delis and Lucas, 1996; Sechi and Serra, 2007).

Lateral hypothalamic zone and medial forebrain bundle

The lateral zone contains several groups of cells, the largest of which is the tuberomammillary nucleus, which extends in a posterior direction lateral to and below the mammillary body. The lateral tuberal nuclei consist of two or three sharply delineated cell groups that often produce small visible bumps on the basal surface of the hypothalamus. The medial forebrain bundle courses through the lateral zone and makes delineation of specific nuclei difficult. Axons from the limbic system terminate in the lateral zone, which, in turn, integrates and relays the signals to other parts of the hypothalamus as well as to the midbrain. Of particular significance are projections from the infralimbic area of the cingulate cortex (Chapter 12). This is a key route by which the visceral motor cortex (infralimbic area) influences autonomic tone, and the lateral zone is believed to be important as an integrative center for ingestive behavior (Bernardis and Bellinger, 1996; Saper, 1996).

The lateral zone has been described as the hunger center. A lesion placed in this zone will eliminate an animal's motivation to seek food, and the animal will lose weight and will eventually die. Electrical stimulation of the medial forebrain bundle seems to induce pleasure in the animal. The rate of self-stimulation (and thus the amount of pleasure induced) is maximal when the stimuli are delivered directly to the lateral hypothalamus. Indeed, if the lateral region is destroyed, the experience of pleasure and emotional responsiveness is almost completely attenuated (Saver et al., 1996). Electrical stimulation or the infusion of acetylcholine into the posterior lateral hypothalamus produces aggressive attack behavior in animals (Kruck, 1991). The lateral hypothalamic zone is important in the cardiovascular response to fearful stimuli. Neurons in the lateral zone project to the lower brainstem, which directly controls alterations in blood pressure (LeDoux, 1996). Signals arrive in the lateral zone of the hypothalamus from the amygdala and from other regions.

The medial forebrain bundle (fasciculus telencephalicus medialis) is a complex collection of fibers that resembles a freeway with many on and off ramps (no. 18, Figure 13.5). It extends from the midbrain to the frontal cortex and passes through the lateral hypothalamus. Fibers representing many different functions enter the medial forebrain bundle, course through it for a short or long distance, and then exit. Mesolimbic and mesocortical fibers are part of the medial forebrain bundle (Chapter 7). Descending fibers from the hypothalamus extend caudally to the brainstem. Raphe serotonergic nuclei (Chapter 10) and basal forebrain acetylcholinergic nuclei (Chapter 13) both project through the medial forebrain bundle.

Lesions of the lateral hypothalamus have been responsible for anorexia in humans (Martin and Riskind, 1992). Significant neuronal loss has been reported in the lateral tuberal nucleus in Huntington disease, adult-onset dementia (Braak and Braak, 1989), and in a patient with severe depressive illness (Horn et al., 1988). The loss of neurons in the lateral hypothalamus may be responsible for the weight loss that commonly accompanies these disorders (Kremer, 1992).

Connections of the hypothalamus

Neural signals reach the hypothalamus over many pathways. Two major pathways that carry signals to and from the hypothalamus are the medial forebrain bundle and dorsal longitudinal fasciculus. The dorsal longitudinal fasciculus connects the hypothalamus with the brainstem and spinal cord. Much of the information is of a visceral nature and includes signals related to taste, blood pressure, and other autonomic functions. The medial forebrain bundle provides connections between the hypothalamus, brainstem tegmentum, limbic structures and cortex of the forebrain. It contains fibers of the mesolimbic pathway and has been nicknamed the "hedonic highway."

Inputs

Ascending input to the hypothalamus includes fibers from the locus ceruleus and raphe nuclei (Chapter 10). These inputs provide signals that have a general alerting effect on the hypothalamus. In particular, fibers to the lateral hypothalamus from the locus ceruleus and the amygdala have been implicated in the sympathetic activation and hormonal release associated with fear and anxiety (Charney et al., 1996). Fibers from the brainstem solitary nucleus provide specific information from visceral afferents, including taste, as well as signals from the thoracic and abdominal viscera.

Descending influences to the hypothalamus include signals from the limbic system, especially from the hippocampus and amygdala (Figures 11.2 and 11.8). The prefrontal cortex projects directly to the hypothalamus via the medial forebrain bundle. The cingulate gyrus influences the hypothalamus by way of the septal nuclei and hippocampus (Figure 12.5).

Clinical vignette

A 19-year-old man sustained a fall with head injury and underwent neurosurgical evacuation of a right-sided epidural hematoma. Two months after the head trauma and surgery, he began eating excessively, particularly a great many sweets, and gained about 176 lb. During the following 18 months, he had periodic episodes lasting six to ten weeks where he would sleep up to 16 hours a night with continued drowsiness during the rest of the day. He was periodically irritable and aggressive, with mood alterations and an increased interest in pornographic material. The patient developed the Kleine–Levin syndrome probably consequent to hypothalamic injury. His magnetic resonance imaging showed a posttraumatic lesion in the right hypothalamus (Figure 8.7). The Kleine–Levin syndrome includes hypersomnolence, hyperphagia and sexual disinhibition or other behavioral disorders.

Outputs

Efferent signals from the hypothalamus tend to leave by way of long axons that arise from cell bodies located in the medial and lateral hypothalamic zones. The hypothalamus has reciprocal (back-and-forth) connections with most of the structures that provide afferents, including the periaqueductal gray, the locus ceruleus, and the raphe nuclei in the brainstem. Descending fibers to the brainstem are responsible for the direct control of the sympathetic and parasympathetic systems. Efferent fibers to the limbic system include connections with the septal nuclei, amygdala, and hippocampus. Some fibers project directly from the hypothalamus to the prefrontal cortex via the medial forebrain bundle. The hypothalamus influences the cingulate cortex indirectly by way of signals relayed in the anterior thalamic nucleus. Other efferent fibers terminate in the mediodorsal thalamic nucleus, which relays information to the prefrontal lobe.

Other behavioral considerations

The hypothalamus lies in a position between the "thinking brain" (neocortex) and the "emotional brain" (limbic system) on the one hand, and the body systems that are controlled by the autonomic and endocrine systems on the other hand. Mental state can operate through the hypothalamus to alter endocrine function and autonomic tone.

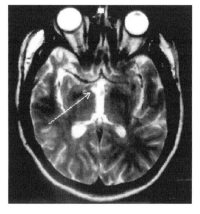

Figure 8.7. A magnetic resonance image (T2-weighted) demonstrating a high-intensity lesion in the right hypothalamus (arrow). (Reprinted with permission from Kostic *et al.*, 1998.)

Tonkonogy and Geller (1992) reported two cases of craniopharyngioma presenting with and meeting *Diagnostic and Statistical Manual of Mental Disorders-III-R* criteria for intermittent explosive disorder.

In the first case, a 21-year-old man presented with frequent episodes of explosive behavior and threats to cut himself or to kill his mother. He complained of insomnia, depressed mood, periodic hypnagogic visual and auditory hallucinations, and periods of 15–20 minutes of spacing out. He had a family history of alcoholism and personality disorder, and he grew up in foster homes. A decline in his IQ, progressive weight loss, dizziness, and fatigue prompted a medical examination. Polydipsia, polyuria, lack of pigmentation, and diabetes insipidus eventually developed. Removal of the tumor did not lead to behavioral improvement.

In the second case, a 24-year-old woman presented with episodes of explosive behavior, including threats to start fires and a history of assaults on staff. She complained of depressed mood and had attempted suicide a number of times. She was markedly obese. At age 11, she had shown signs of growth retardation, weight loss, and other signs of hypopituitarism. A craniopharyngioma was removed at that time. After surgery, her assaultive and self-threatening behavior manifested itself. She did not respond to neuroleptics, antidepressants, or substitute hormonal therapy. An abnormal encephalogram led to treatment with carbamazepine, to which the patient responded with a marked improvement in behavior.

Emotional stress can induce ulcers. In women, stress can block the menstrual cycle. Normally the milk ejection reflex is induced by the infant suckling at the nipple. An experienced nursing mother can sometimes cause milk to trickle from her nipples by forming a mental image of her infant. There is some evidence that mental processes can operate through the hypothalamus to influence the immune system (Michaelson and Gold, 1998; Petrovich, *et al.*, 2005).

The hypothalamus is in a position to control the outward manifestations of emotion. Heart rate, blood pressure, pupil size, and vasoconstriction are all controlled by the hypothalamus. Other behaviors that involve striated muscles are also controlled by the hypothalamus. Shivering for heat conservation, piloerection during rage and facial expression reflecting emotion are all under hypothalamic influence. It is thought that much of the autonomic and somatic expression of emotion is controlled by the hypothalamus. It is believed that emotional expression is controlled by the hypothalamus, whereas the feelings of emotion lie elsewhere, particularly within the limbic system. Sham rage in experimental animals can be seen when the hypothalamus is electrically stimulated. The animal's rage is nondirected and dies out quickly. For example, cats exhibiting sham rage may alternately growl and purr when lapping warm milk (DeMoranville and Jackson, 1996).

Delville *et al.* (1998) found that social subjugation of hamsters during puberty resulted in males that were more aggressive toward intruders and were significantly more likely to bite smaller males than were control males. This behavior is not unlike that of schoolyard bullies. Delville and colleagues' analysis revealed a 50% decrease in the level of vasopressin in the anterior hypothalamus of the subjugated hamsters but an increase in the number of serotonin-containing fibers. The number of vasopressin fibers suggested that less vasopressin is produced and released in the subjugated hamsters. The increase in serotonin fibers suggested to the authors that the capacity to release serotonin was increased. An increase in serotonin is consistent with reduced aggression and may account for the fact that the subjected hamsters were less aggressive than controls when in the presence of males of equal or greater size.

Many case reports of intermittent explosive disorders associated with hypothalamic lesions appear in the literature. A number of these are remarkable since the patients were diagnosed with behavioral disorders, sometimes years before the underlying tumor was discovered. Visual hallucinations have been reported by these patients (Tonkonogy and Geller, 1992). An association between precocious puberty and hypothalamic lesions (particularly hamartomas) has been repeatedly noted (Takeuchi *et al.*, 1979). An even more interesting association is between hypothalamic hamartomas, precocious puberty, and gelastic (laughing) seizures (Breningstall, 1985). It is suggested that the area of the hypothalamus that is critical for the expression of intermittent explosive disorder is the posterior lateral hypothalamic region. This region was at one time surgically destroyed for the treatment of aggressive behavior (Tonkonogy and Geller, 1992).

In summary, at the hypothalamic level, the emotional states elicited are primitive, undirected, and unrefined. Higher-level emotions such as love or hate require the involvement of other limbic, as well as neocortical, regions.

Epithalamus

Pineal (epiphysis)

The pineal is found in the midline, above the third ventricle, and in front of the superior colliculus (P in Figure 13.5). It is glandular in appearance and contains a unique cell called the pinealocyte. It is richly vascular with its rate of blood flow second only to that of the kidney. In lower forms the pineal forms the parietal eye, a photosensitive organ important in circadian rhythms. The prominent pinealocytes synthesize serotonin and melatonin, both of which are released into the extracellular space.

The pineal has been called a "tranquilizing organ" due to the hypnotic properties of melatonin (Romijn, 1978) and is described as a neuroendocrine transducer that transforms a neural signal into an endocrine signal (Reuss, 1996). Exposure to light blocks the transmission of neural signals to the pineal gland from the hypothalamus and therefore blocks the production of melatonin. The synthesis of melatonin and release into the bloodstream are normally observed to take place only during the nighttime hours. Blinded animals continue to produce melatonin in rhythm with the day–night cycle. However, a lesion of the suprachiasmatic nucleus of the hypothalamus abolishes the rhythm. Pinealocytes found in the deep portion of the pineal give rise to long, beaded processes that terminate in the pretectum and in the medial nucleus of the habenula (see the following section). (The pretectum is part of the visual system and is found in the midbrain in front of the superior colliculus.) The ends of these processes form neuron-like connections with neurons located in these two sites (Figure 8.8). The pineal is usually considered an endocrine organ; however, the axon-like processes and point-to-point organization suggest that it may have neuronal connections as well (Korf *et al.*, 1990).

The pineal is the most influential component of the melatonin system. However, melatonin is also synthesized in photoreceptors of the retina. Retinal melatonin is secreted locally, whereas pineal melatonin is released into the bloodstream. A well-recognized pathway to the pineal originates with the retinohypothalamic tract to the suprachiasmatic nucleus, paraventricular nucleus of the hypothalamus, medial forebrain bundle, lateral horn of the upper thoracic spinal cord, superior cervical ganglion, and sympathetic pre- and postganglionic nerves to the pineal (Figure 8.8). This route includes the sympathetic innervation of the pineal from the superior cervical ganglion. A second pathway

149

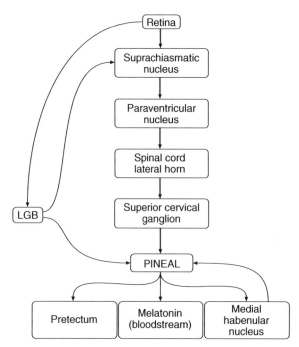

Figure 8.8. The connections of the pineal include afferents from the retina and lateral geniculate body (LGB). Exposure to light inhibits melatonin production by the pinealocytes. The lines leaving the pineal represent cytoplasmic extensions of the pinealocytes. Feedback from the pineal to the suprachiasmatic nucleus is by way of melatonin in the bloodstream.

involves the lateral geniculate nucleus, which sends efferent fibers to both the suprachiasmatic nucleus and to the pineal (Reuss, 1996).

The suprachiasmatic nucleus and the anterior pituitary are two regions where melatonin exerts its major effects. Melatonin feedback to the suprachiasmatic nucleus regulates the output of melatonin by the pineal. The effect of melatonin in the anterior pituitary is to regulate neuroendocrine and gonadal function (Morgan *et al.*, 1994). Melatonin synchronizes daily activity/inactivity with daily changes in light/dark. It also synchronizes other body functions and is responsible for maternal entrainment of fetus activity (Reppert *et al.*, 1989). The pain threshold is raised by melatonin. Since this effect is blocked by naloxone, it appears that melatonin acts through opiate mechanisms (Golombek *et al.*, 1991). Melatonin has also been demonstrated to have anticonvulsant properties and anxiolytic effects in laboratory animals (Golombek *et al.*, 1996). It increases the turnover of the inhibitory neurotransmitter γ-aminobutyric acid (GABA) in the hypothalamus, cerebral cortex, and cerebellum, suggesting that

a melatonin–GABA interaction is responsible for some of its behavioral effects (Golombek *et al.*, 1996).

Parenchymatous pinealomas are associated with depression of gonadal function and delayed pubescence. Destruction of the pineal is associated with precocious puberty. The pineal is frequently calcified in schizophrenia, and the melatonin system may be involved in SAD (Sandyk, 1992).

The level of melatonin normally rises at night. Melatonin given during the day, when levels are normally low, induces fatigue. Exposure to bright light at night suppresses the normal nocturnal elevation of circulating melatonin (Dollins *et al.*, 1993). It has been suggested that melatonin or melatonin analogs may be therapeutic for the control of circadian clock dysfunctions such as jet lag, shift-work syndrome, and sleep disorders. Melatonin has been used effectively for treatment of insomnia to correct the sleep–wake cycle (Tzichinsky *et al.*, 1992). However, it has not always proved effective in the treatment of SAD (Wehr, 1991). Sleep patterns are often affected by depression, although it is believed that there is no primary disturbance of the circadian rhythm system in this disease (Moore, 1997).

Habenula

The habenula (habenular nucleus) is located in the wall of the third ventricle anterior to the pineal (Figure 9.3, and nos. 9 and 23, Figure 13.5). It consists of a smaller medial nucleus, which contains small cells, and a larger lateral nucleus, which contains larger cells. Both may be further divided into multiple subnuclei (Andres *et al.*, 1999). The stria medullaris is the major afferent bundle serving the habenular nucleus, and brings signals from the medial forebrain and septum, limbic lobe hypothalamus, and ventral striatum. The fasciculus retroflexus (habenulointerpeduncular tract; no. 11, Figure 13.5) is the major efferent pathway that projects primarily to the nigral complex (ventral tegmental area and substantia nigra; see Chapter 7) and to brainstem nuclei, including the raphe nuclei and locus ceruleus (Chapter 10). The habenular nucleus is part of a dorsal pathway connecting cortex with brainstem that parallels the ventral medial forebrain bundle. It is positioned to link limbic structures with nuclei in the upper brainstem (Figure 8.9).

Lateral habenular nucleus

The lateral habenular nucleus has been described as the "crossroad between the basal ganglia and the

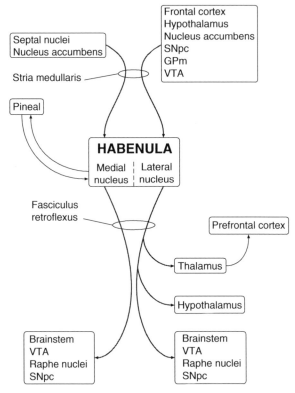

Septal nuclei
Nucleus accumbens

Stria medullaris

Pineal

Frontal cortex
Hypothalamus
Nucleus accumbens
SNpc
GPm
VTA

HABENULA

Medial | Lateral
nucleus | nucleus

Fasciculus
retroflexus

Prefrontal cortex

Thalamus

Hypothalamus

Brainstem
VTA
Raphe nuclei
SNpc

Brainstem
VTA
Raphe nuclei
SNpc

Figure 8.9. The medial habenula links the septal nuclei with the thalamus. The lateral habenula links the frontal cortex, hypothalamus, and dopaminergic nuclei to the brainstem and allows for feedback to the medial preoptic area of the hypothalamus and to the frontal cortex. GPm, medial segment of globus pallidus; SNpc, substantia nigra pars compacta (dopamine); VTA, ventral tegmental area (dopamine).

of the dopaminergic mesocortical, mesolimbic, and mesostriatal systems. The animals exhibited impulsive responding, represented by a large increase in premature responding and a decline in accuracy.

Dopamine from the ventral tegmental area is important through the mesolimbic and mesocortical pathways for reward and cognition. Dopamine from the substantia nigra is important for motor activity. Dopamine is critical in its role for maximizing reward potential resulting from anticipated motor behavior (Matsumoto and Hikosaka, 2007). It is also important in support of spatial memory (declarative memory) and attention. These represent cognitive activity (Lecourtier et al., 2006).

The lateral habenula also inhibits serotonin neurons in the raphe nuclei and the dopamine neurons of the ventral tegmental area (Park, 1987; Ji and Shepard, 2007). Lateral habenula neurons are strongly activated in response to stress and food deprivation and in animal models of depression (Shumake et al., 2004; Yang et al., 2008), but this effect is reduced by antidepressant drugs or lesions of the lateral habenula (Yang et al., 2008). Hikosaka et al., 2008 hypothesize that increased activity in the habenula can result in depressed mood through its control of dopamine and serotonin (Geisler, 2008). There is some human evidence to support this hypothesis (Morris et al., 1999). These findings have led to the suggestion that inactivation of the lateral habenula by deep brain stimulation may be effective in treatment-resistant depression (Sartorius and Henn, 2007; Hauptman et al., 2008).

Medial habenular nucleus

The medial habenular nucleus shares many of the same incoming afferent fibers with its lateral counterpart. It also receives melatonin-containing axons from the pinealocytes of the pineal. The septum is an especially rich source of incoming fibers to the medial habenula. The majority of outgoing fibers from the medial habenular nucleus terminate in the interpeduncular nucleus and median raphe of the midbrain where they regulate sleep-wakefulness and food intake in response to stress (Smith and Lonstein, 2008).

The habenular nucleus has been observed to be significantly more calcified in schizophrenic patients than in normal individuals. It is hypothesized that the calcification may be correlated with the enlargement of the third ventricle. Calcification of the habenular nucleus may disrupt its role in providing a link between the limbic system and the upper brainstem (Ellison, 1994).

limbic system" (Hikosaka et al., 2008). It receives fibers from the frontal cortex, the basal forebrain (substantia innominata and bed nucleus of the stria terminalis of the extended amygdala), the preoptic area, and lateral hypothalamus as well as the basal ganglia (medial segment of the globus pallidus). It has reciprocal connections (back-and-forth) with the raphe nuclei (serotonin) (Chapter 10) and the ventral tegmental area (dopamine).

Matsumoto and Hikosaka (2007) showed that in monkeys and humans activity in the lateral habenula increased in unrewarded trials and decreased in rewarded trials. In another study, electrical stimulation of the lateral habenula in rats resulted in almost complete and long-lasting suppression of the dopamine neurons of the ventral tegmental area and substantia nigra pars compacta (Ji and Shepard, 2007). In contrast, Lecourtier and Kelly (2005) showed that lesions of the habenula nuclei in rats resulted in an activation

Select bibliography

Arendt, J. *Melatonin and the Mammalian Pineal Gland*. (New York: Chapman & Hall, 1995.)

Buijs, R.M., Kalsbeek, A., Romijn, H.J., Pennartz, C.M.A., and Mirmiran, M. Hypothalamic integration of circadian rhythms. *Progress in Brain Research* (vol. 111). (Amsterdam: Elsevier, 1996.)

Carter, C.S., Lederhendler, I.I., and Kirkpatrick, B. The integrative neurobiology of affiliation. *Annals of the New York Academy of Sciences* (vol. 807). (New York: The New York Academy of Sciences, 1997.)

Joseph, R. *Neuropsychology, Neuropsychiatry, and Behavioral Neurology*. (New York: Plenum Press, 1989.)

Swaab, D.F., Hofman, M.A., Mirmiran, M., Ravid, R., and van Leeuwen, F.W. The human hypothalamus in health and disease. *Progress in Brain Research* (vol. 93). (Amsterdam: Elsevier, 1992.)

References

Abelson, J.L., and Curtis, G.C. 1996. Hypothalamic-pituitary-adrenal axis activity in panic disorder. *Arch. Gen. Psychiatry* **53**:323–331.

Andres, K.H., During, M.V., and Veh, R.W. 1999. Subnuclear organization of the rat habenular complexes. *J. Comp. Neurol.* **407**:130–150.

Bernardis, L.L., and Bellinger, L.L. 1996. The lateral hypothalamic area revisited: Ingestive behavior. *Neurosci. Biobehav. Rev.* **20**:189–287.

Braak, H., and Braak, E. 1989. Cortical and subcortical argyrophilic grains characterize a disease associated with adult onset dementia. *Neuropathol. Appl. Neurobiol.* **15**:13–26.

Bray, G.A. 1992. Genetic, hypothalamic and endocrine features of clinical and experimental obesity. In: D.F.Swabb, M.A.Hofman, M.Mirmiran, R.Ravid and F.W. vanLeeuwen (eds.) *The Human Hypothalamus in Health and Disease*. *Prog. Brain Res.* **93**:333–341.

Breningstall, G.N. 1985. Gelastic seizures, precocious puberty, and hypothalamic hamartomas. *Neurology* **35**:1180–1183.

Burstein, R. 1996. Somatosensory and visceral input to the hypothalamus and limbic system. In: G.Holstege, R.Bandler, and C.B.Saper (eds.) *The Emotional Motor System*. *Prog. Brain Res.* **107**:257–267.

Charney, D.S., Nagy, L.M., Bremner, J.D., Goddard, A.W., Yehuda, R., and Southwick, S.M. 1996. Neurobiological mechanisms of human anxiety. In: B.S.Fogel, R.B.Schiffer, and S.M.Rao (eds.) *Neuropsychiatry*. Baltimore: Williams & Wilkins, pp. 257–286.

Corodimas, K.P., Rosenblatt, J.S., Canfield, M.E., and Morrell, J.I. 1993. Neurons in the lateral subdivision of the habenular complex mediate the hormonal onset of maternal behavior in rats. *Behav. Neurosci.* **107**:827–843.

Delis, D.C., and Lucas, J.A. 1996. Memory. In: B.S.Fogel, R.B.Schiffer, and S.M.Rao (eds.) *Neuropsychiatry*. Baltimore: Williams & Wilkins, pp. 365–399.

Delville, Y.U., Melloni, R.H. Jr., and Ferris, C.F. 1998. Behavioral and neurobiological consequences of social subjugation during puberty in golden hamsters. *J. Neurosci.* **18**:2667–2672.

Demitrack, M.A., and Gold, P.W. 1988. Oxytocin: Neurobiologic considerations and their implications for affective illness. *Prog. Neuropsychopharmacol.* **12**:S23–S51.

Demitrack, M.A., Lesem, M.D., Listwak, S.J., Brandt, H.A., Jimerson, D.C., and Gold, P.W. 1990. Cerebrospinal fluid oxytocin in anorexia nervosa and bulimia nervosa: Clinical and pathophysiological considerations. *Am. J. Psychiatry* **147**:882–886.

DeMoranville, B.M., and Jackson, I.M.D. 1996. Psychoneuroendocrinology. In: B.S.Fogel, R.B.Schiffer, and S.M.Rao (eds.) *Neuropsychiatry*. Baltimore: Williams & Wilkins, pp. 173–192.

DeVries, G.J., and Villalba, C. 1997. Brain sexual dimorphism and sex differences in parental and other social behaviors. In: C.S.Carter, I.I.Lederhendler, and B.Kirkpatrick (eds.) The Integrative Neurobiology of Affiliation. *Ann. N. Y. Acad. Sci.* **807**:273–286.

Dollins, A.B., Lynch, H.J., Wurtman, R.J., Deng, M.H., and Lieberman, H.R. 1993. Effects of illumination on human nocturnal serum melatonin levels and performance. *Physiol. Behav.* **53**:153–160.

Ellison, G. 1994. Stimulant-induced psychosis, the dopamine theory of schizophrenia and the habenula. *Brain Res. Rev.* **19**:223–239.

Friedman, R.C., and Downey, J. 1993. Neurobiology and sexual orientation. *J. Neuropsychiatry Clin. Neurosci.* **5**:147–148.

Geisler, S. 2008. The lateral habenula: No longer neglected. *CNS Spectr.* **13**:484–489.

Gjerris, A. 1990. Studies on cerebrospinal fluid in affective disorders. *Pharmacol. Toxicol.* **66**(Suppl. 3):133–138.

Goldstein, J.M., Seidman, L.J., Makris, N., Ahern, T., O'Brien, L.M., Caviness, V.S. Jr., Kennedy, D.N., Faraone, S.V., and Tsuang, M.T. 2007. Hypothalamic abnormalities in schizophrenia: Sex effects and genetic vulnerability. *Biol. Psychiatry* **61**:935–945.

Golombek, D.A., Pevet, P., and Cardinali, D.P. 1996. Melatonin effects on behavior: Possible mediation by the central GABAergic system. *Neurosci. Biobehav. Rev.* **20**:403–412.

Golombek, D.A., Escolar, E., Burin, L., Brito Sanchez, M.G., and Cardinali, D.P. 1991. Time-dependent melatonin analgesia in mice: inhibition by opiate or benzodiazepine antagonism. *Eur. J. Pharmacol.* **194**:25–30.

Hamann, S., Herman, R.A., Nolan, C.L., and Wallen, K. 2004. Men and women differ in amygdala response to visual sexual stimuli. *Nat. Neurosci.* **7**:411–416.

Hansen, S., and Ferreira, A. 1986. Food intake, aggression, and fear behavior in the mother rat: Control by neural systems concerned with milk ejection and maternal behavior. *Behav. Neurosci.* **100**:64–70.

Hauptman, J.S., DeSalles, A.A., Espinoza, R. Sedrak, M., and Ishida, W. 2008. Potential surgical targets for deep brain stimulation treatment-resistant depression. *Neurosurg. Focus* **25**:E3.

Hennessy, M.B. 1997. Hypothalamic-pituitary-adrenal responses to brief social separation.*Neurosci. Biobehav. Rev.* **21**:11–29.

Herman, J.P., Adams, D., and Prewitt, C. 1995. Regulatory changes in neuroendocrine stress-integrative circuitry produced by a variable stress paradigm. *Neuroendocrinology* **61**:180–190.

Hikosaka, O., Sesack, S.R., Lecourtier, L., and Shepard, P.D. 2008. Habenula: Crossroad between the basal ganglia and the limbic system. *J. Neurosci.* **28**:11825–11829.

Hofman, M.A., Puirba, J.S., and Swaab, D.F. 1993. Annual variation in the vasopressin neuron population of the human suprachiasmatic nucleus. *Neuroscience* **53**:1103–1112.

Holsboer-Trachsler, E., Stohler, R., and Hatzinger, M. 1991. Repeated administration of the combined dexamethasone–human corticotropin releasing hormone stimulation test during treatment of depression. *Psychiatry Res.* **38**:163–171.

Horn, E., Lach, B., Lapierre, Y., and Hrdina, P. 1988. Hypothalamic pathology in the neuroleptic malignant syndrome. *Am. J. Psychiatry* **145**:617–620.

Horvath, T.L. 2005. The hardship of obesity: A soft-wired hypothalamus. *Nat. Neurosci.* **8**:561–565.

Ji, H., and Shepard, P.D. 2007. Lateral habenula stimulation inhibits rat midbrain dopamine neurons through a GABA(A) receptor-mediated mechanism. *J. Neurosci.* **27**:6923–6930.

Katter, J.T., Burstein, R., and Giesler, G.J. 1991. The cells of origin of the spinohypothalamic tract in cats. *J. Comp. Neurol.* **303**:101–112.

Korf, H.W., Sato, T., and Oksche, A. 1990. Complex relationship between the pineal organ and the medial habenular nucleus–pretectal region of the mouse as revealed by S-antigen immunocytochemistry. *Cell* **261**:493–500.

Kostic, V.S., Stefanova, E., Svetel, M., and Kozic, D. 1998. A variant of the Kleine–Levin syndrome following head trauma. *Behav. Neurol.* **11**:105–108.

Kremer, H.P.H. 1992. The hypothalamic lateral tuberal nucleus: Normal anatomy and changes in neurological diseases. In: R.M.Buijs, A.Kalsbeek, H.J.Romijn, C.M.A.Pennartz, and M.Mirmiran (eds.) Hypothalamic Integration of Circadian Rhythms. *Prog. Brain Res.* **111**:249–261.

Kruck, M.R. 1991. Ethology and pharmacology of hypothalamic aggression in the rat. *Neurosci. Biobehav. Rev.* **15**:527–538.

Kupfermann, I. 1991. Hypothalamus and limbic system: Peptidergic neurons, homeostasis, and emotional behavior. In: E.R.Kandel, J.H.Schwartz, and T.M.Jessell (eds.) *Principles of Neural Science* (3rd ed.). New York: Elsevier, pp. 735–749.

Lecourtier, L., and Kelly, P.H. 2005. Bilateral lesions of the habenula induce attentional disturbances in rats. *Neuropsychopharmacology* **30**:484–496.

Lecourtier, L., Deschaux, O., Arnaud, C., Chessel, A., Kelly, P.H., and Garcia, R. 2006. Habenula lesions alter synaptic plasticity within the fimbria-accumbens pathway in the rat. *Neuroscience* **141**:1025–1032.

LeDoux, J. 1996. Emotional networks and motor control: A fearful view. In: G.Holstege, R.Bandler, and C.B.Saper (eds.) The Emotional Motor System. *Prog. Brain Res.* **107**:437–446.

Legros, J.J., Ansseau, M., and Timsit-Berthier, M. 1993. Neurohypophyseal peptides and psychopathology. *Prog. Brain Res.* **93**:455–461.

LeVay, S. 1991. A difference in hypothalamic structure between heterosexual and homosexual men. *Science* **253**:1034–1037.

LeVay, S., and Hamer, D.H. 1994. Evidence for a biological influence in male homosexuality. *Sci. Am.* **270**:44–49.

Lewy, A.J., and Sack, R.L. 1996. The role of melatonin and light in the human circadian system. In: R.M.Buijs, A.Kalsbeek, H.J.Romijn, C.M.A.Pennartz, and M.Mirmiran (eds.) Hypothalamic Integration of Circadian Rhythms. *Prog. Brain Res.* **111**:205–216.

Marson, L., and McKenna, K.E. 1994. Stimulation of the hypothalamus initiates the urethrogenital reflex in male rats. *Brain Res.* **638**:103–108.

Martin, J.H. 1996. *Neuroanatomy: Text and Atlas*. Stamford, CT: Appleton & Lange, p. 434.

Martin, J.B., and Riskind, P.N. 1992. Neurologic manifestations of hypothalamic disease. In: D.F.Swabb, M.A.Hofman, M.Mirmiran, R.Ravid and F.W. vanLeeuwen (eds.) *The Human Hypothalamus in Health and Disease. Prog. Brain Res.* **93**:31–42.

Matsumoto, M., and Hikosaka, O. 2007. Lateral habenula as a source of negative reward signals in dopamine neurons. *Nature* **447**:1111–1115.

Michaelson, D., and Gold, P.W. 1998. Pathophysiologic and somatic investigations of hypothalamic-pituitary-adrenal axis activation in patients with depression. *Ann. N. Y. Acad.Sci.* **840**:717–722.

Michelson, D., Stratakis, C., Hill, L., Reynolds, J., Galliven, E., Chrousos, G., and Gold, P. 1996. Bone mineral density in women with depression. *N. Engl. J. Med.* **335**:1176–1181.

Moore, R.Y. 1997. Circadian rhythms: Basic neurobiology and clinical applications. *Annu. Rev. Med.* **48**:253–266.

Morgan, P.J., Barrett, P., Howell, H.E., and Helliwell, R. 1994. Melatonin receptors: localization, molecular pharmacology and physiological significance. *Neurochem. Int.* **24**:101–146.

Morris, J.S., Smith, K.A., Cowen, P.J., Friston, K.J., and Dolan, R.J. 1999. Covariation of activity in habenula and dorsal raphe nuclei following tryptophan depletion. *Neuroimage* **10**:163–172.

Nadvornik, P., Sramka, M., and Patoprsta, G. 1975. Transventricular anterior hypothalamotomy in stereotactic treatment of hedonia. In: W.H.Sweet, S.Obrador, and J.G.Martin-Rodriguez (eds.) *Neurosurgical Treatment in Psychiatry, Pain and Epilepsy.* Baltimore: University Park Press, pp. 445–450.

Numan, M., and Smith, H.G. 1984. Maternal behavior in rats: Evidence for the involvement of preoptic projections to the ventral tegmental area. *Behav. Neurosci.* **98**: 712–727.

Numan, M., and Sheenan, T.P. 1997. Neuroanatomical circuitry for mammalian maternal behavior. In: C.S.Carter, I.I.Lederhendler, and B.Kirkpatrick (eds.) *The Integrative Neurobiology of Affiliation. Ann. N. Y. Acad. Sci.* **807**:101–125.

Park, M.R. 1987. Monosynaptic inhibitory postsynaptic potentials from lateral habenula recorded in dorsal raphe neurons. *Brain Res. Bull.* **19**:581–586.

Pedersen, C.A. 1997. Oxytocin control of maternal behavior: Regulation by sex steroids and offspring stimuli. *Ann. N. Y. Acad. Sci.* **807**: 126–145.

Pedersen, C.A., and Prange, A.J. Jr. 1979. Induction of maternal behavior in virgin rats after intracerebroventricular administration of oxytocin. *Proc. Natl. Acad. Sci. USA.* **76**:6661–6665.

Petrovich, G.D., Holland, P.C., and Gallagher, M. 2005. Amygdalar and prefrontal pathways to the lateral hypothalamus are activated by a learned cue that stimulates eating. *J. Neurosci.* **25**:8295–8302.

Pevet, P., Pitrosky, B., Vuillez, P., Jacob, N., Teclemariam-Mesbah, R., Kirsch, R., Vivien-Roels, B., Lakhdar-Ghazal, N., Canguilhem, B., and Masson-Pevet, M. 1996. The suprachiasmatic nucleus: The biological clock of all seasons. In: R.M.Buijs, A.Kalsbeek, H.J.Romijn, C.M.A.Pennartz, and M.Mirmiran (eds.) Hypothalamic Integration of Circadian Rhythms. *Prog. Brain Res.* **111**:369–384.

Pfaff, D.W., Schwartz-Giblin, S., McCarthy, M.M., and Kow, L.-M. 1994. Cellular mechanisms of female reproductive behavior. In: E.Knobil, and J.Neill (eds.) *The Physiology of Reproduction* (2nd ed.). New York: Raven Press, pp. 107–220.

Purba, J.S., Hoogendijk, W.J.G., Hofman, M.A., and Swaab, D.F., 1996. Increased number of vasopressin- and oxytocin-expressing neurons in the paraventricular nucleus of the hypothalamus in depression. *Arch. Gen. Psychiatry* **53**:137–143.

Raadsheer, F.C., Hoogendijk, W.J.G., Stam, F.C., Tilders, F.J.H., and Swaab, D.F. 1994. Increased number of corticotropin-releasing hormone neurons in the hypothalamic paraventricular nuclei of depressed patients. *Neuroendocrinology* **60**:436–444.

Rance, N.E. 1992. Hormonal influences on morphology and neuropeptide gene expression in the infundibular nucleus of post-menopausal women. In: D.F. Swabb, M.A. Hofman, M. Mirmiran, R. Ravid, and F.W. van Leeuwen (eds.) *The Human Hypothalamus in Health and Disease. Prog. Brain Res.* **93**:221–236.

Reppert, S.M., Rivkees, S.A., and Weaver, D.R. 1989. Prenatal entrainment of a circadian clock. In: S.M.Reppert (ed.) *The Development of Circadian Rhythmicity and Photoperiodism in Mammals.* New York: Perinatology Press, pp. 25–44.

Reuss, S. 1996. Components and connections of the circadian timing system in mammals. *Cell Tissue Res.* **285**:353–378.

Romijn, H. 1978. The pineal: A tranquilizing organ? *Life Sci.* **3**:2257–2274.

Ross, E.D., and Stewart, R.M. 1981. Akinetic mutism from hypothalamic damage: Successful treatment with dopamine agonists. *Neurology* **31**:1435–1439.

Sandyk, R. 1992. Pineal and habenula calcification in schizophrenia. *Int. J. Neurosci.* **67**:19–30.

Saper, C.B. 1996. Role of the cerebral cortex and striatum in emotional motor response. In: G.Holstege, R.Bandler, and C.B.Saper (eds.) *The Emotional Motor System. Prog. Brain Res.* **107**:537–550.

Sartorius, A., and Henn, F.A. 2007. Deep brain stimulation of the lateral habenula in treatment resistant major depression. *Med. Hypotheses* **69**:1305–1308.

Saver, J.L., Salloway, S.P., Devinsky, O., and Bear, D.M. 1996. Neuropsychiatry of aggression. In: B.S.Fogel, R.B.Schiffer, and S.M.Rao (eds.) *Neuropsychiatry.* Baltimore: Williams & Wilkins, pp. 523–548.

Schwartz, M.W., and Seeley, R.J. 1997. The new biology of body weight regulation. *J. Am. Diet. Assoc.* **97**:558.

Sechi, G., and Serra, A., 2007. Wernicke's encephalopathy: New clinical settings and recent advances in diagnosis and management. *Lancet Neurol.* **6**:442–455.

Segraves, R.T. 1996. Neuropsychiatric aspects of sexual dysfunction. In: B.S.Fogel, R.B.Schiffer, and S.M.Rao (eds.) *Neuropsychiatry.* Baltimore: Williams & Wilkins, pp. 757–770.

Shipley, M.T., Murphy, A.Z., Rizvi, T.A., Ennis, M., and Behbehani, M.M. 1996. Olfaction and brainstem circuits of reproductive behavior in the rat. In: G.Holstege, R.Bandler, and C.B.Saper (eds.) *The Emotional Motor System. Prog. Brain Res.* **107**:353–377.

Shumake, J., Conejo-Jiminez, N., Gonzalez-Pardo, H., and Gonzalez-Lima, F. 2004. Brain differences in newborn rats predisposed to helpless and depressive behavior. *Brain Res.* **1030**:267–276.

Smith, C.D., and Lonstein, J.S. 2008. Contact with infants modulates anxiety-generated c-fos activity in the brains of postpartum rats. *Behav. Brain Res.* **190**:193–200.

Sofroniew, M.W. 1983. Vasopressin and oxytocin in the mammalian brain and spinal cord. *Trends Neurosci.* **6**:467–472.

Swaab, D.F., Gooren, L.J., and Hofman, M.A. 1995. Brain research, gender and sexual orientation. *J. Homosex.* **28**:283–301.

Takeuchi, J., Handa, H., and Miki, Y. 1979. Precocious puberty due to hypothalamic hamartoma. *Surg. Neurol.* **11**:456–460.

Tonkonogy, J.M., and Geller, J.L. 1992. Hypothalamic lesions and intermittent explosive disorder. *J. Neuropsychiatry Clin. Neurosci.* **4**:45–50.

Tzichinsky, O., Pal, I., Epstein, R., Dagan, Y., and Lavie, P. 1992. The importance of timing in melatonin administration in a blind man. *J. Pineal Res.* **12**: 105–108.

Uvnas-Moberg, K. 1997. Physiological and endocrine effects of social contact. *Ann. N. Y. Acad. Sci.* **807**:146–163.

Van de Poll, N.E., and Van Goozen, S.H.M. 1992. Hypothalamic involvement in sexuality and hostility: Comparative psychological aspects. In: D.F.Swabb, M.A.Hofman, M.Mirmiran, R.Ravid, and F.W. vanLeeuwen (eds.) *The Human Hypothalamus in Health and Disease. Prog. Brain Res.* **93**:343–361.

Wehr, T.A. 1991. The duration of human melatonin secretion and sleep respond to changes in daylength (photoperiod). *J. Clin. Enocrinol. Metab.* **73**:1276–1280.

Weinstock, M. 1997. Does prenatal stress impair coping and regulation of hypothalamic-pituitary-adrenal axis? *Neurosci. Biobehav. Rev.* **21**:1–10.

Wiegant, V.M., Ronken, E., Kovacs, G., and DeWied, D. 1992. Endorphins and schizophrenia. In: D.F. Swabb, M.A.Hofman, M.Mirmiran, R.Ravid and F.W. vanLeeuwen (eds.) *The Human Hypothalamus in Health and Disease. Prog. Brain Res.* **93**:433–453.

Witt, D.W. 1997. Regulatory mechanisms of oxytocin-mediated sociosexual behavior. *Ann. N. Y. Acad. Sci.* **807**: 287–301.

Yang, L.M., Hu., B., Xia, Y.H., Zhang, B.L., and Zhao, H. 2008. Lateral habenula lesions improve the behavioral response in depressed rats via increasing the serotonin level in dorsal raphe nucleus. *Behav. Brain Res.* **188**:84–90.

Introduction

The thalamus functions as the principal relay station for sensory information destined for the cerebral cortex. It is made up of a number of nuclei, which can be grouped into relay nuclei and diffuse-projection nuclei (Table 9.1). Each relay nucleus is associated with a single sensory modality or motor system and projects to a specific region of the cerebral cortex with which it has reciprocal connections. The diffuse-projection group of nuclei has more widespread connections with the cortex. They also interact with other thalamic nuclei. It is believed that the diffuse-projection group is involved with regulating the level of arousal of the brain. The limbic thalamus consists of a number of the thalamic nuclei that project to the limbic cortex and includes both relay and diffuse-projection nuclei.

Anatomy and behavioral considerations

The thalamus consists of a symmetrical pair of ovoid structures located above (dorsal to) the hypothalamus. The left thalamus and right thalamus are separated medially by the third ventricle and bounded laterally by the posterior limb of the internal capsule (Figures 9.1, 9.2, and 9.3). The massa intermedia (interthalamic adhesion) is a bridge of cells that spans the third ventricle and joins the left with the right thalamus. The thalamus is bounded in front (anteriorly) by the head of the caudate nucleus and the genu of the internal capsule and behind (posteriorly) by the midbrain. The subthalamic nucleus (subthalamus) lies immediately below (ventral to) the thalamus and is sandwiched between the thalamus, internal capsule, and pretectal area (Figures 9.2 and 9.3).

The internal medullary lamina is a sheet of fibers that runs through the center of the thalamus, dividing it into three subdivisions (Figures 9.2 and 9.3). The anterior subdivision is embraced within the split anterior leaves of the internal medullary lamina and consists of the anterior group of thalamic nuclei. The medial subdivision lies medial to the internal medullary lamina and consists of the midline and medial nuclear groups. The lateral subdivision lies lateral to the internal medullary lamina and consists of the lateral, ventral, and reticular nuclei, as well as the medial and lateral geniculate bodies. The intralaminar nuclei represent a fourth subdivision, and these nuclei are found encapsulated within the fibers of the internal medullary lamina. The most prominent of the intralaminar nuclei is the centromedian nucleus (CM in Figure 9.3).

Thalamic nuclei

Anterior thalamic nuclei

The anterior group of thalamic nuclei consists of the anterodorsal, the anteroventral, and the anteromedial nuclei. The anterior thalamic nuclei receive input from the mammillary body of the hypothalamus by way of the mammillothalamic tract. The anterior group projects to the cingulate gyrus. The anterior thalamic nuclear group is part of the limbic circuitry and constitutes the original "limbic thalamus". It is part of the circuit of Papez (Figures 9.2 and 13.8). Disorientation has been seen following lesions of the anterior thalamic nuclei (Graff-Radford et al., 1984). Zubieta et al. (2002) found that the anterior thalamus was activated during pain processing, more so in men than in women. A decrease in volume has been reported in the anterior nucleus in patients with schizophrenia but this was not significant (Young et al., 2000; Byne et al., 2002, 2006). Decreases in the number of projection neurons and oligodendrocytes have also been reported in schizophrenia (Danos et al., 1998; Jakary et al., 2005; Byne et al., 2006).

Midline and medial nuclei

Two groups of thalamic nuclei lie medial to the internal medullary lamina. These are the medial nuclei and the midline nuclei (Figures 9.2 and 9.3). The midline nuclei are continuous with the periaqueductal gray

Table 9.1. Major connections of the thalamic nuclei that make up the four nuclear groups found in the human thalamus.

Nucleus	Functional class	Major input from	Major output to	Function
Anterior group				
Anterior*	Relay	Hypothalamus (mammillary body)	Cingulate gyrus	Learning, emotion, memory
Medial group				
Midline*	Diffuse-projecting	Reticular formation, hypothalamus	Cerebral cortex including cingulate gyrus, amygdala	Regulation forebrain excitability
Mediodorsal*	Relay	Basal ganglia, amygdala, hypothalamus, nucleus accumbens, olfactory system	Prefrontal cortex, cingulate gyrus, nucleus basalis	Emotion, cognition, learning, memory
Lateral group				
Ventral anterior*	Relay	Basal ganglia	Supplementary motor cortex, cingulate gyrus	Movement planning
Ventral lateral	Relay	Cerebellum	Premotor and primary motor cortex	Movement planning and control
Ventral posterior	Relay	Spinal cord, brainstem, ascending discriminative touch systems	Parietal cortex	Touch, limb position sense
Lateral dorsal*	Relay	Hippocampus	Cingulate gyrus, parietal cortex	?
Lateral posterior	Relay	Superior colliculus, pretectum, occipital lobe	Posterior parietal cortex	Sensory integration
Pulvinar	Relay	Superior colliculus; parietal, temporal, and occipital lobes	Parietal, temporal, occipital association cortex; cingulate gyrus	Sensory integration, perception, eye movement control, language
Lateral geniculate	Relay	Retina	Primary visual cortex	Vision
Medial geniculate	Relay	Inferior colliculus	Primary auditory cortex	Hearing
Reticular	Diffuse-projecting	Thalamus, cortex	Thalamus	Regulation of thalamic activity
Intralaminar*	Diffuse-projecting	Brainstem, spinal cord, basal ganglia	Cerebral cortex, basal ganglia	Regulation of cortical activity

*Nuclei that are considered to be part of the limbic thalamus.

of the midbrain reticular formation (Chapter 10). They are the target of dopaminergic fibers and express dopamine receptors. These are two criteria that qualify them as part of the ascending dopaminergic system (Chapter 7). Fibers from the midline nuclei project diffusely. Targets include the amygdala and the anterior cingulate gyrus. The midline nuclei provide an indirect link from the brainstem to these limbic structures.

A bilateral surgical lesion placed in the anterior portion of the internal capsule (anterior capsulotomy) disconnects the orbital frontal cortex from the midline thalamic nuclei and is thought to decrease symptoms of obsessive-compulsive disorder (OCD) (Chapter 12; Martuza et al., 1990).

The medial nuclear group is dominated by the mediodorsal nucleus. It is a very large nucleus that occupies most of the space between the midline nuclei and the internal medullary lamina and can be divided into as many as seven subdivisions. The most common division describes a medially located magnocellular and laterally located parvocellular part. The medial part projects to medial prefrontal cortex and the lateral part

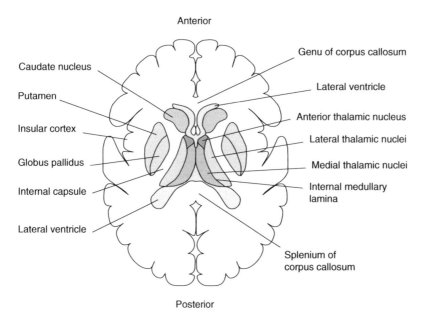

Anterior

Caudate nucleus

Putamen

Insular cortex

Globus pallidus

Internal capsule

Lateral ventricle

Genu of corpus callosum

Lateral ventricle

Anterior thalamic nucleus

Lateral thalamic nuclei

Medial thalamic nuclei

Internal medullary lamina

Splenium of corpus callosum

Posterior

Figure 9.1. The brain section in this view is cut perpendicular to the long axis of the body and parallel to the horizontal limb of the neuraxis (see Figure 1.1). It is as if we are standing at the foot of the bed and looking at the patient. This diagram is identical to that of the insert on the left-hand side of Figure 9.2. Anterior refers to the front of the head, posterior to the back of the head.

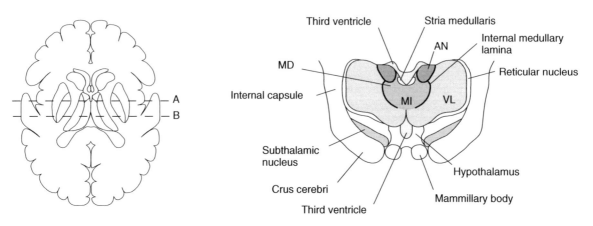

Third ventricle

Stria medullaris

Internal medullary lamina

AN

MD

Reticular nucleus

Internal capsule

MI

VL

Subthalamic nucleus

Crus cerebri

Third ventricle

Hypothalamus

Mammillary body

Figure 9.2. The level of this cross section is indicated by A in the inset. The massa intermedia (MI) contains the midline nuclei. MD, mediodorsal nucleus; AN, anterior group of nuclei; VL, ventrolateral nuclei.

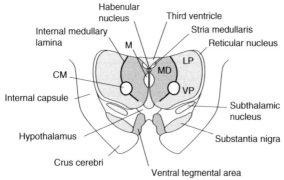

Habenular nucleus

Third ventricle

Internal medullary lamina

Stria medullaris

M

Reticular nucleus

LP

CM

MD

Internal capsule

VP

Hypothalamus

Subthalamic nucleus

Substantia nigra

Crus cerebri

Ventral tegmental area

Figure 9.3. The level of this cross section is indicated by B in the inset in Figure 9.2. The centromedian nucleus (CM) lies within the internal medullary lamina. M, midline nuclei; MD, mediodorsal nucleus; LP, lateral posterior nucleus; VP, ventral posterior nuclei.

to lateral prefrontal cortex. Dopamine D_2 receptors are found concentrated in the magnocellular part (Alelú-Paz and Giménez-Amaya, 2008).

The mediodorsal nucleus is described as the thalamic relay nucleus for association areas in the frontal lobe. It receives input from the amygdala, the nucleus accumbens, the olfactory region, the hypothalamus, and the basal ganglia. It projects to the nucleus basalis (of Meynert), the frontal eye fields, the prefrontal cortex, and the cingulate gyrus (Baleydier and Mauguiere, 1987). The mediodorsal nucleus relays limbic system information to the prefrontal cortex and to the cingulate cortex. It has been subdivided into several regions. The magnocellular portion of the mediodorsal nucleus,

A lesion of the ventral lateral nucleus along with the intralaminar nuclei and the mediodorsal nucleus on the right side was postulated to be the cause of a disinhibition syndrome that appeared in a 72-year-old woman (Bogousslavsky *et al.*, 1988b). The patient, who had no prior psychiatric history, developed a syndrome of increased speech, jokes, laughing, inappropriate comments, and confabulations. The authors suggested that this behavioral syndrome was produced by interrupting the link provided by the mediodorsal nucleus between the limbic system and the prefrontal lobe. Mania following thalamic lesions is associated with damage to the right side (Cummings and Mendez, 1984).

which lies medially, has close connections with the pyriform cortex, the amygdala, and the neocortex of the temporal lobe, as well as with the cingulate cortex. The parvicellular portion is much larger and lies laterally. It projects heavily to the prefrontal cortex.

Thalamic dementia presents with amnesia, speech disturbances, confusion, apathy, flattened affect, and aspontaneity of motor acts. It often results from bilateral paramedian infarction of the thalamus (Clarke *et al.*, 1994). The lesion apparently interrupts reciprocal connections between the thalamus and areas of the frontal cortex. In contrast, some patients with bilateral paramedian thalamic infarction exhibit thalamic pseudodementia (robot syndrome), in which they act in a manner similar to patients with thalamic dementia but can act normally if they are constantly stimulated by other people who show them what to do. It is suggested that both syndromes result from damage to the mediodorsal nucleus but that only the nonmagnocellular portions are involved in the robot syndrome. The magnocellular portion of the mediodorsal nucleus appears to be important in memory (Graff-Radford *et al.*, 1990; Bogousslavsky, 1991; Bogousslavsky *et al.*, 1991).

In a report of eight patients with bilateral thalamic tumors who exhibited personality change, memory loss, inattention, confusion, and hallucinations, in each case, the tumor involved the medial aspect of the left and right thalamus (Partlow *et al.*, 1992). Personality changes often are severe enough to result in institutional care. Most symptoms seen following an infarct improve over time with the exception of amnesia.

It has been hypothesized that the magnocellular portion of the mediodorsal nucleus may be released (disinhibited) in OCD. The release in behavior is similar

to that seen in the involuntary motor activity following lesions in other parts of the basal ganglia responsible for Parkinson and Huntington diseases (Baxter, 1990).

The mediodorsal nucleus has been implicated in schizophrenia. It has been reported to be reduced in size in early-onset schizophrenia (Pakkenberg, 1992). However, a study of late-onset schizophrenia demonstrated that the thalamus was increased in size (Corey-Bloom *et al.*, 1995), leading to the speculation that the thalamus compensates for abnormalities and delays the onset of symptoms in some individuals (Jeste *et al.*, 1996).

Ventral thalamic nuclei

The ventral thalamic group contains three major nuclei: the ventral anterior nucleus, the ventral lateral nucleus, and the ventral posterior nucleus. The border between the ventral anterior and the ventral lateral nucleus is indistinct, making it difficult to clearly separate the function of these two nuclei, which relay signals from the cerebellum and basal ganglia to the cortex. A small number of cells in the ventral anterior nucleus project to the cingulate cortex. These cells are located in the region of the nucleus that receives input from the globus pallidus and substantia nigra.

The ventral anterior nucleus is the most common lesion site in the thalamus associated with aphasia (Nadeau *et al.*, 1994). Mild transient hemiparesis and hemiataxia may be present following damage to the ventral lateral nucleus (Bogousslavsky *et al.*, 1986; Melo and Bogousslavsky, 1992). Hemineglect may be observed in right-sided lesions (Graff-Radford *et al.*, 1985).

Touch (somesthetic) signals are relayed from the head and body to the somesthetic (parietal) cortex through the ventral posterior nucleus. This nucleus is frequently subdivided into the ventral posterolateral nucleus (VPL), which mediates touch from the body to the parietal cortex, and the ventral posteromedial nucleus (VPM), which mediates touch from the head region to the parietal cortex (Chapter 4).

A lesion of the ventral posterior nucleus produces sensory loss on the contralateral side without major cognitive deficits. Paresthesias, including pain, may be the first symptoms. The patient may exhibit contralateral neglect. In some cases pain may develop only after several weeks. The thalamic pain syndrome is now more accurately called the central poststroke pain syndrome. It can occur after thalamic lesions as well as lesions in the spinal cord, brainstem, or cerebral hemispheres (Bovie *et al.*, 1989).

Neuropathic pain has been treated with varying degrees of success with electrical stimulation of VPM/VPL. It is theorized that the pain results from lack of proprioceptive stimuli reaching the thalamus (Head and Holmes, 1911). Stimulation correlates with increased blood flow to the region including VPM/VPL contralateral to the painful body site. Increased blood flow has also been reported in the anterior insula ipsilateral to the thalamic stimulation (Duncan *et al.*, 1998).

Lesions of the posterolateral thalamus can result in thalamic astasia, the inability to stand unsupported. This is distinguished from pusher syndrome, in which patients actively push away from the nonparetic side (Karnath *et al.*, 2000; Karnath 2007). Patients with pusher syndrome have a misperception of the body's orientation. Pusher syndrome is seen following lesions involving the posterior thalamus and less frequently, the insula. The lesion, which usually includes the ventral posterior and lateral posterior thalamic nuclei, may disrupt projections associated with somesthetic information (Pérennou *et al.*, 2002).

The ventral intermediate (ventrointermedial) nucleus forms the posterior and ventral portion of the ventrolateral nucleus. Deep brain stimulation of this nucleus is effective in treating essential tremor. While using electrodes to record tremors, Münte and Kutas (2008) and Wahl *et al.* (2008) found that the thalamus is sensitive to semantic and syntactic speech errors. The authors suggested that the nearby centromedian nucleus is the source of the signals representing speech error detection.

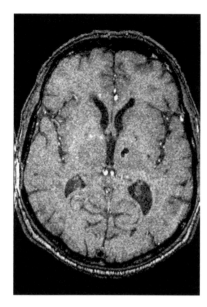

Figure 9.4. A magnetic resonance image (T1-weighted) demonstrated a strategic stroke in the left thalamus in a patient with cognitive deficits, particularly in working memory and calculations. (Reprinted with permission from Mendez *et al.*, 2003.)

Clinical vignette

A 61-year-old right-handed carpet salesman became acutely unable to perform the calculations needed to determine the amount of carpet for a floor area. He underwent tests of his calculation ability. On 16 written problems, he made the following errors: 5 + 6 = 36, 26 + 17 = 53, 621 − 72 = 541, 5 × 13 = 75, 78/13 = 5.5. On a word problem ("18 books on 2 shelves, put twice as many on the top shelf), he stated, "18 on the top and none on the bottom." Further testing revealed difficulties related to working memory, a frontal-executive function. This patient had cognitive difficulties from a thalamic stroke (Figure 9.4). On magnetic resonance imaging, he had a new lacunar infarct in the left thalamus. Infarction in the territory of the left tuberothalamic artery, with injury to the medial group of thalamic nuclei and their prefrontal connections, can produce difficulty in the working memory necessary to perform calculations.

Lateral thalamic nuclei

The lateral thalamic nuclear group makes up the largest of the thalamic nuclear groups. It consists of three nuclei. The lateral dorsal nucleus, the most anterior of the group, is functionally related to the anterior thalamic nuclear group and lies immediately behind the anterior nuclei. The major connections of the lateral dorsal nucleus are with the cingulate and parietal cortex. The larger and more posterior lateral posterior nucleus projects to the inferior parietal lobule.

The pulvinar forms the most posterior portion of the thalamus and overhangs the dorsal surface of the midbrain. The medial pulvinar has projections to the frontal lobe similar to those of the mediodorsal nucleus. Targets of fibers from the medial pulvinar include the dorsolateral and orbital prefrontal cortex as well as the insula and posterior cingulate gyrus (Romanski *et al.*, 1997). The mediodorsal nucleus and medial pulvinar may represent components of a single nuclear continuum (Romanski *et al.*, 1997; Byne *et al.*, 2009). In contrast, the lateral pulvinar has connections with the visual cortex and is believed to be involved in the control of eye movements. The pulvinar contains several nuclei that are retinotopically organized and implicated in processing behaviorally salient visual targets. It has direct projections to the lateral amygdala and is proposed to form part of a secondary extrageniculostriate visual system (Morris *et al.*, 2001; Vuilleumier *et al.*, 2003).

Significant volume reductions in autopsy material from schizophrenia patients have been reported for the pulvinar bilaterally (Danos *et al.*, 2003) and on the right side (Highley *et al.*, 2003). A volume reduction in the pulvinar but not the mediodorsal nucleus was reported in schizotypal personality disorder (Byne *et al.*, 2001).

The pulvinar has been implicated in "blindsight" (Chapter 4). An increase in bilateral pulvinar relative cerebral blood flow (rCBF) has been reported following alleviation of chronic pain by anesthetic blocks and by direct thalamic stimulation (Kupers *et al.*, 2000) and an increase in rCBF in the left pulvinar in response to sub-occipital stimulation for relief of the pain of migraine headache (Matharu *et al.*, 2003). Pulvinotomy and electrical stimulation of the pulvinar have been used successfully in the past for the control of chronic pain (Yoshii *et al.*, 1980). The pulvinar receives nociceptive input and projects to the superior parietal lobule but it is unknown whether the pulvinar mediates pain or is just associated with it (Matharu *et al.*, 2003).

Medial and lateral geniculate bodies

The medial geniculate body relays auditory signals from the inferior colliculus to the temporal cortex. The lateral geniculate body relays visual signals from the retina to the occipital cortex. Damage to the lateral geniculate body can result in visual field disturbances (Bogousslavsky *et al.*, 1988a).

Reticular nucleus

A sheet of myelinated fibers called the external medullary lamina covers the lateral, anterolateral, and ventrolateral surfaces of the thalamus and lies between the thalamus and the internal capsule. Embedded within the external medullary lamina is a group of small nuclei, collectively called the reticular nuclei, or more simply the reticular nucleus. Neurons of the reticular nucleus are γ-aminobutyric acid (GABA) ergic and make extensive reciprocal connections with all the nuclei of the dorsal thalamus. They receive fibers from, but do not project fibers to, the cerebral cortex. The reticular nucleus receives collateral input from the thalamocortical, corticothalamic, thalamostriate, and pallidothalamic fibers.

The reticular nucleus is believed to serve as an attentional valve or gate for thalamocortical transmission. There appear to be as many gates as there are sensory modalities with individual cell groups within the reticular nucleus that are sensitive to specific sensory modalities or to portions of sensory modalities. The reticular nucleus is believed to mediate the inhibitory influences from the frontal lobes as well as excitatory impact of the brainstem reticular formation. It provides a possible mechanism for autohypnosis and voluntary pain control (Mesulam, 1985; Scheibel, 1997).

Intralaminar nuclei

The intralaminar nuclei represent an anterior continuation of the brainstem reticular formation (Chapter 10). In addition to reticular afferents, projections from spinal and brainstem pain systems are important inputs to the intralaminar nuclei. The pattern of projection from the intralaminar nuclei is diffuse and widespread, and reaches all areas of the cerebral cortex. The intralaminar nuclei provide significant input to the basal ganglia as well as to cells located in the thalamus itself.

The centromedian nucleus is the largest of the intralaminar nuclei. It receives fibers from the basal ganglia, brainstem reticular formation, vestibular nuclei, and superior colliculus. It projects diffuse excitatory projections to broad cortical areas. It has connections with the basal ganglia, primarily the putamen, and is part of sensorimotor and limbic loops. The centromedian and parafascicular nuclei make up the caudal group of intralaminar nuclei. The two are sometimes grouped together as the centromedian–parafascicular complex.

The diffusely projecting intralaminar nuclei are part of a system that governs the level of arousal of the brain. The system is believed to play a role in selective attention. It becomes activated when going from a relaxed to an attention-demanding state (Kinomura *et al.*, 1996).

Lesions placed in the medial portion of the centromedian nucleus produce a reduction in aggression. Lesions located laterally in this nucleus are less effective in reducing aggression (Andy *et al.*, 1975). Transient loss of consciousness usually seen after a paramedian infarction may be due to involvement of the intralaminar nuclei (Karabelas *et al.*, 1985).

Significant centromedian volume reduction has been reported in autopsy studies in schizophrenia. One study reported a nonsignificant 13.5% reduction and a second found a significant reduction when corrected for brain weight (Byne *et al.*, 2002). Findings suggested that volume is increased by exposure to neuroleptic drugs (Kemether *et al.*, 2003). It was speculated that this is due to the high density of D_2-like receptors in the centromedian nucleus (Rieck, *et al.*, 2004; Lieberman *et al.*, 2005; Byne *et al.*, 2009).

161

The centromedian–parafascicular complex exhibits a marked decrease in cell numbers in Huntington disease. Because of the suspected role played by the centromedian nucleus in oculomotor control, it is speculated that the cell loss is the basis of abnormal saccadic eye movement seen in Huntington disease (Heinsen *et al.*, 1999).

Limbic thalamus

The limbic thalamus is defined as that portion of the thalamus that serves the limbic cortex (Bentivoglio *et al.*, 1993). Based on this definition, the limbic thalamus originally was made up of only the anterior thalamic nuclear group. Results of more recent studies have broadened the content of the limbic thalamus to include parts of a number of thalamic nuclei (Table 9.1). The lateral dorsal nucleus projects to the cingulate cortex. In addition, the diffuse group of nuclei that project to many areas of the cortex include cell groups that project to the cingulate cortex. The midline and intralaminar nuclei, in particular, contain cells that project to the cingulate cortex. The ventral anterior nucleus is generally considered one of the motor nuclei and is associated with the basal ganglia and cerebellum. However, the ventral anterior nucleus also projects to the cingulate cortex, thus establishing a close link between motor systems and the limbic cortex (Vogt *et al.*, 1987). The mediodorsal nucleus projects heavily to the prefrontal cortex. It also sends fibers to the cingulate cortex and is included by some as part of the limbic thalamus (Bentivoglio *et al.*, 1993). The cingulate cortex projects back to all of the components of the limbic thalamus. Anterior, mediodorsal, and midline nuclei project to the ventral anterior portion of the cingulate cortex. These thalamic nuclei receive much of their information from brainstem and hypothalamic nuclei that are recognized as autonomic centers. The regulation of visceral and autonomic function is one of the prominent roles of the ventral anterior cingulate cortex (Chapter 12).

Other behavioral considerations

A number of studies have shown decreased thalamic volume in schizophrenia. Several have compared it with total brain volume, which is known to be decreased in schizophrenia, and found the thalamic decrease significant (Konick and Friedman, 2001; Kemether *et al.*, 2003). Thalamic volume may be sensitive to neuroleptics. Several studies have reported that thalamic volume correlates positively with dosage of neuroleptic drugs (Gur *et al.*, 1998; Khorram *et al.*, 2006). A link has been proposed between thalamus volume and clinical response to drugs (Strungas *et al.*, 2003).

One of the primary functions of the thalamus is to filter or gate sensory input. A defect in this function could explain difficulties in the interpretation of sensory input, which may include some of the symptoms of schizophrenia.

Distractibility, loss of associations, and shifting attentional focus commonly seen in schizophrenia patients may result from sensory overload. The inability to screen out irrelevant stimuli may be a failure of the gating function of the thalamus (Braff, 1993). Regional blood flow to the thalamus increases bilaterally during auditory hallucinations (but not during visual hallucinations) experienced by schizophrenia patients (Silversweig *et al.*, 1995).

One hypothesis advanced to explain the variety of symptoms of schizophrenia is that the midline neural circuits which mediate attention and information processing are dysfunctional. When magnetic resonance (MR) images of normal individuals were averaged together and then compared with the averaged MR images of schizophrenia patients, specific regional abnormalities were observed in the thalamus and adjacent white matter. The lateral and ventrolateral areas of the thalamus, which project to the cingulate gyrus, parietal cortex, and temporal cortex, were seen to be most involved (Andreasen *et al.*, 1994). The reduction in size of the thalamus may produce an abnormality in the normal gating and filtering function of the thalamus and allow a bombardment of the cortex by sensory stimuli, resulting in difficulty in distinguishing "self" from "nonself." Figure 9.5 illustrates a decrease in blood flow in the thalamus seen in schizophrenia (Andreasen, 1997).

The thalamus is involved in many functions, including the storage and retrieval of memory. As stated by Silversweig and associates (1995), "The thalamus is believed to generate an internal representation of reality, in the presence or absence of sensory input." The anterior nuclei and the lateral dorsal nucleus in particular are involved in memory. Memory disturbance in Korsakoff disease corresponds with loss of cells in the medial portion of the dorsal medial nucleus as well as cells in the nearby midline nuclei.

It has been hypothesized that there exists a medial and a lateral pain system (Albe-Fessard *et al.*, 1985). The medial pain system includes the periaqueductal gray of the midbrain and the intralaminar and midline thalamic nuclei, which project to the cingulate

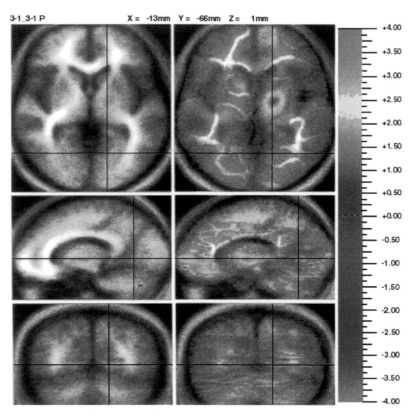

Figure 9.5. Difference in cerebral blood flow between schizophrenic patients and control subjects using positron emission tomography (PET) while they recalled Story A from the Weschler Memory Scale. Three orthogonal views are shown, with transaxial at the top, sagittal in the middle, and coronal on the bottom. The crosshairs show the location of the slice. Structures are as if standing at the foot of the bed (transaxial view) or facing the patient (coronal view). The left column shows differences using the "peak map." The right column demonstrates differences using the "t map." Significantly higher blood flow corresponds with lighter areas and is seen in the anterior frontal pole, thalamus, and cerebellum of control subjects. (Reproduced by permission from Andreasen, N.C. 1997. The role of the thalamus in schizophrenia. Can. J. Psychiatry 42:27–30.)

cortex and to the prefrontal cortex. The medial pain system is responsible for the affective component of pain. Ablation of the midline and intralaminar nuclei has been used to relieve chronic pain. The lateral pain system involves the ventral posteromedial and ventral posterolateral nuclei, which project onto the parietal cortex. The lateral system is responsible for the localization of pain.

Select bibliography

Jones, E.G. *The Thalamus.* (New York: Cambridge University Press, 2007.)

Kultas-Ilinsky, K., and Ilinsky, I.A. eds. *Basal Ganglia and Thalamus in Health and Movement Disorders.* (New York: Kluwer Academic/Plenum Publishers, 2000.)

Sherman, S.M., and Guillery, R.W. *Exploring the Thalamus.* (San Diego: Academic Press, 2001.)

References

Albe-Fessard, D., Berkeley, K.J., Kruger, L., Ralston, H.J. III, and Willis, W.D., Jr. 1985. Diencephalic mechanisms of pain sensation. *Brain Res.* **356**:217–296.

Alelú-Paz, R., and Giménez-Amaya, J.M. 2008. The mediodorsal thalamic nucleus and schizophrenia. *J. Psychiatry Neurosci.* **33**:489–498.

Andreasen, N.C. 1997. The role of the thalamus in schizophrenia. *Can. J. Psychiatry* **42**:27–33.

Andreasen, N.C., Arndt, S., Swayze V., Cizadlo, T., Flaum, M., O' Leary, D., Ehrhardt, J.C., and Yuh, W.T.C. 1994. Thalamic abnormalities in schizophrenia visualized through magnetic resonance image averaging. *Science* **266**:294–297.

Andy, O.J., Jurko, M.F., and Giurintano, L.P. 1975. Behavioral changes correlated with thalamotomy site. *Confin. Neurol.* **36**:106–112.

Baleydier, C., and Mauguiere, F. 1987. Network organization of the connectivity between parietal area 7, posterior cingulate cortex and medial pulvinar nucleus: A double fluorescent tracer study in monkey. *Exp. Brain Res.* **66**:385–393.

Baxter, L.R. 1990. Brain imaging as a tool in establishing a theory of brain pathology in obsessive compulsive disorder. *J. Clin. Psychiatry* **51**(Suppl.):22–26.

Bentivoglio, M., Kultas-Llinsky, D., and Llinsky, I. 1993. Limbic thalamus: Structure, intrinsic organization, and connections. In: B.A.Vogt and M.Gabriel (eds.) *Neurobiology of Cingulate Cortex and Limbic Thalamus: A Comprehensive Handbook.* Boston: Birkhauser.

Bogousslavsky, J. 1991. Thalamic dementia and pseudo-dementia. In: A.Hartmann, W.Kuschinsky, and S.Hoyer (eds.) *Cerebral Ischemia and Dementia.* Berlin: Springer.

Bogousslavsky, J., Regli, F., and Assal, G. 1986. The syndrome of unilateral tuberothalamic artery territory infarction. *Stroke* **17**:434–441.

Bogousslavsky, J., Regli, F., and Uske, A.1988a. Thalamic infarcts: Clinical syndromes, etiology, and prognosis. *Neurology* **38**:837–848.

Bogousslavsky, J., Ferrazzini, M., Regli, F., Assal, G., Tanabe, H., and Delaloye-Bischof, A.1988b. Manic delirium and frontal-like syndrome with paramedian infarction of the right thalamus. *J. Neurol. Neurosurg. Psychiatry* **51**:116–119.

Bogousslavsky, J., Regli, F., Delaloye, B., Delaloye-Bischof, A., Assal, G., and Uske, A. 1991. Loss of psychic self activation with bithalamic infarction: Neurobehavioural, CT, MRI and SPECT correlates. *Acta Neurol. Scand.* **83**:309–316.

Bovie, J., Leijon, G., and Johansson, I. 1989. Central post-stroke pain –a study of the mechanisms through analyses of the sensory abnormalities. *Pain* **37**:173–185.

Braff, D.L. 1993. Information processing and attention dysfunctions in schizophrenia. *Schizophr. Bull.* **19**:233–259.

Byne, W., Buchsbaum, M.S., Kemether, E., Hazlett, E.A., Shinwari, A., Mitropoulou, V., and Siever, L.J. 2001. Magnetic resonance imaging of the thalamic mediodorsal nucleus and pulvinar in schizophrenia and schizotypal personality disorder. *Arch. Gen. Psychiatry* **58**:133–140.

Byne, W., Buchsbaum, M.S., Mattiace, L.A., Hazlett, E.A., Kemether, E., Elhakem, S.L., Purohit, D.P., Haroutunian, V., and Jones, L. 2002. Postmortem assessment of thalamic nuclear volumes in subjects with schizophrenia. *Am. J. Psychiatry* **159**:59–65.

Byne, W., Kidkardnee, S., Tatusov, A., Yiannoulos, G., Buschbaum, M.S., and Haroutunian, V. 2006. Schizophrenia-associated reduction of neuronal and oligodendrocyte numbers in the anterior principal thalamic nucleus. *Schizophr. Res.* **85**:245–253.

Byne, W., Hazlett, E.A., Buchsbaum, M.S., and Kemether, E. 2009. The thalamus and schizophrenia: Current status of research. *Acta Neurpathol.* **117**:347–368.

Clarke, W., Assal, G., Bogousslavsky, J., Regli, F., Townsend., D.W., Leenders, K.L., and Blecic, S. 1994. Pure amnesia after unilateral left polar thalamic infarct: topographic and sequential neuropsychological and metabolic (PET) correlations. *J. Neurol. Neurosurg. Psychiatry* **57**:27–34.

Corey-Bloom, J., Jernigan, T., Archibald, S., Harris, M.J., and Jeste, D.V. 1995. Quantitative magnetic resonance imaging in late-life schizophrenia. *Am J. Psychiatry* **152**:447–449.

Cummings, J.L., and Mendez, M.F. 1984. Secondary mania with focal cerebrovascular lesions. *Am. J. Psychiatry* **141**:1084–1087.

Danos, P., Baumann, B., Bernstein, H.G., Franz, M., Stauch, R., Northoff, G., Krell, D., Falkai, P., and Bogerts, B. 1998. Schizophrenia and anteroventral thalamic nucleus: Selective decrease of parvalbumin-immunoreactive thalamocortical projection neurons. *Psychiatry Res.* **82**:1–10.

Danos, P., Baumann, B., Kramer, A., Bernstein, H.G., Stauch, R., Krell, D., Falkai, P., and Bogerts, B. 2003. Volumes of association thalamic nuclei in schizophrenia: A postmortem study. *Schizophr. Res* **60**:141–155.

Duncan, G.H., Kupers, R.C., Marhand, S., Villemure, J-G., Gybels, J.M., and Bushnell, M.C. 1998. Stimulation of human thalamus for pain relief: possible modulatory circuits revealed by positron emission tomography. *J. Neurophysiol.* **80**:3326–3330.

Graff-Radford, N.R., Eslinger, P.J., Damasio, A.R., and Yamada, T. 1984. Nonhemorrhagic infarction of the thalamus: Behavioral, anatomic, and physiologic correlates. *Neurology* **34**:14–23.

Graff-Radford, N.R., Damasio, H., Yamada, T., Eslinger, P.J., and Damasio, A.R. 1985. Nonhaemorrhagic thalamic infarction: Clinical, neuropsychological and electrophysiological findings in four anatomical groups defined by computerized tomography. *Brain* **108**:485–516.

Graff-Radford, N.R., Tranel, D., Van Hoesen, G., and Brandt, J.P. 1990. Diencephalic amnesia. *Brain* **113**:1–25.

Gur, R.E., Maany, V., Mozley, P.D., Swanson, C., Bilker, W., and Gur, R.C. 1998. Subcortical MRI volumes in neuroleptic-naïve and treated patients with schizophrenia. *Am. J. Psychiatry* **155**:1711–1717.

Head, H., and Holmes, G. 1911. Sensory disturbances from cerebral lesions. *Brain* **34**:102–254.

Heinsen, H., Rub, W., Bauer, M., Ulmar, G., Bethke, B., Schuler, M., Bocker, F., Eisenmenger, W., Gotz, M., Korr, H., and Schmitz, C., 1999. Nerve cell loss in the thalamic mediodorsal nucleus in Huntington's disease. *Acta Neuropathol.* 97:613–622.

Highley, J.R., Walker, M.A., Crow, T.J., Esiri, M.M., and Harrison, P.J. 2003. Low medial and lateral right pulvinar volumes in schizophrenia: A postmortem study. *Am. J. Psychiatry* 162:2233–2245.

Jakary, A., Vinogradov, S., Feiwell, R., and Deicken, R.F. 2005. N-acetylaspartate reductions in the mediodorsal and anterior thalamus in men with schizophrenia verified by tissue volume corrected proton MRSI. *Schizophr. Res.* 76:173–185.

Jeste, D.V., Galasko, D., Corey-Bloom, J., Walens, S., and Granholm, E. 1996. Neuropsychiatric aspects of the schizophrenias. In: B.S.Fogel, R.B.Schiffer, and S.M.Rao (eds.) *Neuropsychiatry*. Baltimore: Williams & Wilkins.

Karabelas, T., Kalfakis, N., Kasvikis, I., and Vassilopoulos, D. 1985. Unusual features in a case of bilateral paramedian thalamic infarction. *J. Neurol. Neurosurg. Psychiatry* 48:186.

Karnath, H.O. 2007. Pusher syndrome – A frequent but little-known disturbance of body orientation perception. *J. Neurol.* 254:415–424.

Karnath, H.O., Ferber, S., and Dichgans, J. 2000. The neural representation of postural control in humans. *Proc. Natl. Acad. Sci. USA.* 97:13931–13936.

Kemether, E.M., Buchsbaum, M.S., Byne, W., Hazlett, E.A., Haznedar, M. Brickman, A.M., Platholi, J., and Bloom, R. 2003. Magnetic resonance imaging of mediodorsal, pulvinar, and centromedian nuclei of the thalamus in patients with schizophrenia. *Arch. Gen. Psychiatry* 60:983–991.

Khorram, B., Lang, D.J., Kopala, L.C., Vandorpe, R.A., Rui, Q., Goghari, V.M., Smith, G.N., and Honer, W.G. 2006. Reduced thalamic volume in patients with chronic schizophrenia after switching from typical antipsychotic medications to olanzaprine. *Am. J. Psychiatry* 163:2005–2007.

Kinomura, S., Larsson, J., Gulyas, B., and Roland, P.E. 1996. Activation by attention of the human reticular formation and thalamic intralaminar nuclei. *Science* 271:512–515.

Konick, L.C., and Friedman, L. 2001. Meta-analysis of thalamic size in schizophrenia. *Biol. Psychiatry* 49:28–38.

Kupers, R.C., Gybels, J.M., and Gjedde, A. 2000. Positron emission tomography study of a chronic pain patient successfully treated with somatosensory thalamic stimulation. *Pain* 87:295–302.

Lieberman, J.A., Tollefson, G.D., Charles, C., Zipursky, R., Sharma, T., Kahn, R.S., Keefe, R.S., Green, A.I., Gur, R.E., McEvoy, J., Perkins, D., Hamer, R.M., Gu, H., and Tohen, M. 2005. Antipsychotic drug effects on brain morphology in first-episode psychosis. *Arch. Gen. Psychiatry* 62:361–370.

Martuza, R.L., Chiocca, E.A., and Jenike, M.A. 1990. Stereotactic radiofrequency thermal cingulotomy for obsessive compulsive disorder. *J. Neuropsychiatry Clin. Neurosci.* 2:331–336.

Matharu, M.S., Bartsch, T., Ward, N., Frackowiak, R.S.J., Weiner, R., and Goadsby, P.J. 2003. Central neuromodulation in chronic migraine patients with suboccipital stiulators: a PET study. *Brain* 127:220–230.

Melo, T.P., and Bogousslavsky, J. 1992. Hemiataxia-hypesthesia: A thalamic stroke syndrome. *J. Neurol. Neurosurg. Psychiatry* 55:581–584.

Mendez, M.F., Papasian, N.C., Lim, G.T., and Swanberg, M. 2003. Thalamic acalculia. *J. Neuropsychiatry Clin. Neurosci.* 15:115–116.

Mesulam, M.M. 1985. Attention, confusional states and neglect. In: M.M.Mesulem (ed.) *Principles of Behavioral Neurology*. Philadelphia: Davis, pp.125–168.

Morris, J.S., DeGelder, B., Weiskrantz, L, and Dolan, R.J. 2001. Differential extrageniculostriate and amygdala response to presentation of emotional faces in a cortically blind field. *Brain* 124:1241–1252.

Münte, T.F., and Kutas, M., 2008. Capitalizing on deep brain stimulation: Thalamus as a language monitor. *Neuron* 59:667–679.

Nadeau, S.E., Roeltgen, D.P., Sevush, S., Ballinger, W.E., and Watson, R.T. 1994. Apraxia due to a pathologically documented thalamic infarction. *Neurology* 44:2133–2137.

Pakkenberg, B. 1992. The volume of the mediodorsal thalamic nucleus in treated and untreated schizophrenics. *Schizophr. Res.* 7:95–100.

Partlow, G.D., Carpio-O ' Donovan, R., Melanson, D., and Peters, T.M. 1992. Bilateral thalamic glioma: Review of eight cases with personality change and mental deterioration. *A.J.N.R. Am. J. Neuroradiol.* 13:1225–1230.

Pérennou, D.A., Amblard, B., Laassel, E.M., Benaim, C., Herisson, C., and Pélissier, J. 2002. Understanding the pusher behavior of some stroke patients with spatial deficits: A pilot study. *Arch. Phys. Med. Rehabil.* 83:570–575.

Rieck, R.W., Ansari, M.S., Whetsell, W.O. Jr., Deutch, A.Y., and Kessler, R.M. 2004. Distribution of dopamine D2-like receptors in the human thalamus: Autoradiographic and PET studies. *Neuropsychopharmacology* 29:362–372.

Romanski, L.M., Giguere, M., Bates, J.F., and Goldman-Rakic, P.S. 1997. Topograpic organization of medial pulvinar connections with the prefrontal cortex in the rhesus monkey. *J. Comp. Neurol.* 379:313–332.

Scheibel, A.B. 1997. The thalamus and neuropsychiatric illness. *J. Neuropsychiatry Clin. Neurosci.* 9:342–353.

Silversweig, D.A., Stern, E., Frith, C., Cahill, C., Holmes, A., Groutoonik, S., Seaward, J., McKenna, P., Chua,

S.E., Schnorr, L, Jones, T., and Frackowiak, R.S.J. 1995. A functional neuroanatomy of hallucinations in schizophrenia. *Nature* **378**:176–179.

Strungas, S., Christensen, J.D., Holcomb, J.M., and Garver, D.L. 2003. State-related thalamic changes during antipsychotic treatment in schizophrenia: Preliminary observations. *Psychiatry Res.* **124**:121–124.

Vogt, B.A., Pandya, D.N., and Rosene, D.L. 1987. Cingulate cortex of the rhesus monkey: I. Cytoarchitecture and thalamic afferents. *J. Comp. Neurol.* **262**:256–270.

Vuilleumier, P., Armony, J.L., Driver, J., and Dolan, R.J. 2003. Distinct spatial frequency sensitivities for processing faces and emotional expressions. *Nat. Neurosci.* **6**:624–631.

Wahl, M., Marzinzik, F., Friederici, A.D., Hahne, A., Kupsch, A., Schneider, G-H., Saddy, D., Curio, G., and Klostermann, F. 2008. The human thalamus processes syntactic and semantic language violations. *Neuron* **59**:695–707.

Yoshii, N., Mizokami, T., Ushikubo, T., Kuramitsu, T., and Fukuda, S. 1980. Long-term follow-up study after pulvinotomy for intractable pain. *Appl. Neurophysiol.* **43**:128–132.

Young, K.A., Manaye, K.F., Liang, C.L., Hicks, P.B., and German, D.C. 2000. Reduced number of mediodorsal and anterior thalamic neurons in schizophrenia. *Biol. Psychiatry* **47**:944–953.

Zubieta, J-K., Smith, Y.R., Bueller, J.A., Xu, Y., Kilbourn, M.R., Jewett, D.M., Meyer, C.R., Koeppe, R.A., and Stohler, C.S. 2002. μ-Opioid receptor-mediated antinociceptive responses differ in men and women. *J. Neurosci.* **22**:5100–5107.

Chapter 10 — Brainstem

Introduction

The brainstem is the connection between the spinal cord, the cerebellum, and the cerebrum. It has only recently been implicated in behavior. The brainstem anatomically comprises three areas: the medulla, the pons, and the midbrain (Figure 2.1). The medulla, the most inferior segment of the brainstem, represents a conical, expanded continuation of the upper cervical spinal cord. The pons lies between the medulla and the midbrain. The midbrain is the smallest and least differentiated division of the brainstem. The nuclei of cranial nerves III through XII are located in the brainstem along with long sensory and motor tracts that pass between the brain and spinal cord. Several regions of the brainstem, however, seem to be significantly involved in behavior. These behaviorally active regions include: the reticular formation, the parabrachial nucleus, the raphe nuclei, the periaqueductal gray (PAG), the nucleus locus ceruleus, the lateral tegmental nucleus, the ventral tegmental area (VTA), and the inferior olive. The VTA is considered to be one of the basal ganglia (Chapter 7).

Anatomy and behavioral considerations

Reticular formation

The reticular formation is one of the oldest portions of the brain and represents the core of the brainstem. It is composed of complex collections of cells that form both diffuse cellular aggregations and more defined nuclei.

The ascending reticular activating system (ARAS) is a physiological concept. It is represented anatomically by the central core region of the brainstem (Figure 10.1), including the raphe nuclei (Figure 10.2). This region contains a number of nuclei. The ARAS receives collateral fibers from the surrounding specific sensory systems. The main long ascending pathway of the brainstem reticular formation is the central tegmental tract (Figure 10.3). This tract projects to the

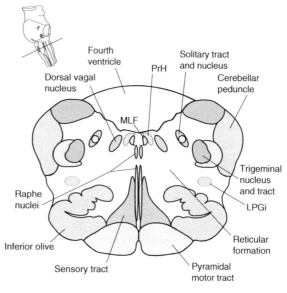

Figure 10.1. A cross section typical of the medulla. The brainstem inset in the upper left indicates the level of the cross section. PrH, nucleus prepositus hypoglossi; LPGi, caudal extent of nucleus paragigantocellularis lateralis (positions approximate); MLF, medial longitudinal fasciculus.

intralaminar nuclei of the thalamus (Table 9.1, Chapter 9). The reticular formation extends rostrally from the brainstem into the hypothalamus. Ascending reticular fibers to the hypothalamus are distinct from those that go to the thalamus.

The continuous bottom-up sensory input into the ARAS plays an important role in wakefulness, alertness, and arousal. Lesions in the rostromedial midbrain tegmentum abolish the electroencephalographic (EEG) arousal reaction elicited by sensory stimulation even though the long ascending sensory pathways remain intact. The cerebral cortex acts in a top-down manner to alter the state of consciousness by influencing the reticular neurons. Such a role has been suggested by the well-known arousing effect of psychic stimuli. Areas of the cerebral cortex from which the arousing effect can be obtained by electrical stimulation include

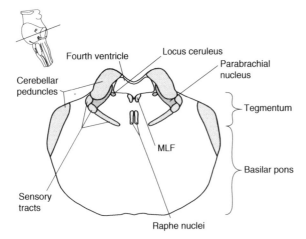

Figure 10.2. A cross section typical of the pons. The sensory tracts from medial to lateral are the medial lemniscus, the spinal lemniscus, and the lateral lemniscus. MLF, medial longitudinal fasciculus.

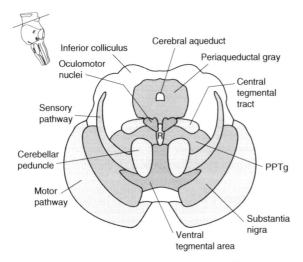

Figure 10.3. A cross section typical of the caudal midbrain at the level of the inferior colliculus. PPTg, pedunculopontine tegmental nucleus; R, raphe nucleus.

the orbital prefrontal cortex, the lateral surface of the frontal lobe, the sensory motor cortex, the superior temporal gyrus, and the cingulate gyrus. The reticular formation has three more important functions: regulation of muscle reflexes, coordination of autonomic functions, and modulation of pain sensation. It is of interest that reticular formation neurons involved in the control of breathing and cardiac function are influenced by higher centers, including the hypothalamus and prefrontal association areas.

The pedunculopontine tegmental nucleus (PPTg) is a cholinergic nucleus of the ARAS that is involved

in sleep mechanisms (Figure 10.3). It is recognized as important in the induction and maintenance of rapid eye movement (REM) sleep (Semba, 1993). It is considered to be a striatal output station and is a component of the "mesencephalic locomotor region" (Mogenson *et al.*, 1989; Winn *et al.*, 1997). A decrease in choline acetyltransferase has been reported in this nucleus in schizophrenia patients, which suggests a reduction in brainstem acetylcholine activity in this disorder (Karson *et al.*, 1993). See Chapter 7 for a more complete discussion of the importance of the pedunculopontine tegmental nucleus in the regulation of behavior.

Parabrachial nucleus

The parabrachial nucleus lies medial to the superior cerebellar peduncle and medial to the sensory (lemniscal) tracts in the pons and midbrain (Figure 10.3). It receives visceral sensory information from the spinal cord and brainstem. It gives rise to ascending fibers that project to the hypothalamus (Chapter 8) and amygdala (Chapter 11) and to the raphe nuclei (Holstege, 1988).

The parabrachial nucleus is a general integrative site for visceral information, including taste, cardio-respiratory signals, and visceral pain (Craig, 1996; Chamberlin, 2004). It links these sensations with the central nucleus of the amygdala and the hypothalamus (see "autonomic sensory nuclei" in Figure 11.5 and 11.6). It is proposed that the parabrachial nucleus is important in the emotional and autonomic responses to incoming visceral signals, especially visceral pain (Bernard *et al.*, 1996; Norgren *et al.*, 2006).

Raphe nuclei

Several groups of cells that are situated along the midline of the medulla, pons, and midbrain are collectively called the raphe nuclei (Figures 10.1, 10.2, 10.3, and 10.4). They are part of the brainstem reticular formation, but produce a particular neurotransmitter, serotonin [5-hydroxytryptamine (5-HT)]. Neurons from different raphe nuclei contain specific cotransmitters (peptides). Areas that project fibers to the raphe nuclei include the amygdala, hypothalamus, and PAG, as well as other brainstem nuclei (Figure 10.5).

Rostral pontine and midbrain raphe nuclei project to the PAG and to structures in the cerebrum. Most pontine raphe nuclei have long ascending projections that are located in the medial forebrain bundle. Fibers project to the hypothalamus, nigral complex, intralaminar thalamic nuclei, stria terminalis, septum, hippocampus, amygdala, and cerebral cortex. Of particular interest are raphe projections to the ventral tegmental area and to the nucleus accumbens. Cortical projections are confined largely to the frontal lobe, although fibers to other neocortical areas have been demonstrated.

Medullary and caudal pontine raphe nuclei project to other parts of the brainstem and to all levels of the cord. Targets include the trigeminal nuclei and the dorsal and ventral spinal cord gray matter. These descending projections of the raphe nuclei are ideally situated to regulate incoming sensory stimuli. The raphe spinal tract, which terminates in the spinal trigeminal nucleus and in the spinal cord dorsal horn, regulates (inhibits) incoming pain signals (Mason and Leung, 1996). The nucleus raphe magnus, which gives rise to the raphe spinal tract, is controlled by neurons in the PAG. They, in turn, receive input from the limbic system, thus providing a link between emotion, pain, and defense behaviors (see the following section on PAG). Other raphe spinal projections that terminate in the ventral horn are thought to function in a neuromodulatory role to facilitate locomotion.

Serotonin and the raphe nuclei have been implicated in the regulation of sleep, aggressive behavior, pain, and a variety of visceral and neuroendocrine functions. Raphe neurons decrease their firing rate from waking to sleep and cease firing during REM sleep. Destruction of serotonin neurons or blockade of serotonin receptors produces an animal that is

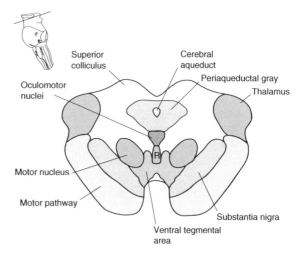

Figure 10.4. A cross section typical of the rostral midbrain at the level of the superior colliculus. R, raphe nucleus.

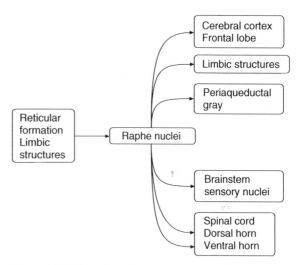

Figure 10.5. The raphe nuclei are a major source of serotonin. Descending influences can block pain stimuli (dorsal horn) and facilitate motor activity (ventral horn). Ascending projections inhibit nonmeaningful stimuli and facilitate meaningful signals.

hypersensitive to virtually all environmental stimuli and is hyperactive in all situations. Serotonin inhibits sensory stimuli that have a waking effect (see the section later on locus ceruleus and lateral tegmental nucleus). It may help to facilitate meaningful sensory stimuli and to inhibit nonmeaningful sensory stimuli. Serotonin in this way aids in maintaining behavior within specific limits.

Serotonergic neurons may have a priming effect on the cells of the nucleus locus ceruleus, which are responsible for triggering the REM sleep stage (Jacobs, 1994). In contrast to locus ceruleus neurons, which increase their firing rate during periods of intense environmental stimuli, the serotonergic neurons fire more rapidly during periods of quiet, rhythmical behaviors such as grooming or chewing, behaviors associated with a relaxed state (Jacobs and Fornal, 1993).

Activity in the dorsal raphe nuclei raises the threshold that activates defensive behaviors controlled by the PAG of the midbrain. Medullary raphe nuclei play a similar role in the modulation of cardiovascular responses to stress (Lovick, 1996). Projections from the raphe nuclei to the mesolimbic structures (ventral tegmental area and nucleus accumbens) provide a link between serotonin and dopamine. It is hypothesized that the raphe nuclei play an important regulatory role in the control of dopamine release. Because of this relationship the raphe nuclei may play a role in schizophrenia (Mylecharane, 1996).

A loss of the serotonergic neurons of the raphe nuclei has been documented in Alzheimer disease (Aletrino *et al.*, 1992). However, the concentration of cortical serotonin was found to be in the normal range, suggesting that sprouting of raphe axon terminals in the cortex makes up for the deficiency of serotonin due to raphe neuron loss (Chen *et al.*, 1996).

Blood levels of serotonin are elevated in autistic and in some mentally retarded individuals. The significance of this finding is obscure since cerebrospinal fluid levels do not correlate with blood levels. It has been suggested that the abnormal serotonin levels may reflect a role played by serotonin in brain development (McNamara *et al.*, 2008).

Uncontrolled crying is a behavior commonly seen after stroke (one-year incidence is 20%). Successful treatment by selective serotonin reuptake inhibitor drugs has led to the suggestion that this behavior results from stroke-induced partial destruction of raphe nuclei or of their ascending projections to the cerebral hemispheres (Andersen, 1995).

Periaqueductal gray

The PAG surrounds the cerebral aqueduct in the midbrain (Figures 10.2 and 10.4). It is connected with many forebrain structures above as well as with brainstem structures below. It has reciprocal connections with the central nucleus of the amygdala. Descending fibers from the PAG include those to the raphe nuclei involved in the suppression of incoming pain signals. The PAG is centrally located between the limbic system and somatic and visceral motor control centers. The central nucleus of the amygdala of the limbic

Clinical vignette

A 59-year-old man was found dead from a self-inflicted gunshot wound. Three years before his death he had developed left-sided hemianesthesia. A computed tomographic (CT) scan taken at the time showed a lesion in the tegmentum of the upper pons on the right side. Over the following few months other neurological deficits developed but he was not incapacitated. Five months after the initial episode he developed severe depression with paranoid ideations. The patient had no past or family history of affective disorders. He failed to respond to a number of antidepressants that were tried over a period of two years. Postmortem examination revealed a cavernous hemangioma impinging on the upper pontine region of the raphe nuclei on the right side and extending to partially involve the raphe on the left side. It was believed that the lesion caused depletion of the ascending serotonergic system to the forebrain (Kline and Oertel, 1997).

Clinical vignette

A 55-year-old right-handed man presented with acute, uncontrolled crying spells and numbness over his left face and arm. Around 6:00 am he awoke with a diffuse pressure headache and suddenly started crying for no apparent reason. After five minutes, the crying abruptly ceased. Over the next two to three hours, he had five more crying spells, each lasting five to ten minutes, occurring out of context, without precipitating factors or sadness, with an acute onset and offset, and without alteration of consciousness. The patient's left face and arm numbness persisted during and between these crying spells but abruptly resolved shortly after his last crying spell.

After an extensive neurological evaluation, a diagnosis of transient ischemic attacks with crying spells was made. The transient ischemic attacks could have involved the right brainstem and the raphe nuclei. This patient may have had a temporary activation or stimulation of ischemic areas or alterations in serotonergic neurons (Mendez and Bronstein, 1999).

system is also an important source of fibers to the PAG (Chapter 11, Figure 11.5).

The PAG is important in eliciting many somatic and visceral stereotypical behaviors. It is the major center through which the hypothalamus enacts behaviors critical to the survival of the self and of the species. These behaviors include regulation of heart rate and respiration, urination, grooming, and basic elements of defensive and reproductive behaviors (Craig, 1996). Other behaviors elicited by stimulating the PAG include threat, freezing, escape, and vocalization (Bandler and Keay, 1996; Schenberg *et al.*, 2005).

Nashold *et al.* (1974) found that stimulation of the PAG evoked "feelings of fear and death". Facial blushing, sweating, and other autonomic responses were noted. It has been suggested that the PAG plays a key role in triggering panic (Gorman *et al.*, 1989: Chapter 11).

Locus ceruleus and lateral tegmental nucleus

The locus ceruleus is represented by a group of distinct nerve cell bodies that make up a nucleus near the ventrolateral corner of the fourth ventricle in the pontine tegmentum (Figure 10.3). It extends rostrally into the PAG of the midbrain. Cells of the locus ceruleus are rich in norepinephrine (NE), and the locus ceruleus contains half the NE neurons found in the brain.

Input to the LC is provided largely by two reticular nuclei, the nucleus prepositus hypoglossi and the nucleus paragigantocellularis (see PrH and LPGi, Figures 10.1 and 10.6; Aston-Jones *et al.*, 1995). The nucleus prepositus hypoglossi provides inhibitory input whereas the nucleus paragigantocellularis provides strong excitatory input (Aston-Jones *et al.*, 1990, 1991a). The prepositus hypoglossi nucleus receives input from the nucleus of the solitary tract, which conveys information about the vegetative state of the body. The prepositus also receives input from other brainstem sensory nuclei and from the spinal cord (Aston-Jones *et al.*, 1991a). The nucleus paragigantocellularis receives signals from diverse sites throughout the brainstem and spinal cord that are associated with autonomic and integrative functions (Aston-Jones *et al.*, 1991b). Other fibers to the locus ceruleus arrive from the parabrachial nucleus, the PAG, and the hypothalamus. It has been suggested that one or more of these sources are important in the inhibition of neuron discharge seen in the locus ceruleus during paradoxical sleep (Luppi *et al.*, 1995).

The ascending projection from the locus ceruleus represents the majority of its output. This group of fibers passes rostrally through the midbrain, lateral to the medial longitudinal fasciculus. The fibers accompany the medial forebrain bundle to and through the lateral hypothalamus. This ascending pathway continues rostrally to levels of the anterior commissure, where it divides into fibers that innervate midline portions of the thalamus, the amygdala, the hippocampus, and vast regions of the cortex (Foote *et al.*, 1983). Other fibers from the locus ceruleus pass via the fornix to

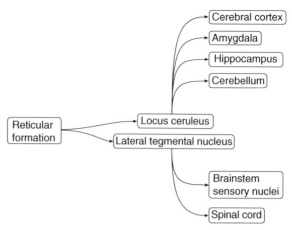

Figure 10.6. The locus ceruleus and lateral tegmental nucleus provide norepinephric projections to the entire neuraxis. Novel environmental stimuli act through norepinephrine to direct the brain to alert, orient, and attend to selective stimuli. The two specific reticular nuclei that contact the locus ceruleus are nucleus hypoglossi prepositus and nucleus paragigantocellularis.

the hippocampal formation and as a component of the cingulum to the cingulate cortex. A contingent of fibers even terminates in the cerebellum (Chapter 2). Descending fibers from the locus ceruleus are relatively sparse. Efferent fibers from the locus ceruleus to the caudal brainstem terminate on sensory nuclei. Fibers to the spinal cord end in both the dorsal and the ventral horns (Holets, 1988).

One of the most profuse projections of the locus ceruleus is to the thalamus, where terminals are found in the intralaminar and anterior nuclei (Table 9.1). These thalamic nuclei are included as part of the limbic thalamus. The limbic thalamus projects to all cortical areas and has been linked to arousal and selective attention. The norepinephrine system that arises in the LC "is unique in the brain in that it innervates more CNS areas than any other single nucleus" (Aston-Jones *et al.*, 1995). The remarkable feature of the locus ceruleus projection is its wide distribution throughout the brain. Each locus ceruleus neuron may contact thousands of cortical neurons. The most rostrally projecting fibers of the locus ceruleus exit from the medial forebrain bundle and distribute to the rostral, dorsal, and lateral cortex of the frontal lobe, where they terminate in the most superficial cortical layer, which is considered an important site for cortical integration.

The lateral tegmental nucleus is represented by scattered NE neurons that extend ventrolaterally from the locus ceruleus to the ventral aspect of the brainstem. Although these cells may appear to be only a ventrolateral extension of the locus ceruleus, the connections of the lateral tegmental nucleus differ from those of the locus ceruleus. Targets of the fibers from the lateral tegmental nucleus generally do not overlap those of the locus ceruleus, thus justifying the recognition of the lateral tegmental nucleus as more than just an extension of the locus ceruleus. Major projections descend and terminate in the spinal cord and brainstem. More diffuse projections terminate in the thalamus, hypothalamus, amygdala, and cerebellar cortex (Burstein, 1996). Like the NE neurons of the locus ceruleus, the lateral tegmental nucleus neurons also cease firing during sleep.

The LC operates in a bimodal fashion: phasic and tonic. In the phasic mode it produces a short lasting, widespread release of norepinephrine. This functions to increase gain of cortical processing to enhance focus on task-appropriate behavior while at the same time inhibiting attention to distracting stimuli. The phasic response is believed to be driven by activity in the orbital prefrontal cortex and anterior cingulate gyrus (Rajkowski et al., 2000, 2004; Aston-Jones et al., 2002). The orbital prefrontal cortex and anterior cingulate are also responsible for transitions between tonic and phasic modes (Corbetta et al., 2008).

Locus ceruleus neurons in the tonic mode increase baseline activity and at the same time decrease phasic activity. The tonic mode allows the brain when not engaged in a specific task, to operate in a search mode to explore alternative behaviors (Aston-Jones and Cohen, 2005). In contrast, abnormally elevated tonic baseline activity of the locus ceruleus is believed to be associated with high distractibility. A high tonic level of locus ceruleus activity is associated with labile attention and poor task performance –behavior often seen in attention-deficit hyperactivity disorder (Aston-Jones and Gold, 2009).

Operation in either tonic or phasic mode has been recognized in the regulation of arousal, attention, and related autonomic tone. Locus ceruleus neurons respond with increased rates of firing to novel environmental stimuli but not to routine environmental stimuli (Jacobs, 1990). Stimuli that are effective in producing a response in the neurons of the locus ceruleus are stimuli that disrupt ongoing behavior and elicit an orienting response. The largest response in locus ceruleus activity occurs during an abrupt transition from sleep to waking (Aston-Jones et al., 1996).

The ascending locus ceruleus system is believed to function in arousal. It determines the salience of a target and is speculated to facilitate some types of learning.

A relatively low tonic level of locus ceruleus activity is associated with inattention.

Norepinephrine facilitates long-term potentiation of hippocampal neurons, indicting that it can influence memory. NE functions in the cortex to inhibit ongoing random neuron activity and to potentiate neuron response to selective stimuli, thus increasing the signal-to-noise ratio for incoming sensory signals. Actions of NE on the thalamus and cortex enhance the signal processing ability of the forebrain (Berridge, 1993). Norepinephrine produces a slow excitatory postsynaptic potential (EPSP) in neurons of the hippocampus and over a wide area of the cerebral cortex (Nicoll et al., 1987).

The locus ceruleus is believed to play an important role in the initiation of REM sleep. Locus ceruleus neurons are inactive during sleep, and electrical stimulation of the locus ceruleus and subsequent release of NE produce an increase in the state of arousal (Aston-Jones and Bloom, 1981). The administration of NE is known to increase the state of arousal and also to increase the level of anxiety. Both arousal and anxiety, therefore, may be linked to the locus ceruleus. Monoamine oxidase (MOA) inhibitors and tricyclic agents, which are clinically effective in treating depression in humans, inhibit the firing of locus ceruleus neurons in experimental animals. The high level of anxiety and loss of pleasure reported by depressed patients may be related to the loss of regulation of NE by locus ceruleus neurons.

Acute exposure to opiates inhibits the action of locus ceruleus neurons by binding μ receptors that are coupled to G-protein (Chapter 3) (Williams et al., 2001). In contrast, chronic exposure to opiates increases the excitability of the locus ceruleus neurons by upregulation of the intracellular cyclic adenosine monophosphate (cAMP) pathway (Nestler and Aghajanian, 1997). This is an expected response that brings the locus ceruleus firing rate back toward a normal level. When opiates are withdrawn, the locus ceruleus is activated. This activation is responsible for some of the behavioral signs of withdrawal.

A loss of cells is seen in the locus ceruleus of patients with Parkinson disease or Alzheimer disease (Zweig et al., 1993). These individuals are often diagnosed with depression, and cell loss in the locus ceruleus correlates with depressive signs and symptoms (Forstl et al., 1992). One model of depression recognizes the degeneration or retraction, or both, of locus ceruleus neurons as part of the pathophysiology of this disorder (Kitayama et al., 1994). Locus ceruleus neurons are sensitive to corticotropin-releasing factor (CRF), and the hypothalamic-pituitary-adrenal (HPA) axis is activated in depression and altered in panic disorder (Chapter 8). The increase in CRF production during activation of the HPA axis may involve the LC in these disorders. Some antidepressant drugs may act by blocking CRF activation of the locus ceruleus (Curtis and Valentino, 1994). In contrast, loss of cells in the locus ceruleus has been reported in patients with Alzheimer disease, but with no additional loss of locus ceruleus neurons in patients with both Alzheimer disease and depression (Hoogendijk et al., 1999).

Alcohol activates the norepinephrine system through a system that involves serotonin (Blum and Kozlowski, 1990). The number of locus ceruleus neurons is reduced in alcoholics (Halliday and Baker, 1996). The mechanism remains in question (Karolewicz et al., 2008). Locus ceruleus neurons increase their firing rate during opiate withdrawal (Self and Nestler, 1995). Karson et al. (1991) reported no change in the number of locus ceruleus neurons in patients with schizophrenia, but they found a significant reduction in neuron size.

A model has been proposed that an increase in LC activity is involved in attention-deficit hyperactivity disorder. The model proposes that LC neurons fire at an abnormally high level as a result of a biochemical defect in the brainstem systems that regulate the locus ceruleus (Mefford and Potter, 1989).

Inferior olive

The inferior olive (inferior olivary complex) is located in the medulla and forms an olive-shaped prominence on the ventrolateral surface of the brainstem (Figure 10.1). It receives input from the cerebral cortex, red nucleus, and spinal cord. The bulk of the afferent fibers descends in the central tegmental tract and arises in the red nucleus.

The inferior olive gives rise to the climbing fibers that terminate on cells in the deep cerebellar nuclei and Purkinje cells of the cortex. Climbing fibers provide a strong excitatory signal when activated. It is believed they play a role in timing and error detection (McKay et al., 2007). There is also a projection of GABAergic fibers from the deep nuclei of the cerebellum. Thus there exists a loop between the inferior olive and cerebellum similar to those seen between the basal ganglia and cerebral cortex.

Neurons in the inferior olive are electrotonically coupled and generate synchronous oscillations when activated. Their action is modulated through GABA-receptor-controlled gap junctions. Animal models indicate that inferior olive neurons may be involved in essential tremor (Miwa, 2007). Patients with essential tremor are reported to exhibit hypermetabolism in the inferior olive (Hallett and Dubinsky, 1993; Wills et al., 1994). It is hypothesized that sub-threshold oscillations in the inferior olive form the basis of essential tremor (Loewenstein, 2002).

Select bibliography

Arango, V., Underwood, M.D., and Mann, J.J. Biological alterations in the brainstem of suicides. In: J.J.Mann (ed.) Suicide. Psychiatric Clinics of North America (vol. 20). (Philadelphia: Saunders, 1997, pp. 581–594.)

Carpenter, M.B., and Sutin, J. Human Neuroanatomy. (Baltimore: Williams & Wilkins, 1983.)

Hales, R.E., and Ydofsky, S.C. Textbook of Neuropsychiatry. (Washington D.C.: American Psychiatric Association Press, 1987.)

Holstege, G., Bandler, R., and Saper, C.B. The emotional motor system. Progress in Brain Research (vol 107). (Amsterdam: Elsevier, 1996.)

References

Aletrino, M.A., Vogels, D.J.M., Van Doinburg, P.H.M.F., and Ten Donkelaar, H.J. 1992. Cell loss in the nucleus raphe dorsalis in Alzheimer's disease. Neurobiol. Aging 13:461–468.

Andersen, G. 1995. Treatment of uncontrolled crying after stroke. Drugs Aging 6:105–111.

Aston-Jones, G., and Bloom, F.E. 1981. Norepinephrine containing locus coeruleus neurons in behaving rats exhibit pronounced responses to non-noxious environmental stimuli. J. Neurosci. 1:887–900.

Aston-Jones, G., and Cohen, J.D., 2005. Adaptive gain and the role of the locus ceruleus-norepinephrine system in optimal performance. J. Comp. Neurol. 493:99–110.

Aston-Jones, G., and Gold, J.I. 2009. How we say no: Norepinephrine, inferior frontal gyrus, and response inhibition. Biol. Psychiatry 65:548–549.

Aston-Jones, G., Shipley, M.T., Ennis, M., Williams, J.T., and Pieribone, V.A. 1990. Restricted afferent control of locus coeruleus neurons revealed by anatomical, physiological, and pharmacological studies. In: D.J.Heal and C.A.Marsden (eds.) The Pharmacology of Noradrenaline in the Central Nervous System. Oxford: Oxford Medical Press, pp. 187–247.

Aston-Jones, G., Chiang, C., and Alexinsky, T. 1991a. Discharge of noradrenergic locus coeruleus neurons in behaving rats and monkeys suggests a role in vigilance. Prog. Brain Res. 88:501–520.

Aston-Jones, G., Shipley, M.T., Chouvet, G., Ennis, M., van Bockstaele, E., Pieribone, V., Shiekhattar, R., Akaoka, H., Drolet, G., Astier, B., Charlety, P., Valentino, R.J., and Williams, J.T.1991b. Afferent regulation of locus coeruleus neurons: Anatomy, physiology and pharmacology. *Prog. Brain Res.* **88**:47–75.

Aston-Jones, G., Shipley, M.T., and Grzanna, R. 1995. The locus coeruleus, A5 and A7 noradrenergic cell groups. In: G.Paxinos (ed.) *The Rat Nervous System* (2nd ed.). San Diego: Academic Press, pp. 183–213.

Aston-Jones, G., Rajkowski, J., Kubiak, P., Valentino, R.J., and Shipley, M.T. 1996. Role of the locus coeruleus in emotional activation. In: G.Holstege, R.Bandler, and C.B.Saper (eds.) *The Emotional Motor System.Prog. Brain Res.* **107**:379–402.

Aston-Jones, G., Rajkowski, J., Lu, W., Zhu, Y., Cohen, J.D., and Morecraft, R.J. 2002. Prominent projections from the orbital prefrontal cortex to the locus ceruleus in monkey. *Soc. Neurosci. Abstr.* **28**:86–89.

Bandler, R., and Keay, K.A. 1996. Columnar organization in the midbrain periaqueductal gray and the integration of emotional expression. In: G.Holstege, R.Bandler, and C.B.Saper (eds.) The Emotional Motor System. *Prog. Brain Res.* **107**:285–300.

Bernard, J.F., Bester, H., and Besson, J.M. 1996. Involvement of the spino-parabrachio-amydaloid and -hypothalamic pathways in the autonomic and affective emotional aspects of pain. In: G.Holstege, R.Bandler, and C.B.Saper (eds.) The Emotional Motor System. *Prog. Brain Res.* **107**:243–255.

Berridge, D.W. 1993. Noradrenergic modulation of cognitive function: Clinical implications of anatomical, electrophysiological and behavioural studies in animal models. *Psychol. Med.* **23**:557–564.

Blum, K., and Kozlowski, G.P. 1990. Ethanol and neuromodulator interactions: A cascade model of reward. *Prog. Alcohol Res.* **2**:131–149.

Burstein, R. 1996. Somatosensory and visceral input to the hypothalamus and limbic system. In: G.Holstege, R.Bandler and C.B.Saper (eds.) The Emotional Motor System. *Prog. Brain Res.* 107:257–267.

Chamberlin, N.L. 2004. Functional organization of the parabrachial complex and intertrigeminal region in the control of breathing. *Respir. Physiol. Neurobiol.* **143**:115–125.

Chen, C.P., Adler, J.T., Bowen, D.M., Esiri, M.M., McDonald, B., Hope, T., Jobst, K.A., and Francis, P.T. 1996. Presynaptic serotonergic dysfunction in patients with Alzheimer's disease: Correlations with depression and neuroleptic medication. *J. Neurochem.* **66**:1592–1598.

Corbetta, M., Patel, G., and Shulman, G.L. 2008. The reorienting system of the human brain: From environment to theory of mind. *Neuron* **58**: 306–324.

Craig, A.D. 1996. An ascending general homeostatic afferent pathway originating in lamina I. In: G.Holstege, R. Bandler, and C.B.Saper (eds.) The Emotional Motor System. *Prog. Brain Res.* **107**:226–242.

Curtis, A.L., and Valentino, R.J. 1994. Corticotropin-releasing factor neurotransmission in locus coeruleus: A possible site of antidepressant action. *Brain Res. Bull.* **35**:581–587.

Foote, S.L., Bloom, F.E., and Aston-Jones, G. 1983. Nucleus locus ceruleus: New evidence of anatomical and physiological specificity. *Physiol. Rev.* **63**:844–901.

Forstl, H., Burns, A., Luthert, P., Cairns, N., Lantos, P., and Levy, R. 1992. Clinical and neuropathological correlates of depression in Alzheimer's disease. *Psychol. Med.* **22**:877–884.

Gorman, J.M., Liebowitz, M.R., Fyer, A.J., and Stein, J. 1989. A neuroanatomical hypothesis for panic disorder. *Am. J. Psychiatry* **146**:148–161.

Hallett, M., and Dubinsky, R.M. 1993. Glucose metabolism in the brain of patients with essential tremor. *J. Neurol. Sci.* **114**:45–48.

Halliday, G., and Baker, K. 1996. Noradrenergic locus coeruleus neurons. *Alcohol Clin. Exp. Res.* **20**:191–192.

Holets, V.R. 1988. Locus coeruleus neurons in the rat containing neuropeptide Y, tyrosine hydroxylase or galanin and their efferent projections to the spinal cord, cerebral cortex and hypothalamus. *Neuroscience* **24**:893–906.

Holstege, G. 1988. Anatomical evidence for a strong ventral parabrachial projection to nucleus raphe magnus and adjacent tegmental field. *Brain Res.* **447**:154–158.

Hoogendijk, W.J.G., Sommer, I.E.C., Pool, C.W., Kamphorst, W., Hofman, M.A., Eikelnboom, P., and Swaab, D.F. 1999. Lack of association between depression and loss of neurons in the locus coeruleus in Alzheimer disease. *Arch. Gen. Psychiatry* **56**:45–51.

Jacobs, B.L. 1990. Locus coeruleus neuronal activity in behaving animals. In: D.J. Heal, and C.A.Marsden (eds.) *The Pharmacology of Noradrenaline in the Central Nervous System*. Oxford: Oxford Medical Press, pp. 248–265.

Jacobs, B.L. 1994. Serotonin, motor activity and depression-related disorders. *Am. Sci.* **82**:456–463.

Jacobs, B.L., and Fornal, C.A. 1993. 5-HT and motor control: A hypothesis. *Trends Neurosci.* **16**:346–352.

Karolewicz, B., Johnson, L., Szebeni, K., Craig., A., Stockmeier, C.A., and Ordway, G.A. 2008. Glutamate signaling proteins and tyrosine hydroxylase in the locus ceruleus of alcoholics. *J. Psychiatr. Res.* **42**:348–355.

Karson, C.N., Casanova, M.F., Kleinman, J.E., and Griffin, W.S.T. 1993. Choline acetyltransferase in schizophrenia. *Am. J. Psychiatry* **50**:454–459.

Karson, C.N., Garcia-Rill, E., Biedermann, J., Mrak, R.E., Husain, M.M., and Skinner, R.D. 1991. The brain stem reticular formation in schizophrenia. *Psychiatry Res.* **40**:31–48.

Kitayama, I., Nakamura, S., Yaga, T., Murase, S., Nomura, J., Kayahara, T., and Nakano, K. 1994. Degeneration of locus coeruleus axons in stress-induced depression model. *Brain Res. Bull.* **35**:573–580.

Kline, P., and Oertel, J. **1997**. Depression associated with pontine vascular malformation. *Biol. Psychiatry* **42**:519–521.

Loewenstein, Y. 2002. What does the martini do to the olive? *Mol. Psychiatry* **7**:128–131.

Lovick, T.A. 1996. Midbrain and medullary regulation of defensive cardiovascular functions. In: G.Holstege, R.Bandler, and C.B.Saper (eds.) The Emotional Motor System. *Prog. Brain Res.* **107**:301–313.

Luppi, P.-H., Aston-Jones, G., Akaoka, H., Chouvet, G., and Jouvet, M. 1995. Afferent projections to the rat locus coeruleus demonstrated by retrograde and anterograde tracing with cholera-toxin B subunit and Phaseolus vulgaris leucoagglutinin. *Neuroscience* **65**:119–160.

Mason, P., and Leung, C.G. 1996. Physiological functions of pontomedullary raphe and medial reticular neurons. In: G.Holstege, R.Bandler, and C.B.Saper (eds.) The Emotional Motor System. *Prog. Brain Res.* **107**:269–282.

McKay, B.E., Engbers, J.D.T., Mehaffey, W.H., Gordon, G.R.J., Molineux, M.L., Bains, J.S., and Turner, R.W. 2007. Climbing fiber discharge regulates cerebellar functions by controlling the intrinsic characteristics of Purkinje cell output. *J. Neurophysiol.*2590–2604.

McNamara, I.M., Borella, A.W., Bialowas, L.A., and Whitaker-Azmitia, P.M. 2008. Further studies in the developmental hyperserotonemia mosel (DHS) of autism: Social, behavioral and peptide changes. *Brain Res.* **1189**:203–214.

Mefford, I.N., and Potter, W.Z. 1989. A neuroanatomical and biochemical basis of attention deficit disorder with hyperactivity in children: A defect in tonic adrenaline mediated inhibition of locus coeruleus stimulation. *Med. Hypotheses* **29**:33–42.

Mendez, M.F. 1992. Pavor nocturnus from a brainstem glioma. *J. Neurol. Neurosurg. Psychiatry* **55**:860.

Mendez, M.F., and Bronstein, Y.L. 1999. Crying spells presenting as a transient ischemic attack. *J. Neurol. Neurosurg. Psychiatry* **67**:255.

Miwa, H. 2007. Rodent models of tremor. *Cerebellum* **6**:66–72.

Mogenson, G.J., Wu., M., and Tsai, C.T. 1989. Subpallidal-pedunculopontine projections but not subpallidal-mediodorsal thalamus projections contribute to spontaneous exploratory locomotor activity. *Brain Res.* **485**:396–398.

Mylecharane, E.J. 1996. Ventral tegmental area 5-HT receptors: Mesolimbic dopamine release and behavioural studies. *Behav. Brain Res.* **73**:1–5.

Nashold, B.S. Jr., Wilson, W.P., and Slaugher, G. 1974. The midbrain and pain. In: J.J.Bonica (ed.) International Symposium on Pain. Adv. Neurol. **4**:191–196.

Nestler, E.J., and Aghajanian, G.K. 1997. Molecular and cellular basis of addiction. *Science* **278**:58–63.

Nicoll, R.A., Madison, D.V., and Lancaster, B. 1987. Noradrenergic modulation of neuronal excitability in mammalian hippocampus. In: H.Y.Meltzer (ed.) *Psychopharmacology: The Third Generation of Progress.* New York: Raven Press, pp. 105–112.

Norgren, R., Hajnal, A., and Mungarndee, S.S. 2006. Gustatory reward and the nucleus accumbens. *Physiol. Behav.* **89**:531–535.

Rajkowski, J., Lu, W., Zhu, Y., Cohen, J., and Aston-Jones, G. 2000. Prominent projections from the anterior cingulate cortex to the locus ceruleus in Rhesus monkey. *Soc. Neurosci. Abstr.* **26**:838.15.

Rajkowski, J., Majczynski, H., Clayton, E., and Aston-Jones, G. 2004. Activation of monkey locus ceruleus neurons varies with difficulty and behavioral performance in a target detection task. *J. Neurophysiol.* **92**:361–371.

Schenberg, L.C., Povoa, R.M.F., Costa, A.L.P., Caldellas, A.V., Tufik, S., and Bitten court, A.S. 2005. Functional specializations within the tectum defense systems of the rat. *Neurosci. Biobehav. Rev.* **29**:1279–1298.

Self, D.W., and Nestler, E.J. 1995. Molecular mechanisms of drug reinforcement and addiction. *Annu. Rev. Neurosci.* **18**:463–495.

Semba, K. 1993. Aminergic and cholinergic afferents to REM sleep induction regions of the pontine reticular formation in the rat. *J. Comp. Neurol.* **330**:543–556.

Williams, J.T., Christie, M.J., and Manszoni, O. 2001. Cellular and synaptic adaptations mediating opioid dependence. *Physiol. Rev.* **81**:299–343.

Wills, A.J., Jenkins, I.H., Thompson, P.D., Findley, L.J., and Brooks, D.J. 1994. Red nuclear and cerebellar but no olivary activation associated with essential tremor: A positron emission tomographic study. *Ann. Neurol.* **36**:636–642.

Winn, P., Brown, V.J., and Inglis, W.L. 1997. On the relationships between the striatum and the pedunculopontine tegmental nucleus. *Crit. Rev. Neurobiol.* **11**:241–261.

Zweig, R.M., Cardillo, J.E., Cohen, M., Giere, S., and Hedreen, J.C. 1993. The locus coeruleus and dementia in Parkinson's disease. *Neurology* **43**:986–991.

175

Anatomy

The temporal lobe can be divided into two parts. The newer lateral portion (neocortical) is responsible for audition, speech, and for the integration of sensory information from a variety of sensory modalities. The neocortical division is the topic of Chapter 5. The other division of the temporal lobe is the ventromedial portion, which is older cortex (archicortex and paleocortex) and consists of regions that have become recognized as components of the limbic system. The limbic system structures that are part of the temporal lobe include the parahippocampal gyrus (Figures 5.4 and 13.1), the entorhinal cortex, the hippocampal formation (Figure 11.1), the uncus (Figure 13.2), and the amygdala (Martin, 1996). The cortex of the temporal pole is sometimes considered limbic but is covered in Chapter 5. All sensory information from the external world passes through unimodal and multimodal association areas before finally converging on the hippocampus and amygdala. These structures can be considered to be supramodal centers. Chapter 13 provides an overall picture of the limbic system.

The hippocampus is important in declarative memory and for learning the importance of specific external stimuli. The amygdala appears to be important in assigning emotions to stimuli. This includes emotional conditioning and learning the relationship between internal and external cues related to emotion and affect (Bechara *et al.*, 1995).

Hippocampal formation

The hippocampal formation occupies a central position in the limbic system (Figures 11.1, 11.2, and 11.3). The hippocampal formation consists of the subiculum, the hippocampus proper, and the dentate gyrus. Viewed from the ventral surface, the cortex medial to the collateral sulcus is the parahippocampal gyrus (Figure 5.4). The anterior end of the parahippocampal gyrus is the entorhinal cortex and corresponds with Brodmann's area (BA) 28 (Figures 13.1 and 13.2). The

parahippocampal gyrus rolls medially deep to the surface to produce the parahippocampal sulcus. The cortex transitions from six layers to three from the entorhinal area to the hippocampal formation. The hippocampal

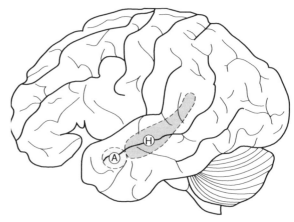

Figure 11.1. The approximate location of the amygdala (A) and hippocampus (H) in the temporal lobe is indicated. Compare with Figure 2.2.

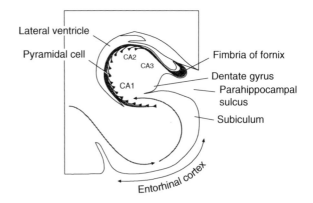

Figure 11.2. A diagrammatic cross section through the ventromedial temporal lobe and the entorhinal cortex of the parahippocampal gyrus. The hippocampal formation consists of the subiculum, the dentate gyrus, and the hippocampus proper. The hippocampus proper is made up of four longitudinal zones, CA1–CA3. Information enters the hippocampal formation via the entorhinal cortex and exits via the fornix.

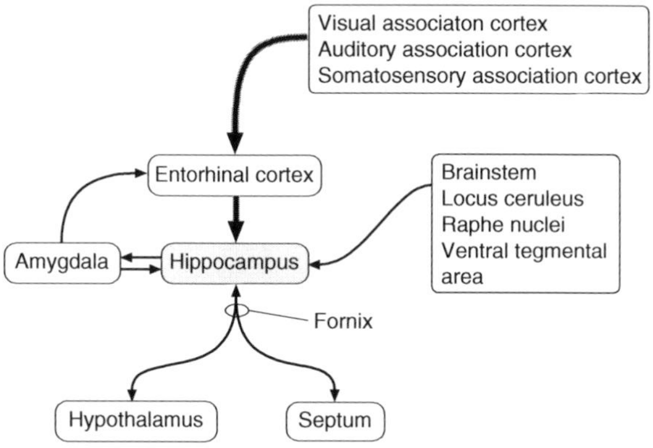

Figure 11.3. A diagram of the major connections of the hippocampus. Processed sensory information arrives at the hippocampus via the entorhinal cortex. Major hippocampal efferents project to the amygdala, hypothalamus, and the septum.

formation lies deep within the parahippocampal sulcus and forms a portion of the medial wall of the temporal horn of the lateral ventricle (Figure 11.2). The subiculum is three-layered cortex that lies between the entorhinal cortex and the hippocampus proper. The presubiculum and parasubiculum are anteroposterior columns that lie between the parahippocampal cortex and the subiculum proper. The hippocampus proper is divided into four major fields represented by cell columns CA1–4 (Figure 11.2). These longitudinally oriented sectors are referred to as CA1, CA2, and CA4. CA refers to cornu ammonis, or Ammon's horn, an early name for the hippocampus. CA1 lies ventrolaterally, and CA4 lies medially near the origin of the fornix. CA1 borders the subiculum and CA4 borders the dentate gyrus. The principal layer of the dentate gyrus is populated by granular cells. It also contains a small population of stem cells.

The entorhinal cortex is the gateway to the hippocampal formation (Figure 11.3). It receives input from the olfactory bulb, prepyriform area, amygdala, and multimodal association areas of the temporal and frontal lobes. The entorhinal cortex differs significantly from that of other six-layered neocortical regions, and it is probably a form of transitional cortex. Two pathways conduct signals from the entorhinal cortex to the hippocampal formation. Axons pass from the medial entorhinal cortex to the hippocampal formation forming the alvear pathway. This pathway terminates in the subiculum and CA1. Axons from the lateral entorhinal cortex make up the perforant pathway. The perforant pathway terminates in the dentate gyrus and all sectors of the hippocampus. The perforant pathway has been

described as the "single most vulnerable circuit in the cerebral cortex" (Morrison and Hof, 1997). Although these two pathways supply input to the hippocampus they also contain a significant number of efferent fibers.

The hippocampus is more primitive than the entorhinal cortex and consists of only three cell layers. The pyramidal cell is the most distinctive cell of the hippocampal formation. Moderate amounts of dopamine, norepinephrine, and acetylcholine are present in the hippocampal formation. In addition to the entorhinal cortex, other sources of input to the hippocampal formation include the septal nuclei, hypothalamus, and thalamus as well as the brainstem (Figure 11.3).

Two functionally separate circuits involve the three hippocampal sectors. A direct entorhinal-CA1 circuit is important for recollection-based recognition memory. The CA3 sector coupled with CA1 is necessary for recall (Brun et al., 2002). Pyramidal cells in CA1 (Sommer's sector) are highly sensitive to anoxia and ischemia, including epileptic seizure-induced damage.

Signals leave the hippocampus by way of the axons of the pyramidal cells (Figure 11.2). These axons accumulate medially to form the fimbria of the fornix (Figures 11.2 and 11.3). Efferent fibers from the hippocampus project to the septal area and to the hypothalamus. Reciprocal (back-and-forth) connections exist between the hippocampus and the amygdala.

The hippocampal formation is well known for its role in declarative memory. Declarative memory is the memory of facts, experiences, and information about events. The hippocampus will retain the memory for weeks to months before it is consolidated elsewhere in the cortex. One hypothesis of memory involving the hippocampal formation is based on the concept of a "cognitive map" (Jacobs and Schenk, 2003). This hypothesis proposes that the original need for memory was for a mechanism that provides for the ability to return home. The hippocampus appears to contain a world-centered map as opposed to the egocentric map found in the posterior parietal lobe (see page 40). Declarative memory grew from the map mechanism and much of declarative memory is based on a stepwise sequence of events similar to those experienced as one journeys away from home. Wilson and McNaughton (1993) reported recording large ensembles of neurons from the CA1 region of the rat during spatial exploration. The investigators could determine the location of the rat by analyzing the pattern of ensemble firing

(Kjelstrup *et al.*, 2008). Sleep is important in consolidating memories. The hippocampus is activated during rapid eye movement (REM) sleep, and is likely to contribute significantly to the REM sleep phenomenon. Changes seen between training sessions are believed to be due to increased synaptic connections formed when sessions were replayed in the hippocampus when the animals slept (Skaggs and McNaughton, 1996).

Clinical vignette

A 40 year-old right-handed man was hospitalized for delirium and generalized seizures. On examination, he was confused, disoriented, and febrile. He was treated for presumed herpes simplex encephalitis with aciclovir and phenytoin. Magnetic resonance imaging showed hyperintense lesions in the left mesial temporal lobe with significant swelling consistent with herpes encephalitis (Figure 11.4). After recovery, the patient was left with a severe amnestic disorder from damage to the left hippocampal formation and parahippocampal gyrus. He had difficulty learning any new information and inability to recall any items on delayed recall tests. His remote memory, however, remained intact.

Maguire *et al.* (2000) found that the posterior hippocampal gray matter volume was greater in experienced London taxi drivers compared with control subjects. The gray matter volume of the right posterior hippocampus volume varied positively with the time driving. This difference appeared to be the result of experience and not innate navigational expertise (Maguire *et al.*, 2003).

Hippocampal structures have been implicated in both cognitive and emotional processes. The hippocampal formation deals with two forms of information. One form arrives from other areas of the cortex, is cognitive in nature, and enters by way of the entorhinal cortex. The other form arrives from the septum, amygdala, hypothalamus, and brainstem, and is related to the behavioral/emotional state. The hippocampal–septal "corridor" is believed to have an important modulatory effect on hypothalamic–brainstem structures involved in various endocrine, autonomic, and somatomotor aspects of emotional behavior (Alheid and Heimer, 1996). Limbic activation may be necessary to bring percepts to a conscious level before they are processed in the temporal lobe.

Lesions restricted to the hippocampus proper, the fornix, the subiculum, or the dentate gyrus each

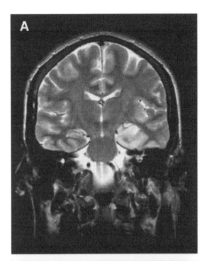
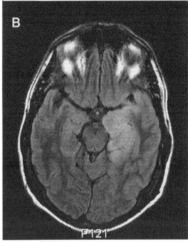

Figure 11.4. A. A coronal cut showed an area of hyperintensity in the left medial temporal lobe on T2-weighted magnetic resonance imaging. B. A horizontal view revealed mass effect from the left medial temporal inflammation. (Reprinted with permission from Mendez and Cummings, 2003.)

produce deficits in declarative memory (Squire *et al.*, 1990). None of these restricted lesions is as disruptive to memory as is a lesion that involves all of the hippocampal formation plus the surrounding temporal cortex (Delis and Lucas, 1996). In addition to temporal lobe structures, lesions involving the fornix, the mammillary body, and the medial thalamus can produce amnesia. Patients who present with severe amnesia without dementia typically have lesions in the medial temporal lobe. The amnesia is anterograde; that is, the ability to store and recall information is lost subsequent to the date of damage to the medial temporal lobe. Events that took place up to several years before the date of the lesion may be hazy. Childhood memories remain intact.

Decreased hippocampal volume has also been reported in other psychiatric disorders such as unipolar depression (Sheline *et al.*, 1996), posttraumatic

A 68-year-old lifelong housewife and mother of four had no psychiatric or neurological problems until approximately three years prior to hospitalization. At that time she noted progressive difficulty with remembering things. On presentation for hospitalization she demonstrated profound memory loss, particularly for recent events. She was unable to care for herself and became agitated at times. A computed tomographic (CT) examination showed a large, left-sided sphenoidal wing meningioma. Amnestic periods resulted from decreased blood flow to the medial temporal regions during a transient ischemic attack. Epileptic activity in this area may also result in similar symptomatology (Pritchard *et al.*, 1985).

stress disorder (PTSD) (Gurvits *et al.*, 1996), bipolar disorder (Hirayasu *et al.*, 1998), and alcohol dependence (DeBellis *et al.*, 2000).

Acetylcholine is important in the operation of the hippocampus. During high cholinergic activity, old memory is recalled. During low cholinergic activity, new memory is formed (Hasselmo *et al.*, 1995). It is proposed that a defect in a cholinergic receptor could result in perceptual difficulties such as those seen in schizophrenia (Adler *et al.*, 1998).

Amygdala

The amygdala is a nuclear complex located inside the temporal lobe, deep to the uncus (Figures 5.4 and 11.1). It is one of the most studied limbic structures, and such a mountain of evidence has accumulated implicating its role in our emotional life that it has been dubbed "the heart and soul of the brain's emotional network" (LeDoux, 1992).

Input to the amygdala allows it to monitor current internal and external sensory cues. It is particularly sensitive to cues that are of a social nature. The amygdala matches sensory input with emotions. Its close ties with the hippocampus help form memory match-ups between particular sensory cues and particular emotions. Although the amygdala has been associated with anxiety and fear we now recognize it is activated equally by positive and negative emotions (Fitzgerald *et al.*, 2006). For example when presented with the face of a new individual the amygdala matches the new individual's facial characteristics with those experienced in the past and assigns an emotion. In this way we prejudge the individual (Figure 6.9).

It is activated in humans during the acquisition of conditioned fear with the magnitude of activation

being greatest during the early stages of acquisition. Simultaneous activation of the amygdala and hippocampus is important in memory formation and recall and inhibits activity in the amygdala (Milad *et al.*, 2007). It is believed that the action of the medial prefrontal cortex suppresses the emotion assigned to the current situation if it is determined that the chosen emotion is incorrect.

A 30-year-old woman with normal IQ had bilateral loss of the amygdala due to calcification resulting from the rare genetic Urbach–Wiethe disease. Testing revealed that she was able to recognize the personal identity of faces and could learn the identity of new faces (Adolphs *et al.*, 1995). She was able to recognize prototypical fear from facial expression but was unable to assess the intensity of the fear expressed. She had experienced failure in social and marital relations and was unable to hold a job but was not a social outcast, as is the case with monkeys with loss of the amygdala (Adolphs *et al.*, 1995).

Connections with the prefrontal cortex and cingulate gyrus allow for appreciation of the emotion, for memory of the emotional situation and for the formulation of appropriate somatic and autonomic responses. Connections with the central nucleus provide the basis of direct control of brainstem motor and autonomic nuclei.

It is convenient to recognize three nuclear areas within the amygdala, although each of these three may be subdivided (Price *et al.*, 1987). These areas are the lateral (basolateral) nuclei, the central nucleus, and the medial (corticomedial) nuclei (11.5).

Lateral (basolateral) nuclei

Sensory input to the lateral nuclei of the amygdala arises from third-order unimodal sensory cortex, especially the visual association cortex of the temporal lobe. Other sensory areas that project to the amygdala include the multimodal sensory areas of the frontal lobe, with those from the temporal lobe being particularly dense (Amaral *et al.*, 1992; Figures 5.2, 11.5 and 11.6). It is via these routes that sensory information from the external environment reaches the amygdala. Other fibers arrive from the insular cortex which provides sensory information from the internal environment (Chapter 5). Sensory fibers from the vagus nerve relay in the solitary nucleus. The solitary nucleus projects directly to

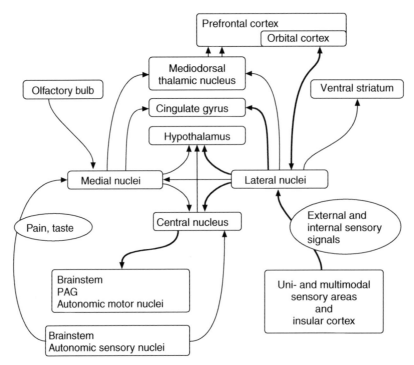

Figure 11.5. The major connections of the individual nuclei of the amygdala (lateral nuclei, central nucleus, and medial nuclei). Behaviorally preeminent pathways are shown with bold lines. The lateral nuclei evaluate integrated sensory information with regard to emotional content and interconnect with the prefrontal cortex, cingulate gyrus, and ventral striatum for somatic response and emotional appreciation. The medial nuclei associate taste and pain signals with emotions. The central nucleus connects with brainstem autonomic centers for motor and autonomic response to emotional stimuli. All three nuclei of the amygdala have connections with the hypothalamus for expression of emotion by way of the autonomic and endocrine systems. PAG, periaqueductal gray.

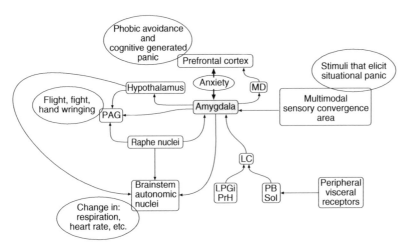

Figure 11.6. Neuroanatomical structures related to panic disorder. The amygdala is believed to play a central role in panic disorder. Sensory cues that trigger panic may originate internally or externally (right side of figure). Anxiety is the result of excitation of the amygdala. Phobic avoidance may originate in the prefrontal lobes. Somatic and motor behaviors typical of panic are effected by the periaqueductal gray (PAG) and brainstem autonomic nuclei. LC, locus ceruleus; MD, mediodorsal thalamic nucleus; PB, parabrachial nucleus; LPGi, nucleus paragigantocellularis lateralis; PrH, nucleus prepositus hypoglossi, Sol, solitary nucleus.

the lateral amygdala providing norepinephrine input. Locus ceruleus also provides norepinephrine projections to the lateral amygdala. Nucleus basalis provides a source of acetylcholine. Corticosterone (cortisol in humans) from the adrenal cortex enters the brain and influences activity in the lateral amygdala.

Two major routes exit the lateral amygdala. The stria terminalis projects to the septal nuclei and hypothalamus. The ventral amygdalofugal pathway projects to the hypothalamus, hippocampus, mediodorsal thalamus, anterior insula, and ventral striatum, which includes the nucleus accumbens. The ventral amygdalofugal pathway also contains direct reciprocal connections with the orbital and medial prefrontal cortex as well as the anterior cingulate gyrus.

The lateral amygdala is important in the acquisition and retention of memories of emotional experiences (Chavez et al., 2009; McGaugh, 2004). Evidence indicates that memory is not stored in the amygdala but that activity within the amygdala consolidates memory elsewhere in the brain. Norepinephrine release within the amygdala appears to be critical for memory formation. Norepinephrine from the adrenal medulla activates vagus nerve receptors, which send signals to the solitary nucleus in the brainstem (Figure 10.1). The solitary nucleus projects noradrenergic fibers to the lateral nuclei of the amygdala. The solitary nucleus also projects to the locus ceruleus which projects its own norepinephrinergic fibers to the amygdala (Williams and Clayton, 2001; Chang et al., 2005; Miyashita and Williams, 2006). The basal nucleus provides cholinergic input. Although cholinergic input may not produce memory consolidation it acts in a modulatory role to enhance memory consolidation initiated by norepinephrinergic activity. Cortisol also plays a role by activating brainstem nuclei such as the solitary nucleus. Cortisol may also act directly on the lateral amygdala (Buchanan and Adolphs, 2003).

Brain regions influenced by the lateral amygdala for memory consolidation include the hippocampus, nucleus accumbens, and caudate nucleus. Efferents from the amygdala influence memory in the caudate nucleus related to visual cues (Packard et al., 1994; Grahn et al., 2009).

Medial nuclei

The most prominent source of fibers that enter into the medial division of the amygdala is the olfactory bulb (Figure 11.5). Other afferents arise from brainstem areas that are related to visceral sensations, taste, and pain. These connections may contribute to the emotional aspects of smell, taste, and pain.

Efferents from the medial nuclei terminate in the hypothalamus, especially in the ventromedial nucleus which is related to feeding behavior. Hypothalamic efferents influenced by the medial amygdala include those that regulate the anterior pituitary (Chapter 8).

Central nucleus

The central nucleus of the amygdala receives input from the lateral and medial amygdala nuclei as well as from brainstem autonomic sensory nuclei (solitary and parabrachial nuclei; Chapter 10). The central nucleus is the predominant output channel for the amygdala (Bohus et al., 1996). Efferents from the central nucleus terminate in the dorsal nucleus of the vagus as well as other brainstem parasympathetic motor nuclei and in the brainstem reticular formation, including the periaqueductal gray (Chapter 10; Figure 10.3). Other efferents also control autonomic activity by way of efferent fibers to the hypothalamus (Figure 11.5).

Signals are processed over parallel pathways through the amygdala. These pathways converge in the central nucleus (Pitkanen et al., 1997). The central nucleus is closely tied with the emotional responsiveness of parasympathetic tone. It copes with environmental challenges by promoting responses that have been successful in the past and by assigning emotional significance to current events (Hatfield et al., 1996). Fight or flight responses or defensive freezing behaviors can be elicited by the central nucleus and its connections with the periaqueductal gray (Chapter 10; Figure 10.3). The central nucleus plays a key role in monitoring the level of autonomic tone by way of feedback from the viscera. Connections with the brainstem autonomic motor nuclei provide a route by which the amygdala directly modifies the autonomic nervous system. Kreindler and Steriade (1964) found that stimulation of the central nucleus in the cat produced electroencephalographic (EEG) changes indicative of arousal. Rats with a lesion in the central nucleus fail to benefit from procedures that normally improve response to conditioned stimuli (Holland and Gallagher, 1993).

Uncus

The uncus is found superficial to the amygdala on the ventromedial aspect of the temporal lobe (Figure 5.4). It is continuous posteriorly with the entorhinal area and is continuous anteriorly with the periamygdaloid area and the prepyriform area. Its dorsal surface is the amygdaloid (semilunar) gyrus. The amygdala lies deep to the surface of the uncus (Figures 11.1 and 13.2). The uncus represents the bulk of the body of the "pear" after which the pyriform (pear-shaped) lobe is named.

Functional and behavioral considerations

The overall function of the amygdala is to assign emotional significance to a current experience (Deakin and Graeff, 1991). It helps focus attention on the critical stimulus at the expense of irrelevant stimuli. The loss of fear seen in the Kluver-Bucy syndrome is attributed to bilateral destruction of the amygdala (see below). The sensation of anxiety is appreciated in the orbital prefrontal cortex and possibly the cingulate gyrus by way of projections from the amygdala. Projections from the amygdala to the hypothalamus as well as reciprocal hypothalamic-prefrontal connections are the basis of the endocrine, autonomic, and behavioral reactions to emotional situations. The location of the amygdala with respect to the prefrontal cortex and autonomic centers is consistent with the role it plays in learning relationships between stimuli and socially important behavior (Aggleton, 1993).

The fifth to the seventh year of age is a critical period for the development of emotion-related facial recognition (Tremblay et al., 2001). As adults age, they pay less attention to negative emotional stimuli than to positive emotional stimuli. Collaborating evidence showed the amygdala of both younger and older adults is activated when viewing emotional images. But compared with younger adults, Mather et al. (2004) reported that activation in older adults was greater for positive than for negative emotional pictures. In contrast, Schwartz et al. (2003) have shown that infants with an inhibited social temperament tend to mature into adults with a similar personality. As adults these socially inhibited individuals showed significantly greater activation of the amygdala bilaterally to novel faces than do uninhibited individuals. Although the amygdala appears to respond preferentially to fearful expressions, left amygdala activation correlated positively with the degree of extraversion of the subject (Canli et al., 2002). The results suggest that the personality of extraversion may influence the brain response to emotionally important stimuli.

The amygdala responds to emotionally expressive faces and other emotionally important images independent of the current focus of attention (Figure 11.7) (Vuilleumier et al., 2001, 2002; Morris et al., 2002). Evidence indicates that it not only detects facially communicated threat, but determines if the threat is directed at the subject or elsewhere (Adams et al., 2003). There appear to be at least two routes by which

sensory signals reach the amygdala. A cortical route involves initial processing in the striate visual cortex. A more direct route involves a subcortical extrastriate pathway that includes the superior colliculus and pulvinar (Chapter 9) (Morris et al., 1999). The direct route allows the amygdala to discriminate between emotional and nonemotional visual targets, even if the image is viewed so quickly that the subject is not consciously aware of having viewed it (Morris et al., 1998; Whalen et al., 1998; Killgore and Yurgelun-Todd, 2004). Activation of the amygdala provides evidence for context enhancement of emotionally important visual targets. It sends feedback projections to the visual pathway that can draw attention to emotionally important targets (Figure 4.6). The left amygdala more than the right responds when sexually explicit visual images are seen and more activation is seen in men than in women (Hamann et al., 2004). The amygdala in cooperation with the hippocampus is responsible for fear conditioning that is the coupling of a neutral stimulus with one that evokes fear (Dolan, 2002). The amygdala does not appear to be critical for species-typical social behavior, but is important in inhibiting social behavior when evaluating new individuals for signs of threat (Amaral, 2003). It is lateralized based on sex. In one experimental setting, enhanced memory for emotional films viewed correlated with increased activity in the right amygdala for men. The same situation correlated with increased activity in the left amygdala for women (Cahill et al., 2001).

Morris et al. (1998) speculated that the right amygdala is more involved in the nonconscious detection of meaningful emotional stimuli, whereas the left amygdala is related to the conscious processing of emotional stimuli. There is evidence that the right amygdala is critical in processing inherent emotional content of stimuli (Phelphs et al., 2001; Nomura et al., 2004). In one study, the right showed more rapid habituation to fearful stimuli than did the left amygdala, especially during processing facial expressions (Hariri et al., 2002).

Electrical stimulation of the amygdala in humans elicits feelings of fear and anxiety as well as autonomic reactions consistent with fear (Gloor et al., 1981). Electrical stimulation of the medial division of the amygdala in female mammals results in ovulation and uterine contraction. It induces penile erection in the male. Exaggerated and indiscriminate sexual activity may result from bilateral damage to the amygdala (Sachs and Meisel, 1994). The descending raphe spinal

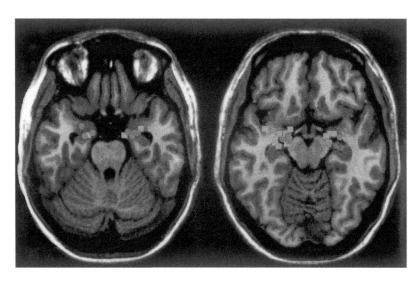

Figure 11.7. Functional magnetic resonance imaging demonstrates activation of both the left and right amygdalae when processing facial expressions of fright (green –see color plate) as well as during conditioned fear (red). Expressions of fright produce activity more in the left side of the upper amygdala than in the right side, whereas the response to conditioned fear is more evenly distributed. (Reproduced with permission from Vass, 2004.) See also color plate.

pathway that regulates incoming pain signals is also a target of fibers from the amygdala.

Projections from the amygdala to brainstem motor and autonomic nuclei mediate the autonomic and facial reactions to emotionally evocative stimuli. Electrical stimulation of the central nucleus of the amygdala in cats results in behavioral and autonomic changes that resemble a state of fear, including an increase in heart and respiration rate and an increase in blood pressure. Chronic stimulation produces stomach ulcers in rats. Electrical stimulation of the medial division also produces an increase in plasma levels of corticosterone, possibly by way of projections to the hypothalamus. Dopaminergic fibers that project from the amygdala to the hippocampus are part of a behaviorally significant reward system (Blum *et al.*, 1996).

Hermann *et al.* (1992) reported that in 13 of 15 patients with ictal (epileptic) fear, the abnormal EEG activity originated from the right temporal lobe limbic structures, especially the amygdala. It is easy to speculate how ictal activity in this region can lead to an increase in anxiety and psychiatric manifestations such as are seen in panic attacks or pathological aggression.

Hallucinations have been experienced during temporal lobe stimulation. The most complex forms of hallucinations are associated with lesions in the anterior portion of the temporal lobe, which contains the amygdala, the uncus, and the anterior hippocampus. Epileptic activity in the different temporal-limbic regions can result in the generation of syndromes that are very similar to many "functional" psychiatric disorders. A "must read" paper by Mesulam (1981) describes 12 such cases in detail. In this series, patients exhibited

multiple personalities, panic-like attacks, and delusions of possession. In most of the cases, structural imaging [computed tomography (CT) or magnetic resonance imaging (MRI)] was normal and EEG revealed the abnormal electrical activity.

Since the highest incidence of psychiatric complications among patients with temporal lobe epilepsy is in those with spike foci in the anterior temporal area, it is assumed that these spikes cause abnormal activation in the amygdaloid complex. It should be noted, however, that the evidence does not support the notion that directed or organized aggression can be a direct consequence or a manifestation of ongoing seizure activity. Surgical amygdalectomy has been performed to alleviate severe and intractable aggression.

Bilateral destruction of the amygdala and surrounding structures in the monkey produces the Kluver–Bucy syndrome (Chapter 13). This disorder is characterized by excessive docility, lack of fear response, and hypersexuality (Delis and Lucas, 1996). Bilateral temporolimbic damage in humans produces a similar behavioral pattern, frequently accompanied by amnesia, aphasia, and visual agnosia (Aggleton, 1992). Patients show few strong responses to provocative stimuli, and aggression is rare (Saver *et al.*, 1996).

Clinical vignette

A 40 year-old man with a history of posttraumatic epilepsy developed hyperoral and other behavioral changes after a period of status epilepticus. On resolution of the abnormal epileptiform activity, he demonstrated a voracious appetite and indiscriminate eating habits, which included eating paper towels, plants, Styrofoam cups, and feces. At one point, he drank urine from a catheter bag. The patient would also wander about the ward and touch many objects. He frequently wandered into the rooms of other patients and touched them inappropriately. Although initially aggressive, he became quite agreeable and docile. The patient had Kluver–Bucy syndrome from damage to both amygdalae. His hyperoral behavior resulted in death from asphyxiation. The patient had a respiratory arrest after stuffing his mouth with surgical gauze. Neuropathology revealed virtual absence of the left amygdaloid complex and atrophy of the right amygdala (Mendez and Foti, 1997).

The degree of craving of cocaine addicts has been shown to parallel an increase in cerebral glucose metabolism in the frontal cortex and the amygdala (London et al., 1996). It is proposed that increased levels of glutamate in the amygdala mediates the craving experienced by cocaine addicts (Kalivas et al., 1998).

Drevets et al. (1992) reported that blood flow to the left amygdala was increased significantly in patients with unipolar major depression. A circuit involving the prefrontal cortex, the amygdala, and related parts of the basal ganglia and medial thalamus has been proposed to describe the functional neuroanatomy of depression. In another study, the amygdala was found to be significantly larger in patients with bipolar disorder than in control subjects. Other structures (thalamus, pallidum, and striatum) showed modest enlargement (Strakowski et al., 1999).

Atrophy of regions of the amygdala containing large neurons which have reciprocal connections with the basal nucleus of Meynert has been reported in Alzheimer disease (Scott et al., 1991). This is consistent with reduced acetylcholine esterase activity in the amygdala in Alzheimer disease (Shinotoh et al., 2000). It is hypothesized that functional changes in the neocortex and amygdala are early and leading events in Alzheimer disease rather than a consequence of degeneration elsewhere (Herholz et al., 2004).

Neurogenesis

Mitotic figures reflecting neuron cell division have been observed in the wall of the lateral ventricle of the rat (Allen, 1912). It is now generally accepted that new neurons (neurogenesis) occur in two regions of the adult brain. One is in the olfactory system. Neurons form in the wall of the anterior forebrain in the subventricular zone which lies just deep to the cavity of the lateral ventricle. As the cells mature they migrate to the olfactory lobe where they differentiate into granule or periglomerular inhibitory neurons (Doetsch et al., 1999). The second neurogenic region is the subgranular zone of the dentate gyrus. This is a thin layer of the dentate gyrus that measures only about three cells deep (Seri et al., 2004). As these cells mature they migrate into the granular cell zone where they differentiate into excitatory granular neurons as well as glia cells in the dentate gyrus as well as CA1 of the hippocampus (Ambrogini et al., 2004; Jin et al., 2004; Verwer et al., 2007). Other areas suspected of supporting neurogenesis include the neocortex (Gould et al., 2001; Dayer et al., 2005), striatum (Bedard et al., 2006; Luzzati et al., 2006), amygdala (Fowler et al., 2002), and hypothalamus (Fowler et al., 2002). Neurogenesis is well established in humans as well as animals (Ericksson, et al., 1998; Manganas et al., 2007).

Jacobs (2002) suggests the new cells may be maintained following a process termed "use it or lose it." It has been estimated that upwards of 10 000 new cells are added each day to the dentate gyrus in the adult rat (Cameron and McKay, 2001). The nascent neurons are excited by γ-aminobutyric acid (GABA) to activate GABAergic receptors that control growth and differentiation of dendrites and synapses (Overstreet-Wadiche et al., 2005; Ge et al., 2006, 2007). A surplus of neurons is produced. Those not used after two to three weeks are lost through programmed cell death (apoptosis) (Biebl et al., 2000; Kempermann et al., 2003). Neurogenesis occurs throughout life as seen in rodents, but decreases significantly with age (Kempermann, 2005). Age-related decline in production has been documented in humans (Manganas et al., 2007).

Several growth factors are associated at different stages of adult neurogenesis. Proliferation, differentiation, and survival of the new neurons is supported by growth factors including fibroblast-growth factor-2 (FGF-2) (Rai et al., 2007), insulin-like growth factor-1 (IGF-1) (Aberg et al., 2003; Trejo et al., 2008), and vascular endothelial growth factor (VEGF) (Jin et al., 2002; Schanzer et al., 2004). Successful neurogenesis also depends on neurotropic factors such as brain-derived neurotropic factor (BDNF) (Scharfman et al., 2005) and nerve growth factor (NGF) (Frielingsdorf et al., 2007). Even electroconvulsive shock has been shown to promote neurogenesis (Madsen et al., 2000).

Neurogenesis in the hippocampus is regulated by glutamatergic fibers that arise in the entorhinal cortex, pass through the perforant path, and terminate in the dentate gyrus. Excitatory input acting on N-methyl-D-aspartate (NMDA) receptors has been shown to inhibit neurogenesis (Bursztain *et al.*, 2007; Nacher *et al.*, 2007). However, stimulation of α-amino-5-hydroxy-3-methyl-4-isoxazole propionic acid (AMPA) and kainite receptors enhances hippocampal neurogenesis (Bai *et al.*, 2003; Jessberger *et al.*, 2007). The effect of activation of other neurotransmitter pathways is being examined and the results of published studies have been comprehensively reviewed by Balu and Lucki (2009).

Stress is documented to affect learning and memory (Stranahan *et al.*, 2008). It may operate through several mechanisms, but stress is also shown to have a strong negative affect on adult hippocampal neurogenesis (Mirescu and Gould, 2006; Airan *et al.*, 2007). Several experimental studies have found that voluntary exercise and an enriched environment increased hippocampal neurogenesis in animals (van Praag *et al.*, 1999; Brown *et al.*, 2003; Bruel-Jungerman *et al.*, 2005, 2007).

Learning and memory are impaired in patients with depression (Austin *et al.*, 2001; Fossati *et al.*, 2002). Depressed patients exhibit reduced hippocampal volume (Bremner *et al.*, 2000; Sheline *et al.*, 2003). Evidence indicates that the reduction is due to reduced dendritic arborization and glial cell number rather than neuron loss (Reif *et al.*, 2006). Neuron loss may not contribute to depression, but neurogenesis corresponds with the beneficial effects of affective antidepressant drug therapy. The time course of action of antidepressant drugs corresponds with the time required for increase of neurogenesis in mice (Nakagawa *et al.*, 2002).

Neurogenesis is decreased in patients with schizophrenia (Reif *et al.*, 2006. The administration of antipsychotic drugs shows mixed effects on enhancing neurogenesis (Halim *et al.*, 2004; Kodama *et al.*, 2004; Schmitt *et al.*, 2004; Wang *et al.*, 2004).

Schizophrenia

Ventricular enlargement of up to 33% has been reported in schizophrenia (Pakkenberg, 1987). The greatest enlargement is seen in the temporal horn of the lateral ventricle (Brown *et al.*, 1986). Ventricular enlargement is a reflection of brain tissue loss. The greatest loss of tissue in schizophrenia is seen in the hippocampal formation, the amygdala, and the parahippocampal gyrus (Bogerts *et al.*, 1985; Nelson *et al.*, 1998; Velakoulis *et al.*, 1999). Lower volumes have been reported in the temporal lobes of patients with schizophrenia when compared with normal control subjects. Compared longitudinally over an average of 15 months (schizophrenic patients) and 68 months (controls), the temporal lobe volumes of both groups declined. This decline in volume was viewed as age related and correlated with a decline in neurocognitive performance in the control subjects. Interestingly, the decline in temporal lobe volume in the schizophrenia group correlated with an improvement in delusions and thought disorder (Gur *et al.*, 1998).

The organization of pyramidal cells in the hippocampus is thought to be disturbed in schizophrenia. Guze and Gitlin (1994) reported that the degree of reduction of the tissue volume of both the hippocampus and the amygdala in patients with schizophrenia as compared with normal control subjects correlates with the severity of positive psychotic symptoms. Delusions, hallucinations, and paranoid ideas (positive symptoms of schizophrenia) are associated with temporolimbic dysfunctions (Bogerts, 1998). Reality distortion (delusions and hallucinations) has been shown to correlate with increased blood flow in the left mesiotemporal lobe structures (Liddle *et al.*, 1992).

The glutamatergic hypothesis of schizophrenia proposes that there is a disruption of glutamate-mediated transmission within the hippocampus. Krystal *et al.* (1999) showed that antagonism of the glutamatergic NMDA receptor produced behavioral and cognitive effects in normal subjects similar to schizophrenia. A reduction in excitatory transmission, especially in CA1, is proposed to result in decreased glutamatergic stimulation of the anterior cingulate cortex, nucleus accumbens, and the temporal cortex (Tamminga, 1998, 1999). Hippocampal neurons appear to be particularly vulnerable following traumatic brain injury (McCarthy, 2003).

Imaging studies have revealed differences between control subjects and schizophrenia patients in a number of cortical regions. The most consistent findings are in the region of the medial temporal lobe (Kotrla and Weinberger, 1995). Abnormalities in the histology of the entorhinal cortex have played an important role in discussions of the neuroanatomical substrates of schizophrenia. A bilateral reduction in overall volume of the hippocampus is reported in patients with schizophrenia (Nelson *et al.*, 1998). Decreases in mean hippocampal neuron density have been reported (Krimer *et al.*, 1997) along with disruption of cortical layers and a decrease in mean neuronal size (Heckers and Heinsen, 1991; Jakob and Beckman, 1994). If it is true that the

185

numbers of neurons remain constant while the volume of tissue is reduced, this suggests that there is abnormal connectivity ("wiring"). The areas most affected include the entorhinal area, the subiculum, and the left anterior and mid-regions of CA1 and CA2 in the hippocampus (Arnold *et al.*, 1995; Narr *et al.*, 2004). These abnormalities are compatible with neurodevelopmental models of schizophrenia that describe abnormal synaptic pruning (Figure 6.11) and abnormal embryological migration of neurons (Arnold *et al.*, 1997). However, there is also reported to be a selective decrease in the actual number of nonpyramidal cells of CA2 in schizophrenia and manic depression patients. This indicates that cell loss in the hippocampus may be a contributing factor in the pathophysiology of major psychoses (Benes *et al.*, 1998).

Heckers (2001) summarized hippocampal findings in schizophrenia in three points. First, most studies have found a decrease in hippocampal volume in schizophrenia patients. This reduction is subtle and is in the order of 4% as compared with healthy controls. This is significantly different from the pronounced volume reduction seen in neurodegenerative disorders such as Alzheimer disease. Second, the reduction is seen early in the disease process with evidence of subsequent slow progression of volume loss. Third, volume loss may be affecting certain parts of the hippocampus more than others (some studies report the volume loss to affect mainly the anterior half of the hippocampus). This finding suggests that not all hippocampal functions are impaired in schizophrenia.

Recent studies extended the findings to at-risk children (children of patients with schizophrenia). Pantelis *et al.* (2003) followed 75 high-risk subjects for one year. Subjects with smaller right hippocampal formation, prefrontal, and cingulate cortical regions (23 subjects) developed psychotic symptoms. These subjects had no psychotic symptoms on entry to the study. Fifty-two other subjects with more normal cortical volumes (also high-risk subjects) did not develop psychotic symptoms within the follow-up period.

Depression/bipolar disorder

Major depressive disorder and bipolar disorder have the major depressive episode in common. Anxiety symptoms are common in major depressive episodes. Anxiety is part of panic disorder, social phobia, posttraumatic stress syndrome and obsessive-compulsive disorder (Kessler *et al.*, 2005). Mood disorders are believed to reflect dysfunction of entire circuits rather than one single brain structure (Drevets *et al.*, 2004). One of these is the limbic-cortical-striatal-pallidal-thalamic circuit. Limbic structures in this circuit include the amygdala and hippocampal subiculum (Ongür *et al.*, 2003).

Neuroanatomical abnormalities have been seen in limbic structures for early-onset, recurrent major depressive disorder and/or bipolar disorder. Reductions in volume, cell counts, metabolism, and blood flow have all been reported for the amygdala and hippocampus (Ongür *et al.*, 2003; Drevets, 2007; Drevets *et al.*, 2008). Volume reduction in the hippocampus of as much as 19% has been reported and the loss appeared to correlate with time spent depressed (Sheline *et al.*, 2003; Neumeister *et al.*, 2005). Drevets and Price (2005) and Hasler *et al.* (2008) found that the activity of the amygdala as well as that of the subgenual anterior cingulate cortex and ventromedial prefrontal cortex increased proportional to the severity of depression. Hasler *et al.* (2008, 2009), as well as Neumeister *et al.* (2004), also found that the rate of metabolism and blood flow decreased with successful antidepressant treatment but increased again with the return of depressive symptoms. Other researchers reported that activity in the left amygdala was affected in depressed subjects when viewing fearful faces and sad words (Thomas *et al.*, 2001; Siegle *et al.*, 2002; Drevets, 2003). In addition, histopathological studies have shown reduced glial cell number in the amygdala but no loss of neurons or synapses (Eastwood and Harrison, 2000; Cotter *et al.*, 2002); Hamidi *et al.* (2004) stated that the glial loss was due to loss of the myelin-producing oligodendrocytes.

Posttraumatic stress disorder

Studies have found that blood flow to the right limbic and paralimbic structures including the amygdala increased in patients with PTSD under provoked conditions (Figure 11.8). The activation of these brain areas is hypothesized to reflect intense emotions or emotional memory and may not be specific to PTSD (Rauch *et al.*, 1996). There is evidence of reduced hippocampal volume in adults who have been exposed to childhood stress but not in children and adolescents with PTSD (DeBellis *et al.*, 2002; Bremner, 2003).

Hendler *et al.* (2003) and Lindauer *et al.* (2004) reported that patients (versus control subjects) exposed to reminders of traumatic events exhibited greater response in the amygdala and reduced activation of the ventral medial prefrontal cortex. These results

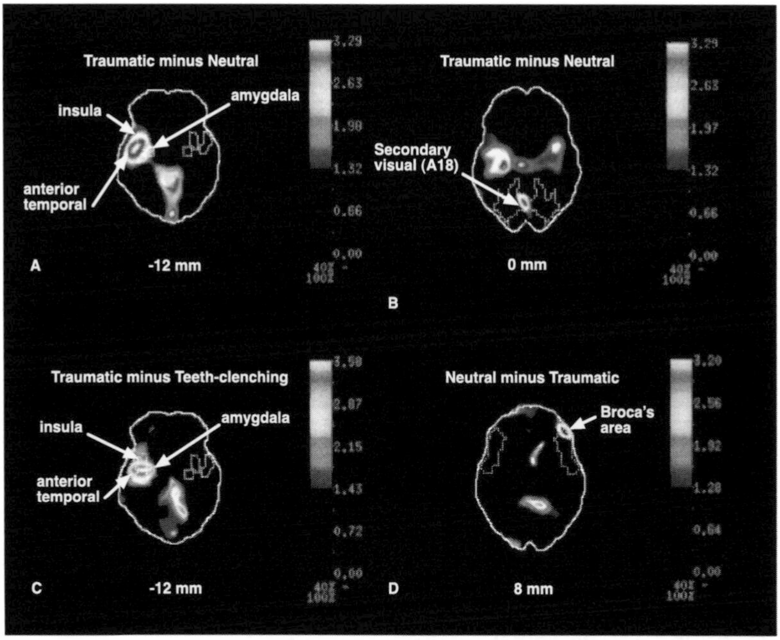

Figure 11.8. A–D. Positron emission tomography statistical parametric maps of traumatic minus control conditions for all subjects (n=8; 16 scans per condition) are displayed with a Sokoloff color scale reproduced in black and white in units of z score. Patients were presented with 30–40 s audio taps of two separated traumatic experiences based on past personal events (traumatic condition) or two neutral scripts (e.g., brushing one's teeth, emptying the dishwasher; neutral condition). Dashed outlines reflecting boundaries of specified brain regions, as defined via a digitized version of the Talairach atlas, are superimposed for anatomical reference. Whole-brain slice outlines are demarcated with solid lines. All images are transverse sections parallel to the intercommissural plane, shown in conventional neuroimaging orientation (top = anterior, bottom = posterior, right = left, left = right). Each transverse section is labeled with its z coordinate, denoting its position with respect to the intercommissural plane (superior > 0). For the traumatic minus neutral condition, activation is located within right anterior temporal and insular cortex, the amygdala (A), and secondary visual cortex (B). C. For the traumatic minus teeth-clenching condition, the pattern of activation shown parallels that are seen in panel B. D. For the neutral minus traumatic condition, activation is located within the left Broca's area (representing a decrease in relative blood flow associated with the traumatic condition). (Modified with permission from Rauch, S.L., van der Kolk, B.A., Fisler, R.E., Alpert, N.M., Orr, S.P., Savage, C.R., Fischman, A.J., Jenike, M.A., and Pitman, R.K. 1996. A symptom provocation study of posttraumatic stress disorder using positron emission tomography and script-driven imagery. Arch. Gen. Psychiatry 53:380–386.)

support a model that involves increased reactivity of the amygdala and associated fear. This is coupled with inadequate suppression of the amygdala by the ventral medial prefrontal cortex (Rauch *et al.*, 2006).

Exposure to stress activates a number of systems (epinephrine, acetylcholine, corticosteroid, etc.) simultaneously. These systems act in concert rather than individually to produce their end results. These systems have mixed effects but for the most part have an excitatory influence on neurons in the amygdala and hippocampus. They not only initiate increased neuronal firing patterns but also facilitate long-term responses [long-term potentiation (Lynch, 2004)]. Long-term potentiation is thought to be important in the process of encoding information (Joëls *et al.*, 2008).

Corticosteroid levels increase over 30–60 minutes as opposed to the almost instantaneous neural response. This results in a late phase of the stress response. Glucocorticoid receptors in CA1 are the most studied (Joëls, 2009). Through a cascade of events the transmission of excitatory signals through CA1 is attenuated along with long-term potentiation in the hippocampus (Wiegert *et al.*, 2006). The initial phase of arousal is terminated and hippocampal activity returns to pre-stress levels (Joëls *et al.*, 2008). This all has a governing effect on the hypothalamo-pituitary-adrenal axis.

Exposure to life-threatening events strongly activates neurons in the amygdala. A model of PTSD proposes that vulnerable individuals have a dysfunction of the pituitary-adrenal axis combined with enhanced sympathetic activity (Yehuda, 2006). These individuals express the early excitatory phase governed by sympathetic drive. They lack the full inhibitory effect of the second phase. As a result central excitation continues and may even be enhanced, unrestrained by the normal adaptive mechanisms mediated by corticosteroid hormones (Joëls *et al.*, 2008).

Borderline personality disorder

Several studies have reported reduced amygdala volume in subjects with borderline personality disorder (BPD) compared with controls (Schmahl *et al.*, 2003; Tebartz *et al.*, 2003). This has not been replicated in other studies (Zetzsche *et al.*, 2006; New *et al.*, 2007). One study found exposure to negative emotion-provoking images produced increased activity in BPD over controls but no difference when presented with neutral images (Herpertz *et al.*, 2001). The amygdala hyperresponsiveness was interpreted to be the result of decreased inhibition by the medial prefrontal cortex (New *et al.*, 2008).

Autism

Volume reductions in the amygdala and hippocampus as well as in the superior temporal gyrus and anterior parietal cortex in children may reflect a genetic vulnerability to schizophrenia and schizotypal disorder. The volume reductions were greatest in the superior temporal gyrus and amygdala (Yuii *et al.*, 2009). Amygdala volume has been reported to be increased in younger (3–4 years) but not in older autistic children (13–19 years) (Sparks *et al.*, 2002; Schumann *et al.*, 2004). Reduced amygdala volumes have been seen in adults with autism (Aylward *et al.*, 1999; Pierce *et al.*, 2001). Munson *et al.* (2006) found that increased right amygdala volume at 3–4 years correlated with poorer social functioning at age 6.

In Mosconi and colleagues' (2009) study, amygdala volume was increased bilaterally by 16% in autism subjects over controls between 2 and 4 years of age; however, the rate of growth did not differ between the two groups, and the right amygdala volume in the autism group was disproportionately enlarged. Scores representing social eye contact showed significant positive association with amygdala volume even though the autistic children expressed less social eye contact. Reduced eye contact has also been reported to associate with reduced amygdala volume in adolescents and adults with autism (Nacewicz *et al.*, 2006). An "allostatic overload" model of autism is proposed that contends that repeated exposure to a highly stimulating event leads to a compensatory response (allostasis) that is seen as increased dendritic arborization in the amygdala. Once a threshold is reached (allostatic overload), excess production of stress hormones results in cell death in the amygdala (Nacewicz, *et al.*, 2006; Schumann and Amaral, 2006).

Bauman and Kemper (1985) found increased neuronal density and reduced neuron size in the hippocampus and portions of the amygdala in children with autism.

Panic disorder

Smaller amygdala volume has been reported in panic disorder (Massana *et al.*, 2003) and early onset bipolar disorder (Dickstein *et al.*, 2005). Dysfunctional neurogenesis may be a contributing factor to these findings (MacKinnon and Zamoiski, 2006). Similar size reductions have not been found in studies with adult patients with bipolar disorder (Strakowski *et al.*, 2005). Sharma *et al.*(2003) reported volume reduction in the medial prefrontal cortex and subgenual anterior cingulate gyrus, which is closely linked to the amygdala.

There is evidence of activation of norepinephrinergic neurons during development of panic attacks (Bailey *et al.*, 2003) and mania as well as in bipolar individuals (Young *et al.*, 1994; Joyce *et al.*, 1995). Activation of prefrontal cortex has been reported to be both enhanced and depressed when bipolar and currently manic individuals were compared with controls (Blumberg *et al.*, 2000).

It is proposed that the onset of manic, depressive and panic episodes results from false or misperception of the emotional importance of familiar objects. The pathological state persists until the deficit can be corrected. This implies that the amygdala overreacts in the assignment of emotions to relatively neutral stimuli. The pathological state persists until the medial prefrontal cortex is able to suppress activity in the amygdala (MacKinnon and Zamoiski, 2006).

Select bibliography

Aggleton, J.P. ed. *The Amygdala: A Functional Analysis.* (Oxford: Oxford University Press, 2000.)

Christianson, S.A. ed. *The Handbook of Emotion and Memory: Research and Theory.* (Hillsdale, N.J.: Lawrence Erlbaum Associates, 1992.)

Ekman, P., Campos, J.J., Davidson, R.J., and deWaal, F.B.M. Emotions inside out. *Annals of the New York Academy of Sciences* (vol. 1000). (New York: The New York Academy of Sciences, 2003.)

Gloor, P. *The Temporal Lobe and Limbic System.* (New York: Oxford University Press, 1997.)

McGinty, J.F. ed. Advancing from the ventral striatum to the extended amygdala. *Annals of the New York Academy of Sciences* (vol. 877). (New York: The New York Academy of Sciences, 1999.)

Trimble, M.R., and Bolwig, T.G. (eds.) *The Temporal Lobes and the Limbic System*. (Petersfield, UK: Wrightson Biomedical Publishing, 1992.)

Whalen, P.J., and Phelps, E.A. eds. *The Human Amygdala*. (New York: Guilford Press, 2009.)

References

Aberg, M.A., Aberg, N.D., Palmer, T.D., Alborn, A.M., Carlsson-Skwirut, C., Bang, P., Rosengren, L.E., Olsson, T., Gage, F.H., and Eriksson, P.S. 2003. IGF-1 has a direct proliferative effect in adult hippocampal progenitor cells. *Mol. Cell. Neurosci.* **24**:23–40.

Adams, R.B. Jr., Gordon, H.L., Baird, A.A., Ambady, N., and Kleck, R.E. 2003. *Science* **300**:1536.

Adler, L.E., Olincy, A., Waldo, M., Harris, J.G., Griffith, J., Stevens, K., Flach, K., Nagamoto, H., Bickford, P., Leonard, S., and Freedman, R. 1998. Schizophrenia, sensory gating, and nicotinic receptors. *Schizophr. Bull.* **24**:189–202.

Adolphs, R., Tranel, D., Damasio, H., and Damasio, A.R. 1995. Fear and the human amygdala. *J. Neurosci.* **15**:5879–5891.

Aggleton, J.P. 1992. The functional effects of amygdala lesions in humans: A comparison with findings from monkeys. In: J.P.Aggleton (ed.) *The Amygdala: Neurobiological Aspects of Emotion, Memory, and Mental Dysfunction*. New York: Wiley-Liss, pp. 485–503.

Aggleton, J.P. 1993. The contribution of the amygdala to normal and abnormal emotional states. *Trends Neurosci.* **16**:328–333.

Airan, R.E., Meltzer, L.A., Roy, M., Gong, Y., Chen, H., and Deisseroth, K. 2007. High-speed imaging reveals neurophysiological links to behavior in an animal model of depression. *Science* **317**:819–823.

Alheid, G.F., and Heimer, L. 1996. Theories of basal forebrain organization and the "emotional motor system". *Prog. Brain Res.* **107**:461–484.

Allen, E. 1912. The cessation of the mitosis in the central nervous system of the albino rat. *J. Comp. Neurol.* **22**:547–568.

Amaral, D.G. 2003. The amygdala, social behavior, and danger detection. *Ann. N. Y. Acad. Sci.* **1000**:337–347.

Amaral, D.G., Price, J.L., Pitkanen, A., and Carmichael, S.T. 1992. Anatomical organization of the primate amygdaloid complex. In: J.P.Aggleton (ed.) *The Amygdala*. New York: Wiley, pp.1–66.

Ambrogini, P., Lattanzi, D., Ciuffoli, S., Agostini, D., Bertini, L., Stocchi, V., Santi, S., and Cuppini, R. 2004. Morpho-functional characterization of neuronal cells at different stages of maturation in granule cell layer of adult rat dentate gyrus. *Brain Res.* **1017**:21–31.

Arnold, S.E., Franz, B.A., Gur, R.C., Gur, R.E., Shapiro, R.M., Moberg, P.J., and Trojanowski, J.Q. 1995. Smaller neuron size in schizophrenia in hippocampal subfields that mediate cortico-hippocampal interactions. *Am. J. Psychiatry* **152**:738–748.

Arnold, S.E., Ruscheinsky, D.D., and Han, L.-Y. 1997. Further evidence of abnormal cytoarchitecture of the entorhinal cortex in schizophrenia using spatial point pattern analyses. *Biol. Psychiatry* **42**:639–647.

Austin, M.P., Mitchell, P., and Goodwin, G.M. 2001. Cognitive deficits in depression: Possible implications for functional neuropathology. *Br. J. Psychiatry* **178**:200–206.

Aylward, E.H., Minshew, N.J., Goldstein, G., Honeycutt, N.A., Augustine, A.M., Yates, K.O., Barta, P.E., and Pearlson, G.D. 1999. MRI volumes of amygdala and hippocampus in non-mentally retarded autistic adolescents and adults. *Neurology* **53**:2145–2150.

Bai, F., Bergeron, M., and Nelson, D.L. 2003. Chronic AMPA receptor potentiator (LY451646) treatment increases cell proliferation in adult rat hippocampus. *Neuropharmacology* **44**:1013–1021.

Bailey, J.E., Argyropoulos, S.V., Lightman, S.L., and Nutt, D.J. 2003. Does the brain noradrenaline network mediate the effects of the CO2 challenge? *J. Psychopharmacol.* **17**:252–259.

Balu, D.T., and Lucki, I. 2009. Adult hippocampal neurogenesis: Regulation, functional implications, and contribution to disease pathology. *Neurosci. Biobehav. Rev.* **33**:232–252.

Bauman, N.M., and Kemper, T. 1985. Histoanatomic observations of the brain in early infantile autism. *Neurology* **35**:866–874.

Bechara, A., Tranel, D., Damasio, H., Adolphs, R., Rockland, C., and Damasio, A.R. 1995. Double dissociation of conditioning and declarative knowledge relative to the amygdala and hippocampus in humans. *Science* **269**:1115–1118.

Bedard, A., Gravel, C., and Parent, A. 2006. Chemical characterization of newly generated neurons in the striatum of adult primates. *Exp. Brain Res.* **170**: 501–512.

Benes, F.M., Kwok, E.W., Vincent, S.L., and Todtenkopf, M.S. 1998. A reduction of nonpyramidal cells in sector CA2 of patients with schizophrenics and manic depressives. *Biol. Psychiatry* **44**:88–97.

Biebl, M. Cooper, C.M., Winkler, J., and Kuhn, H.G. 2000. Analysis of neurogenesis and programmed cell death reveals a self-renewing capacity in the adult rat brain. *Neurosci. Lett.* **291**:17–20.

Blum, K., Cull, J.G., Braverman, E.R., and Comings, D.E. 1996. Reward deficiency syndrome. *Am. Sci.* **84**:132–145.

Blumberg, H.P., Stern, E., Martinez, D., Ricketts, S., de Asis, J., White, T., Epstein, J., McBride, P.A., Eidelberg D., Kocsis, J.H., and Silbersweig, D.A. 2000. Increased anterior cingulate and caudate activity in bipolar mania. *Biol. Psychiatry* **48**:1045–1052.

Bogerts, B. 1998. The temporolimbic system theory of positive schizophrenic symptoms. *Schizophr. Bull.* **23**:423–43.

Bogerts, B., Meertz, E., and Schonfeldt-Bausch, R. 1985. Basal ganglia and limbic system pathology in schizophrenia: A morphometric study of brain volume and shrinkage. *Arch. Gen. Psychiatry* **42**:784–791.

Bohus, B., Koolhaas, J.M., Luiten, P.G.M., Korte, S.M., Roozendaal, B., and Wiersma, A. 1996. The neurobiology of the central nucleus of the amygdala in relation to neuroendocrine and autonomic outflow. In: G. Holstege, R. Bandler, and C.B. Saper (eds.) *The Emotional Motor System. Prog. Brain Res.* **107**: 447–460.

Bremner, J.D. 2003. Long-term effects of childhood abuse on brain and neurobiology. *Child Adolesc. Psychiatr. Clin. North Am.* **12**:271–292.

Bremner, J.D., Narayan, M., Anderson, E.R., Staib, L.H., Miller, H.L., and Charney, D.S. 2000. Hippocampal volume reduction in major depression. *Am. J. Psychiatry* **157**:115–118.

Brown, J., Cooper-Kuhn, C.M., Kempermann, G., Van Praag, H., Winkler, J., Gage, F.H., and Kuhn, H.G. 2003. Enriched environment and physical activity stimulate hippocampal but not olfactory bulb neurogenesis. *Eur. J. Neurosci.* **17**:2042–2046.

Brown, R., Colter, N., Corsellis, J.A.N., Crow, T.J., Frith, C.D., Jagoe, R., Johnstone, E.C., and Marsh, L. 1986. Post-mortem evidence of structural brain changes in schizophrenia: Differences in brain weight, temporal horn area and parahippocampal gyrus compared with affective disorder. *Arch. Gen. Psychiatry* **43**:36–42.

Bruel-Jungerman, E., Laroche, S., and Rampon, C. 2005. New neurons in the dentate gyrus are involved in the expression of enhanced long-term memory following environmental enrichment. *Eur. J. Neurosci.* **21**: 513–521.

Bruel-Jungerman, E., Rampon, C., and Larouche, S. 2007. Adult hippocampal neurogenesis, synaptic plasticity and memory; Facts and hypotheses. *Rev. Neurosci.* **18**:93–114.

Brun, V.H., Otnaess, M.K., Molden, S., Steffenach, H.-A., Witter, M.P., Moser, M.-B., and Moser, E.I. 2002. Place cells and place recognition maintained by direct entorhinal-hippocampal circuitry. *Science* **296**:2243–2246.

Buchanan, T.W., and Adolphs, R. 2003. The neuroanatomy of emotional memory in humans. In D. Reisberg, and P. Hertel (eds.) *Memory and Emotion.* New York: Oxford University Press, pp. 42–75.

Bursztain, S., Falls, W.A., Berman, S.A., and Friedman, M.J. 2007. Cell proliferation in the brains of NMDAR NR1 transgenic mice. *Brain Res.* **1172**:10–20.

Cahill, L., Haier, R.J., White, N.S., Fallon, J., Kilpatrick, L., Lawrence, C., Potkin, S.G., and Alkire, M.T. 2001. Sex-related difference in amygdala activity during emotionally influenced memory storage. *Neurobiol. Learn. Mem.* **75**:1–9.

Cameron, H.A., and McKay, R.D. 2001. Adult neurogenesis produces a large pool of new granule cells in the dentate gyrus. *J. Comp. Neurol.* **435**:406–417.

Canli, T., Sivers, H., Whitfield, S.L., Gotlib, I.H., and Gabrieli, J.D.E. 2002. Amygdala response to happy faces as a function of extraversion. *Science* **296**:2191.

Chang, C.H., Liang, K.C., and Yen, C.T. 2005. Inhibitory avoidance learning altered ensemble activity of amygdaloid neurons in rats. *Eur. J. Neurosci.* **21**: 210–218.

Chavez, C.M., McGaugh, J.L., and Weinberger, N.M. 2009. The basolateral amygdala modulates specific sensory memory representations in the cerebral cortex. *Neurobiol. Learn. Mem.* **91**:382–392.

Cotter, D., Mackay, D., Chana, G., Beasley, C., Landau, S., and Everal, I.P. 2002. Astroglial plasticity in the hippocampus is affected by chronic psychosocial stress and concomitant fluoxetine treatment. *Neuropsychopharmacology* **31**:1616–1626.

Dayer, A.G., Cleaver, K.M., Abouantoun, T., and Cameron, H.A. 2005. New GABAergic interneurons in the adult neocortex and striatum are generated from different precursors. *J. Cell. Biol.* **168**:415–427.

Deakin, J.F.W., and Graeff, F.G. 1991. 5-HT and mechanisms of defense. *J. Psychopharmacol.* **5**:305–315.

DeBellis, M.D., Clark, D.B., Beers, S.R., Soloff, P.H., Boring, A.M., Hall, J., Kersn, A., and Keshavan, M.W. 2000. Hippocampal volume in adolescent-onset alcohol use sdisorders. *Am. J. Psychiatry* **157**:737–744.

DeBellis, M.D., Keshavan, M.S., Shifflett, H., Iyengar, S., Beers, S.R., Hall, J., and Moritz, G. 2002. Brain structures in pediatric maltreatement-related posttraumatic stress disorder: A sociodemographically matched study. *Biol. Psychiatry* **45**:1271–1284.

Delis, D.C., and Lucas, J.A. 1996. Memory. In: B.S.Fogel, R.B.Schiffer, and S.M.Rao (eds.) *Neuropsychiatry.* Baltimore: Williams & Wilkins, pp. 365–399.

Dickstein, D.P., Milham, M.P., Nugent, A.C., Drevets, W.C., Charney, D.S., Pine, D.S., and Leibenluft, E. 2005. Fronto-temporal alterations in paediatric bipolar disorder: Results of a voxel-based morphometry study. *Arch. Gen. Psychiatry* **62**: 734–741.

Doetsch, F., Caille, I., Lim, D.A., Garcia-Verdugo, J.M., and Alvarez-Buylla, A. 1999. Subventricular zone astrocytes are neural stem cells in the adult mammalian brain. *Cell* **97**:703–716.

Dolan, R.J. 2002. Emotion, cognition and behavior. *Science* **298**:1191–1194.

Drevets, W.C. 2003. Neuroimaging abnormalities in the amygdala in mood disorders. *Ann. N. Y. Acad. Sci* **985**:420–444.

Drevets, W.C. 2007. Orbitofrontal cortex function and structure in depression. *Ann. N. Y. Acad. Sci.* **1121**: 499–527.

Drevets, W.C., and Price, J.L. 2005. Neuroimaging and neuropathological studies of mood disorders. In: J.W.M. Licinio (ed.) *Biology of Depression: From Novel Insights to Therapeutic Strategies*. Weinheim:Wiley-VCH Verlag GmbH & Co.

Drevets, W.C., Videen, T.O., Price, J.L., Preskorn, S.H., Carmichael, S.T., and Raichle, M.E. 1992. A functional anatomical study of unipolar depression. *J. Neurosci.* **12**:3628–3641.

Drevets, W.C., Gadde, K., and Krishnan, K.R.R. 2004. Neuroimaging studies of depression. In: D.S.Charney, E.J.Nestler, and B.S.Bunney (eds.) *The Neurobiological Foundation of Mental Illness*, 2nd ed. New York: Oxford University Press.

Drevets, W.C., Price, J.L., and Furey, M.L. 2008. Brain structural and functional abnormalities in mood disorders: implications for neuron circuitry models of depression. *Brain Struct. Funct.* **213**:93–118.

Eastwood, S.L., and Harrison, P.J. 2000. Hippocampal synaptic pathology in schizophrenia, bipolar disorder and major depression: A study of complexin mRNAs. *Mol. Psychiatry* **5**:425–432.

Ericksson, P.S., Perfilieva, E., Bjork-Eriksson, T., Alborn, A.M., Nordborg, C., Peterson, D.A., and Gage, F.H. 1998. Neurogenesis in the adult human hippocampus. *Nat. Med.* **4**:1313–1317.

Fitzgerald, D.A., Angstadt, M., Jelsone, L.M., Nathan, P.J., and Phan, K.L. 2006. Beyond threat: Amygdala reactivity across multiple expressions of facial affect. *Neuroimage* **30**:1441–1448.

Fossati, P., Coyette, F., Ergis, A.M., and Allilaire, J.F., 2002. Influence of age and executive functioning on verbal memory of inpatients with depression. *J. Affect. Disord.* **68**:261–271.

Fowler, C.D., Liu, Y., Ouimer, C., and Wang, Z. 2002. The effects of social environment on adult neurogenesis in the female prairie vole. *J. Neurobiol.* **51**:115–128.

Frielingsdorf, H., Simpson, D.R., Thai, L.J., and Pizzo, D.P. 2007. Nerve growth factor promotes survival of new neurons in the adult hippocampus. *Neurobiol. Dis.* **26**:47–55.

Ge, S., Goh, E.L. Sailor, K.A., Kitabatake, Y., Ming, G.L., and Song, H. 2006. GABA regulates synaptic integration of newly generated neurons in the adult brain. *Nature* **439**:589–593.

Ge, S., Pradhan, D.A., Ming, G.L., and Song, H. 2007. GABA sets the tempo for activity-dependent adult neurogenesis. *Trends Neurosci.* **30**:1–8.

Gloor, P., Olivier, A., and Quesney, L.F. 1981. The role of the amygdala in the expression of psychic phenomena in temporal lobe seizures. In: Y. Ben-Ari (ed.) *The Amygdaloid Complex*. New York: Elsevier, pp. 489–507.

Gould, E., Vail, N., Wagers, M., and Gross, C.G. 2001. Adult-generated hippocampal and neocortical neurons in macaques have a transient existence. *Proc. Natl. Acad. Sci. USA.* **98**:10910–10917.

Grahn, J.A., Parkinson, J.A., and Owen, A.M. 2009. The role of the basal ganglia in learning and memory: Neuropsychological studies. *Behav. Brain Res.* **199**:53–60.

Gur, R.E., Cowell, P., Turetsky, B.I., Gallacher, F., Cannon, T., Bilker, W., and Gur, R.C. 1998. A follow-up magnetic resonance imaging study of schizophrenia. *Arch. Gen. Psychiatry* **55**:145–152.

Gurvits, T.V., Shenton, M.E., Hokama, H., Ohta, H., Lasko, N.B., Gilbertson, M.W., Orr, S.P., Kikinis, R., Jolesz, F.A., McCartey, R.W., and Pitman, R.K. 1996. Magnetic resonance imaging study of hippocampal volume in chronic, combat-related posttraumatic stress disorder. *Biol. Psychiatry* **40**:1091–1099.

Guze, B.H., and Gitlin, M. 1994. The neuropathologic basis of major affective disorders: Neuroanatomic insights. *J. Neuropsychiatry* **6**:114–119.

Halim, N.D., Weickert, C.S., McClintock, B.W., Weinberger, D.R., and Lipska, B.K. 2004. Effects of chronic haloperidol and clozapine treatment on neurogenesis in the adult rat hippocampus. *Neuropsychopharmacology* **29**:1063–1069.

Hamann, S., Herman, R.A., Nolan, C.L., and Wallen, K. 2004. Men and women differ in amygdala response to visual sexual stimuli. *Nat. Neurosci.* **7**:411–416.

Hamidi, M., Drevets, W.C., and Price, J.L. 2004. Glial reduction in amygdala in major depressive disorder is due to oligodendrocytes. *Biol. Psychiatry* **55**:563–569.

Hariri, A.R., Tessitore, A., Matty, V.S., Fera, F., and Weinberger, D.R. 2002. The amygdala response to emotional stimuli: a comparison of faces and scenes. *Neuroimage* **17**:317–323.

Hasler, G., Fromm, S.J., Carlson, P.J., Luckenbaugh, D.A., Waldeck, T., Geraci, M., Roiser, J.P., Neumeister, A., Meyers, N., Charney, D.S., and Drevets, W.C. 2008. Neural response to catecholamine depletion in unmedicated, remitted subjects with major depressive disorder and healthy subjects. *Arch. Gen. Psychiatry* **65**:521–531.

Hasler, G., van der Veen, J.W., Geraci, M., Shen, J., Pine, D., and Drevets, W.C. 2009. Prefrontal cortical gamma-aminobutyric acid levels in panic disorder determined by proton magnetic resonance spectroscopy. *Biol. Psychiatry* **65**: 273–275.

Hasselmo, M.E., Schnett, E., and Barkai, E. 1995. Dynamics of learning and recall at excitatory recurrent synapses and cholinergic modulation in rat hippocampal region CA3. *J. Neurosci.* **15**:5249–5262.

Hatfield, T., Han, J.-S., Conley, M., Gallagher, M., and Holland, P. 1996. Neurotoxic lesions of basolateral, but not central, amygdala interfere with Pavlovian second-order conditioning and reinforcer devaluation effects. *J. Neurosci.* **16**:5256–5265.

Heckers, S. 2001. Neuroimaging studies of the hippocampus in schizophrenia. *Hippocampus* **11**:520–528.

Heckers, S., and Heinsen, H. 1991. Hippocampal neuron number in schizophrenia. A stereological study. *Arch. Gen. Psychiatry* **48**:1002–1008.

Hendler, T., Rotshtein, P., Yeshurun, Y., Weizmann, T., Kahn, I., Ben-Bashat, D., Malach, R., and Bleich, A. 2003. Sensing the invisible: Differential sensitivity of visual cortex and amygdala to traumatic contex. *Neuroimage* **19**:587–600.

Herholz, K., Weisenbach, S., Zündorf, G., Lenz, O., Schröder, Bauer, B., Kalbe, E., and Heiss, W.-D. 2004. In vivo study of acetylcholine esterase in basal forebrain, amygdala, and cortex in mild to moderate Alzheimer disease. *Neuroimage* **21**:136–143.

Hermann, B.P., Wyler, A.R, Blumer, D., and Richey, E.T. 1992. Ictal fear: Lateralizing significance and implications for understanding the neurobiology of pathological fear states. *Neuropsychiatry Neuropsychol. Behav. Neurol.* **5**:203–210.

Herpertz, S., Dietrich, T., Wenning, B., Krings, T., Erberich, S.G., Willmes, K., Thron, A., and Sass, H. 2001. Evidence of abnormal amygdala functioning in borderline personality disorder: A functional MRI study. *Biol. Psychiatry* **50**:292–298.

Hirayasu, Y., Shenton, M.E., Salisbury, D.F., Dickey, C.C., Fioscher, L.A., Mazzoni, P., Kisler, T., Arakaki, H., Kwon, J.S., Anderson, J.E., Yurgelun-Todd, D., Toben, M., and McCartey, R.W. 1998. Lower left temporal lobe MRI volumes in patients with first-episode schizophrenia compared with psychotic patients with first-episode affective disorder and normal subjects. *Am. J. Psychiatry* **155**:1384–1391.

Holland, P.C., and Gallagher, M. 1993. Amygdala central nucleus lesions disrupt increments, but not decrement, in conditioned stimulus processing. *Behav. Neurosci.* **107**:246–253.

Jacobs, B.L. 2002. Adult brain neurogenesis and depression. *Brain Behav. Immun.* **16**:602–609.

Jacobs, L.F., and Schenk, F. 2003. Unpacking the cognitive map: the parallel map theory of hippocampal function. *Psychol. Rev.* **110**:285–315.

Jakob, H., and Beckman, H. 1994. Circumscribed malformation and nerve cell alterations in the entorhinal cortex of schizophrenics. Pathogenetic and clinical aspects. *J. Neural Transm.* **98**:83–106.

Jessberger, S., Zhao, C., Toni, N., Clemenson, G.D. Jr., Li, Y., and Gage, F.H. 2007. Seizure-associated, aberrant neurogenesis in adult rats characterized with retrovirus-mediated cell labeling. *J. Neurosci.* **27**:9400–9407.

Jin, K., Zhu, Y., Sun, Y., Mao, X.O., Xie, L., and Greenbert, D.A. 2002. Vascular endothelial growth factor (VEGF) stimulates neurogenesis in vitro and in vivo. *Proc. Natl. Acad. Sci. USA.* **99**:11946–11950.

Jin, K., Peel, A.L., Mao, X.O., Xie, L., Cottrell, B.A., Henshall, D.C., and Greenberg, D.A. 2004. Increased hippocampal neurogenesis in Alzheimer's disease. *Proc. Natl. Acad. Sci. USA.* **101**:343v347.

Joëls, M. 2009. Stress, the hippocampus, and epilepsy. *Epilepsia* **50**:586–597.

Joëls, M., Krugers, H., and Karst, H. 2008. Stress-induced changes in hippocampal function. *Prog. Brain Res.* **167**:3–13.

Joyce, P.R., Fergusson, D.M., Wollard, G., Abbott, R.M., Horwood, L.J., and Upton, J. 1995. Urinary catecholamines and plasma hormones predict mood state in rapid cycling bipolar affective disorder. *J. Affect. Disord.* **33**:233–243.

Kalivas, P.W., Pierce, R.C., Cornish, J., and Sorg, B.A. 1998. A role for sensitization in craving and relapse in cocaine addiction. *J. Psychopharmacol.* **12**:49–53.

Kempermann, G. 2005. *Adult Neurogenesis: Stem Cells and Neuronal Development in the Adult Brain.* New York: Oxford University Press.

Kempermann, G., Gast, D., Kronenberg, G., Yamaguchi, M., and Gage, F.H. 2003. Early determination and long-term persistence of adult-generated new neurons in the hippocampus of mice. *Development* **130**:391–399.

Kessler, R.C., Chiu, W.T., Demler, O., and Walters, E.E. 2005. Prevalence, severity, and comorbidity of 12-month DSM-IV disorders in the National Comorbidity Survey Replication. *Arch. Gen. Psychiatry* **62**:617–627.

Killgore, W.D.S., and Yurgelun-Todd, D.A. 2004. Activation of the amygdala and anterior cingulate during nonconscious processing of sad versus happy faces. *Neuroimage* **21**:1215–1223.

Kjelstrup, K.B., Solstad, T., Brun, V.H., Hafting, T., Leutgeb, S., Witter, M.P., Moser, E.I., and Moser, M.B. 2008. Finite scale of spatial representation in the hippocampus. *Science* **321**:140–143.

Kodama, M., Fujioka, T., and Duman, R.S. 2004. Chronic olanzapine or fluoxetine administration increases cell proliferation in hippocampus and prefrontal cortex of adult rat. *Biol. Psychiatry* **56**:570–580.

Kotrla, K.J., and Weinberger, D.R. 1995. Brain imaging in schizophrenia. *Annu. Rev. Med.* **46**:113–122.

Krimer, L.S., Herman, M.M., Saunders, R.C., Boyd, J.C., Hyde, T.M., Carter, J.M., Kleinman, J.E., and Winberger, D.R. 1997. Qualitative and quantitative analysis of the entorhinal cortex in schizophrenia. *Cereb. Cortex* 7:732–739.

Kreindler, A., and Steriade, M. 1964. EEG patterns of arousal and sleep induced by stimulating various amygdaloid levels in the cat. *Arch. Ital. Biol.* **102**:576–586.

Krystal, J.H., D'Souza, D.C., Petrakis, I.L., Belger, A., Berman, R., Charney, D.S., Abi-Saab, W., and Madonick, S. 1999. NMDA agonists and antagonists as probes of fglutamatergic dysfunction and pharmacotherapies for neuropsychiatric disorders. *Harv. Rev. Psychiatry* 7:125–133.

Ledoux, J.E. 1992. Brain mechanisms and emotional learning. *Curr. Opin. Neurobiol.* **2**:191–197.

Liddle, P.F., Friston, K.J., Frith, C.D., Hirsch, S.R., Jones, T., and Frackowiak, R.S.J. 1992. Patterns of cerebral blood flow in schizophrenia. *Br. J. Psychiatry* **160**:179–186.

Lindauer, R.J., Booij J., Habraken, J.B., Uylings, H.B., Olff, M., Carlier, I.V., den Heeten, G.J., van Eck-Smit, B.L., and Gersons, B.P. 2004. Cerebral blood flow changes during script-driven imagery in police officers with posttraumatic stress disorder. *Biol. Psychiatry* 56:356–363.

London, E.D., Stapleton, J.M., Phillips, R.L., Grant, S.J., Villemagne, V.L., Liu, X., and Soria, R. 1996. PET studies of cerebral glucose metabolism: Acute effects of cocaine and long-term deficits in brains of drug abusers. *NIDA Res. Monogr.* **163**:146–158.

Luzzati, F., De Marchis, S., Fasolo, A., and Peretto, P. 2006. Neurogenesis in the caudate nucleus of the adult rabbit. *J. Neurosci.* **26**:609–621.

Lynch, M.A. 2004. Long-term potentiation and memory. *Physiol. Rev.* **84**:87–136.

MacKinnon, D.F., and Zamoiski, R. 2006. Panic comorbidity with bipolar disorder: What is the manic-panic connection?*Bipolar Disord.* **8**:648–664.

Madsen, T.M., Treschow, A., Bengzon, J., Bolwig, T. G., Lindvall, O., and Tingström, A. 2000. Increased neurogenesis in a model of electroconvulsive therapy. *Biol. Psychiatry* 47:1043–1049.

Maguire, E.A., Gadian, D.G., Johnsrude, I.S., Good, C.D., Ashburner, J., Frackowiak, R.S.J., and Frith, C.D. 2000. Navigation-related structural change in the hippocampi of taxi drivers. *Proc. Natl. Acad. Sci. USA.* **97**:4398–4403.

Maguire, E.A., Spiers, H.J., Good, C.D., Hartley, T., Frackowiak, R.S.J., and Burgess, N. 2003. Navigational expertise and the human hippocampus: a structural brain imaging analysis. *Hippocampus* **13**:250–259.

Manganas, L.N., Zhang, X., Li, Y., Hazel, R.D., Smith, S.D., Wagshul, M.E., Henn, F., Benveniste, H., Djuric, P.M., Enikolopov, G., and Maletic-Savatic, M. 2007. Magnetic resonance spectroscopy identifies neural progenitor cells in the live human brain. *Science* 318:980–985.

Martin, J.H. 1996. *Neuroanatomy. Text and Atlas* (2nd ed.). Stamford, CT: Appleton & Lange, p. 449.

Massana, G., Serra-Grabulosa, J.M., Salgado-Pineda, P., Gastó, C., Junqué, C., Massana, J., Mercader, J.M., Gómez, B., Tobeñ, A., and Salameroa, M. 2003. Amygdalar atrophy in panic disorder patients detected by volumetric magnetic resonance imaging. *Neuroimage* **19**:80–90.

Mather, M., Canli, T., English, T., Witfiled, S., Wais, P., Ochsner, K., Gabrieli, J.D.E., and Carstensen, L.L. 2004. Amygdala responses to emotionally valenced stimuli in older and younger adults. *Psychol. Sci.* **15**:259–263.

McCarthy, M.M. 2003. Stretching the truth: why hippocampal neurons are so vulnerable following traumatic brain injury. *Exp. Neurol.* **184**:40–43.

McGaugh, J.L., 2004. The amygdala modulates the consolidation of memories of emotionally arousing experiences. Annu. Rev. Neurosci. **27**:1–28.

Mendez, M.F., and Foti, D.J. 1997. Lethal hyperoral behaviour from Kluver–Bucy syndrome. *J. Neural. Neurosurg. Psychiatry* **62**:293–294.

Mendez, M.F., and Cummings, J.L. 2003. *Dementia: A Clinical Approach* (3rd ed.). Philadelphia, P.A.: Butterworth-Heinemann.

Mesulam, M.M. 1981. Dissociative states with abnormal temporal lobe EEG: Multiple personality and the illusion of possession. *Arch. Neurol.* **38**:176–181.

Milad, M.R., Wright, C.I., Orr, S.P., Pitman, R.K., Quirk, G.J., and Rauch, S.L. 2007. Recall of fear extinction in humans activates the ventromedial prefrontal cortex and hippocampus in concert. *Biol. Psychiatry* 62:446–454.

Mirescu, C., and Gould, E., 2006. Stress and adult neurogenesis. *Hippocampus* 16:233–238.

Miyashita, T., and Williams, C.L. 2006. Epinephrine administration increases neural impulses propagated along the vagus nerve: Role of peripheral beta-adrenergic receptors. *Neurobiol. Learn. Mem.* **85**:116–124.

Morris, J.S., Öhman, A., and Dolan, R.J. 1998. Conscious and unconscious emotional learning in the human amygdala. *Nature* 393:467–470.

Morris, J.S., Öhman, A., and Dolan, R.J. 1999. A subcortical pathway to the right amygdala mediating "unseen" fear. *Proc. Natl. Acad. Sci. USA.* **96**:1680–1685.

Morris, J.S., deBonis, M., and Dolan, R.J. 2002. Human amygdala responses to fearful eyes. *Neuroimage* 17:214–222.

Morrison, J.H., and Hof, P.R. 1997. Life and death of neurons in the aging brain. *Science* 278:412–419.

Mosconi, M.W., Cody-Hazlett, H., Poe, M.D., Gerig, G., Gimpel-Smith, R., and Joseph Piven, J. 2009. Longitudinal study of amygdala volume and joint attention in 2- to 4-year-old children with autism. *Arch. Gen. Psychiatry* **66**:509–516.

Munson, J., Dawson, G., Abbott, R., Faja, S., Webb, S.J., Friedman, S.D., Shaw, D., Artru, A., and Dager, D.R. 2006. Amygdalar volume and behavioral development in autism. *Arch. Gen. Psychiatry* **63**:686–693.

Nacewicz, B.M., Dalton, K.M., Johnstone, T., Long, M.T., McAuliff, E.M., Oakes, T.R., Alexander, A.L., and Davidson, R.J. 2006. Amygdala volume and nonverbal social impairment in adolescent an adult males with autism. *Arch. Gen. Psychiatry* **63**:1417–1428.

Nacher, J., Varea, E., Miguel Blasco-Ibanez, J., Gomez-Climent, M.A., Castillo-Gomez, E., Crespo, C., Martinez-Guijarro, F.J., and McEwen, B.S. 2007. N-methyl-D-aspartate receptor expression during adult neurogenesis in the rat dentate gyrus. *Neuroscience* **144**:855–864.

Nakagawa, S., Kim, J.E., Lee, R., Malberg, J.E., Chen, J., Steffen, C., Zhang, Y.J., Nestler, E.J., and Duman, R.S., 2002. Regulation of neurogenesis in adult mouse hippocampus by cAMP and the cAMP response element-binding protein. *J. Neurosci.* **22**:3673–3682.

Narr, K.L., Thompson, P.M., Szeszko, P., Robinson, D., Jang, S., Woods, R.P., Kim, S., Hayashi, K.M., Asunction, D., Toga, A.W., and Bilder, R.M. 2004. Regional specfity of hippocampal volume reductions in first-episode schizophrenia. *Neuroimage* **21**:1563–1575.

Nelson, M.D., Saykin, A.J., Flashman, L.A., and Riordan, H.J. 1998. Hippocampal volume reduction in schizophrenia as assessed by magnetic resonance imaging. *Arch. Gen. Psychiatry* **55**:433–440.

Neumeister, A., Nugent, A.C., Waldeck, T., Geraci, M., Schwarz, M., Bonne, O., Bain, E., Luckenbaugh, D., Herscovitch, P., Charney, D.S., and Drevets, W.C. 2004. Neural and behavioral responses to tryptophan depletion in unmedicated patients with remitted major depressive disorder and controls. *Arch. Gen. Psychiatry* **61**:765–773.

Neumeister, A., Wood, S., Bonne, O., Nugent, A.C., Luckenbaugh, D.A., Young, T., Bain, E.E., Charney, D.S., and Drevets, W.C., 2005. Reduced hippocampal volume in unmedicated, remitted patients with major depression versus control subjects. *Biol. Psychiatry* **57**:935–937, 2005.

New, A.S., Hazlett, E.A., Buchsbaum, M.S., Goodman, M., Mitelman, S.A., Newmark, R., Trisdorfer, R., Haznedar, M.M., Koenigsberg, H.W., Flory, J., and Siever, L.J. 2007. Amygdala-prefrontal disconnection in borderline personality disorder. *Neuropsychopharmacology* **32**:1629–1640.

New, A.S., Goodman, M., Triebwasser, J., and Siever, L.J. 2008. Recent advances in the biological study of personality disorders. *Psychiatr. Clin. North Am.* **31**:441–461.

Nomura, M., Ohira, H., Haneda, K., Iidaka, T., Sadato, N., Okada, T., and Yonekura, Y. 2004. Functional association of the amygdala and ventral prefrontal cortex during cognitive evaluation of facial expressions primed by masked angry faces: an event-related fMRI study. *Neuroimage* **21**:352–363.

Ongür, D., Ferry, A.T., and Price, J.L. 2003. Architectonic subdivision of the human orbital and medial prefrontal cortex. *J. Comp. Neurol.* **460**:425–449.

Overstreet-Wadiche, L., Bromber, D.A., Bensen, A.L., and Westbrook, G.L. 2005. GABAergic signaling to newborn neurons in dentate gyrus. *J. Neurophysiol.* **94**:4528–4532.

Packard, M.G., Cahill, L., and McGaugy, J.L. 1994. Amygdala modulation of hippocampal-dependent and caudate nucleus-dependent memory processes. *Proc. Natl. Acad. Sci. USA.* **91**:8477–8481.

Pakkenberg, B. 1987. Post-mortem study of chronic schizophrenic brains. *Br. J. Psychiatry* **151**:744–752.

Pantelis, C., Velakoulis, D., McGorry, P.D., Wood, S.J., Suckling, J., Phillips, L.J., Yung, A.R., Bullmore, E., Brewer, W., Soulsby, B., Desmond, P., and McGuire, P.K. 2003. Neuroanatomical abnormalities before and after onset of psychosis: a cross sectional and longitudinal MRI comparison. *Lancet* **361**:281–288.

Phelphs, E.A., O'Connor, K.J., Gatenby, J.C., Gore, J.C., Grillon, C., and Davis, M. 2001. Activation of the left amygdala to a cognitive representation of fear. *Nat. Neurosci.* **4**:437–441.

Pierce, K., Muller, R.A., Ambrose, J., Allen, G., and Corchesne, E. 2001. Face processing occurs outside the fusiform "face area" in autism: Evidence from functional MRI. *Brain* **124**:2059–2073.

Pitkanen, A., Savander, V., and LeDoux, J.E. 1997. Organization of intra-amygdaloid circuitries in the rat: An emerging framework for understanding functions of the amygdala. *Trends Neurosci.* **20**:517–523.

Price, J.L., Russchen, F.T., and Amaral, D.G. 1987. The limbic region. II: The amygdaloid complex. In: A. Bjorklund, and T.Hokfelt (eds.) *Handbook of Chemical Neuroanatomy*, volume 5. *Integrated Systems of the CNS, Part I. Hypothalamus, Hippocampus, Amygdala, Retina.* New York: Elsevier.

Pritchard, P.B. III, Holmstrom, V.L., and Roitzsch, J.C. 1985. Epileptic amnestic attacks: Benefits from antiepileptic drugs. *Neurology* **35**:1188–1189.

Rai, K.S., Hattiangady, B., and Shetty, A.K. 2007. Enhanced production and dendritic growth of new dentate granule cells in the middle-aged hippocampus following intracerebroventricular FGF-2 infusions. *Eur. J. Neurosci.* **26**:1765–1779.

Rauch, S.L., van der Kolk, B.A., Fisler, R.E., Alpert, N.M., Orr, S.P., Savage, C.R., Fischman, A.J., Jenike, M.A., and Pitman, R.K. 1996. A symptom provocation study of posttraumatic stress disorder using positron emission tomography and script-driven imagery. *Arch. Gen. Psychiatry* **53**:380–387.

Rauch, S.L., Shin, L.M., and Phelps, E.A. 2006. Neurocircuitry models of posttraumatic stress disorder and extinction: Human neuroimaging research-past, present, and future. *Biol. Psychiatry* **60**:376–382.

Reif, A., Fritzen, S., Finger, M., Strobel, A., Lauer, M., Schmitt, A., and Lesch, K.P. 2006. Neural stem cell proliferation is decreased in schizophrenia, but not in depression. *Mol. Psychiatry* **11**:514–522.

Sachs, B.D., and Meisel, R.L. 1994. The physiology of male sexual behavior. In: E. Knobil, and J.D.Neill (eds.) *The Physiology of Reproduction*. New York: Raven Press, pp. 3–105.

Saver, J.L., Salloway, S.P., Devinsky, O., and Bear, D.M. 1996. Neuropsychiatry of aggression. In: B.S.Fogel, R.B.Schiffer, and S.M.Rao (eds.) *Neuropsychiatry*. Baltimore: Williams & Wilkins, pp. 523–548.

Schanzer, A., Wachs, F.P., Wilhelm, D., Acker, T., Cooper-Kuhn, C., Beck, H., Winkler, J., Aigner, L., Plate, K.H., and Kuhn, H.G. 2004. Direct stimulation of adult neural stem cells in vitro and neurogenesis in vivo by vascular endothelial growth factor. *Brain Pathol.* **14**:237–248.

Scharfman, H., Goodman, J., Macleod, A., Phani, S., Antonelli, C., and Croll, S. 2005. Increased neurogenesis and the ectopic granule cells after intrahippocampal BDNF infusion in adult rats. *Exp. Neurol.* **192**:348–356.

Schmahl, C.G., Vermetten, E., Elzinga, B.M., and Bremner, J.D. 2003. Magnetic resonance imaging of hippocampal and amygdala volume in women with childhood abuse and borderline personality disorder. *Psychiatry Res.* **122**:193–198.

Schmitt, A., Weber, S., Jatzko, A., Braus, D.F., and Henn, F.A. 2004. Hippocampal volume and cell proliferation after acute and chronic clozapine or haloperidol treatment. *J. Neural. Transm.* **111**:91–100.

Schumann, C.M., and Amaral, D.G. 2006. Stereological analysis of amygdala neuron number in autism. *J. Neurosci.* **26**:7674–7679.

Schumann, C.M., Hamstra, J., Goodin-Jones, B.L., Lotspeich, L.J., Kwon, H., Bunocore, M.H., Lammers, C.R., Reiss, A.L., and Amaral, D.G. 2004. The amygdala is enlarged in children but not adolescents with autism: The hippocampus is enlarged at all ages. *J. Neurosci.* **24**:6392–6401.

Schwartz, C.E., Wright, C.I., Shin, L.M., Kagan, J., and Rauch, S.L. 2003. Inhibited and uninhibited infants "grown up": Adult amygdalar response to novelty. *Science* **300**:1952–1954.

Scott, S.A., Dekosky, S.T., and Scheff, S.W. 1991. Volumetric atrophy of the amygdala in Alzheimer's disease: quantitative serial reconstruction. *Neurology* **41**:351–356.

Seri, B., Garcia-Verdugo, J.M., Collado-Morente, L., McEwen, B.S., and Alvarez-Buylla, A. 2004. Cell types, lineage, and architecture of the germinal zone in the adult dentate gyrus. *J. Comp. Neurol.* **478**:359–378.

Sharma, V., Menon, R., Carr, T.J., Densmore, M., Mazmanian, D., and Williamson, P.C. 2003. An MRI study of subgenual prefrontal cortex in patients with familial and non-familial bipolar I disorder. *J. Affect. Disord.* **77**:167–171.

Sheline, Y.I., Wang, P.W., Gado, M.H., Csernansky, J.G., and Vannier, M.W. 1996. Hippocampal atrophy in recurrent major depression. *Proc. Natl. Acad. Sci. USA.* **93**:3908–3913.

Sheline, Y.I., Gado, M.H., and Kraemer, H.C. 2003. Untreated depression and hippocampal volume loss. *Am. J. Psychiatry* **160**:1516–1518.

Shinotoh, H., Namba, H., Fukushi, K., Nagatsuka, S., Tanaka, N., Aotsuka, A., Ota, T., Tanada, S., and Irie, T. 2000. Progressive loss of cortical acetylcholinesterase activity in association with cognitive decline in Alzheimer's disease: a positron emission tomography study. *Ann. Neurol.* **48**:194–200.

Siegle, G.J., Steinhauer, S.R., Thase, M.E., Stenger, V.A., and Carter, C.S. 2002. Can't shake that feeling: Event-related fMRI assessment of sustained amygdala activity in response to emotional information in depressed individuals. *Biol. Psychiatry* **51**:693–707.

Skaggs, W.E., and McNaughton, B.L. 1996. Replay of neuronal firing sequences in rat hippocampus during sleep flowing spatial exposure. *Science* **271**:1870–1873.

Sparks, B.F., Friedman, S.D., Shaw, D.W., Aylward, E.H., Echelard, D., Artru, A.A., Maravilla, K.R., Giedd, J.N., Munson, J., Dawson, G., and Dager, S.R. 2002. Brain structural abnormalities in young children with autism spectrum disorder. *Neurology* **59**:184–192.

Squire, L.R., Amaral, D.G., and Press, G.A. 1990. Magnetic resonance measurements of hippocampal formation and mammillary nuclei distinguish medial temporal lobe and diencephalic amnesia. *J. Neurosci.* **19**:3106–3117.

Strakowski, S.M., DelBello, M.P., Sax, K.W., Zimmerman, M.E., Shear, P.K., Hawkins, J.M., and Larson, E.R. 1999. Brain magnetic resonance imaging of structural abnormalities in bipolar disorder. *Arch. Gen. Psychiatry* **56**:254–260.

Strakowski, S.M., DelBello, M.P., and Adler, C.M. 2005. The functional neuroanatomy of bipolar disorder: A review of neuroimaging findings. *Mol. Psychiatry* **10**:105–116.

Stranahan, A.M., Arumugam, T.V., Cutler, R.G., Lee, K., Egan, J.M., and Mattson, M.P. 2008. Diabetes impairs hippocampal function through glucocorticoid-mediated effects on new and mature neurons. *Nat. Neurosci.* **11**:309–317.

Tamminga, C.A. 1998. Schizophrenia and glutamatergic transmission. *Crit. Rev. Neurobiol.* **12**:21–36.

Tamminga, C.A. 1999. Glutamatergic aspects of schizophrenia. *Br. J. Psychiatry* **174**(Suppl. 37):12–15.

Tebartz van Elsta, L., Hesslingera, B., Thielb, T., Geigera, E., Haegelea, K., Lemieuxc, L., Lieba, K., Bohusa, M., Hennigb, J., and Eberta, D. 2003. Frontolimbic brain abnormalities in patients with borderline personality disorder: A volumetric magnetic resonance imaging study. *Biol. Psychiatry* **54**:163–171.

Thomas, K.M., Drevets, W.C., Dahl, R.E., Ryan, N.D., Birmaher, B., Eccard, C.H., Axelson, D., Whalen, P.J., and Casey, B.J. 2001. Amygdala response to fearful faces in anxious and depressed children. *Arch. Gen. Psychiatry* **58**:1057–1063.

Trejo, J.L., Llorens-Martin, M.V., and Torres-Aleman, I. 2008. The effects of exercise on spatial learning and anxiety-like behavior are mediated by an IGF-I-dependent mechanism related to hippocampal neurogenesis. *Mol. Cell. Neurosci.* **37**:402–411.

Tremblay, C., Kirouac, G., and Dore, F.Y. 2001. The recognition of adults' and children's facial expressions of emotions. *J. Psychol.* **121**:341–350.

van Praag, H. Kempermann, G., and Gage, F.H. 1999. Running increases cell proliferation and neurogenesis in the adult mouse dentate gyrus. *Nat. Neurosci.* **2**:266–270.

Vass, R. 2004. Fear not. *Sci. Am.* **14**:62–69.

Velakoulis, D., Pantelis, C., McGorry, P.E., Dudgeon, P., Brewer, W., Cook, M., Desmond, P., Bridle, N., Tierney, P., Murrie, V., Singh, B., and Copolov, D. 1999. Hippocampal volume in first-episode psychoses and chronic schizophrenia. *Arch. Gen. Psychiatry* **56**:133–140.

Verwer, R.W., Sluiter, A.A., Balesar, R.A., Baayen, J.C., Noske, D.P., Dirven, C.M., Wouda, J., van Dam, A.M., Lucassen, P.J., and Swaab, D.F. 2007. Mature astrocytes in the adult human neocortex express the early neuronal marker doublecortin. *Brain* **130**:3321–3335.

Vuilleumier, P., Armony, J.L., Driver, J., and Dolan, R.J. 2001. Effects of attention and emotion on face processing in the human brain: an event related fMRI study. *Neuron* **30**:829–841.

Vuilleumier, P., Armony, J.L., Clarke, R., Husain, M., Driver, J., and Dolan, R.J. 2002. Neural response to emotional faces with and without awareness: event-related fMRI in a parietal patient with visual extinction and spatial neglect. *Neuropsychologia* **40**:2156–2166.

Wang, H.D., Dunnavant, F.D., Jarman, T., and Deutch, A.Y. 2004. Effects of antipsychotic drugs on neurogenesis in the forebrain of the adult rat. *Neuropsychopharmacology* **29**:1230–1238.

Whalen, P.J., Rauch, S.L., Etcoff, N.L., McInerney, S.C., Lee, M.B., and Jenike, M.A. 1998. Masked presentations of emotional facial expressions modulate amygdala activity without explicit knowledge. *J. Neurosci.* **18**:411–418.

Wiegert, O., Joëls, M., and Krugers, H. 2006. Timing is essential for rapid effects of corticosterone on synaptic potentiation in the mouse hippocampus. *Learn. Mem.* **13**:110–113.

Williams, C.L., and Clayton, E.C. 2001. The contribution of brainstem structures in modulating memory storage processes. In: P.E.Gold, and W.T.Greenough (eds.) *Memory Consolidation: Essays in Honor of James L. McGaugh*. Washington, D.C.: American Psychological Association Press.

Wilson, M.A., and McNaughton, B.L. 1993. Dynamics of the hippocampal ensemble code for space. *Science* **261**:1055–1058.

Yehuda, R. 2006. Advances in understanding neuroendocrine alterations in PTSD and their therapeutic implications. *Ann. N. Y. Acad. Sci.* **1071**:137–166.

Young, L.T., Warsh, J.J., Kish, S.J., Shannak, K., and Hornykeiwicz, O. 1994. Reduced brain 5-HT and elevated NE turnover and metabolites in bipolar affective disorder. *Biol. Psychiatry* **35**:121–127.

Yuii, K., Suzuki, M., and Kurachi, M. 2009. Stress sensitization in schizophrenia. *Ann. N. Y. Acad. Sci.* **1113**:276–290.

Zetzsche, T., Frodl, T., Preuss, U.W., Schmitt, G., Seifert, D., Leinsinger, G., Born, C., Reiser, M., Möller, H-J., and Eva M. Meisenzahl, E.M. 2006. Amygdala volume and depressive symptoms in patients with borderline personality disorder. *Biol. Psychiatry* **60**:302–310.

Chapter 12

Limbic system: Cingulate cortex

Introduction

Several brain regions have emerged relatively recently as major contributors to the human psychological system. A good example is the cingulate cortex. As early as the 1930s, it was observed that cats become mute and akinetic following lesions of the cingulate cortex. However, it was not until the 1950s that the cingulate gyrus was examined more carefully. This gyrus (Figure 12.1) together with the parahippocampal gyrus, which lies below it, form a large arcuate convolution that surrounds the upper brainstem and constitutes what Broca referred to as the *grande lobe limbique* (Figure 13.1).

Anatomy and behavioral considerations

The cingulate cortex lies deep within the longitudinal cerebral fissure and spans the corpus callosum like a great arc (Figure 12.1). It is separated from the frontal and parietal cortex above by the cingulate sulcus, within which much of the cingulate cortex lies. Four major subdivisions of the cingulate cortex and a connecting bundle can be identified.

Early studies divided the cingulate gyrus into just an anterior portion and a posterior portion. Although some current studies report findings using this two-part model, most investigators have now adopted a four-part model. The "old" anterior cingulate gyrus is now divided into the anterior cingulate gyrus and the midcingulate gyrus. The "new" anterior cingulate gyrus is further subdivided into the pregenual anterior cingulate gyrus and subgenual cingulate gyrus. The "old" posterior cingulate gyrus is now divided into the posterior cingulate gyrus and retrosplenial cingulate cortex.

Anterior cingulate cortex

The anterior cingulate cortex (ACC) consists of the cortex of the cingulate gyrus that lies anterior and inferior to the anterior end of the corpus callosum (Figure 12.1). The ACC receives input from the intralaminar and midline thalamic nuclei and has reciprocal connections with the medial and lateral prefrontal cortex. It is remarkable in comparison with the remainder of the cingulate gyrus for massive input from the amygdala. It is affected in major depression (see below).

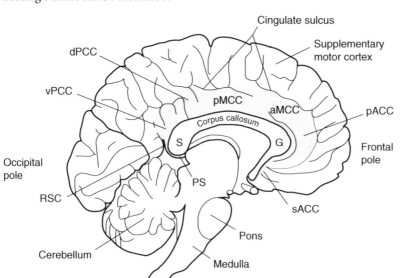

Figure 12.1. The cingulate cortex is shaded. The cingulate cortex consists of the pregenual anterior cingulate cortex (pACC), the subgenual anterior cingulate cortex (sACC), the midcingulate cortex, anterior and posterior (aMCC and pMCC), the posterior cingulate cortex, dorsal and ventral (dPCC and vPCC), the retrosplenial cortex (RSC), and parasplenial area (PS). G, genu of corpus callosum; S, splenium of corpus callosum. See Figure 1.1 for general orientation.

The ACC lies in a position to filter and control the relationship between the emotional limbic system and autonomic portions of the nervous system. Skeletomotor responses may be through connections with the midcingulate cortex. Its close ties with the basal ganglia and orbitofrontal cortex recognize it as part of a cortico-basal ganglia-thalamus-cortical loop (Mega and Cummings, 2001; Middleton and Strick, 2001). It is important in error detection and the appreciation and expression of emotions. It is a key component of the anterior (rostral) limbic system. Studies indicate the ACC receives information about an emotion-evoking stimulus, selects an appropriate response, monitors the action, and adapts behavior if there is a violation of expectancy (Haznedar et al., 2004). The rostral ACC seems to be active after an error commission indicating an error response function. The dorsal ACC is active after both an error commission and feedback suggesting a more evaluative function (Bush et al., 2002; Polli et al., 2005; Taylor et al., 2006). The evaluation is emotional in nature and reflects the degree of distress associated with a certain error (Drevets et al., 1997). Activity in the ACC occurs well in advance of the execution of the behavior, suggesting that it functions in an executive and planning capacity. It plays a central role in shifting attention during working memory. Connections between the ACC and left prefrontal cortex [Brodmann's area (BA) 46, BA 44, and BA 9] are particularly important (Kondo et al., 2004). The ACC recruits conflict control mechanisms that appear to take place in the dorsolateral prefrontal cortex (Figure 12.2) (Kerns et al., 2004).

Thalamic projections carrying signals from the hippocampus and mammillary body of the hypothalamus (Figures 12.3, 12.5 and 12.6) project to portions of both the anterior and posterior cingulate cortex. The ACC is believed to be involved in early acquisition of memory in novel situations (Raichle et al., 1994). The pregenal cortex appears to be particularly important in memory. Grasby et al., (1993) hypothesized that the ACC responds to the attentional demands of response selection to memory tasks and may serve both short-term and long-term memory function. The ACC plays an active role during tasks that require the memorization of words, of faces, or of a series of connected events found in a story.

An increase in regional cerebral blood flow was seen in the ACC of subjects who performed an attention-demanding auditory addition test. It appeared that the increase occurred when internal information stores

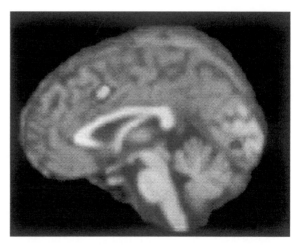

Figure 12.2. Functional magnetic resonance study demonstrates activation of the anterior cingulate gyrus region in the monitoring of conflict (incongruent trials). (Reproduced with permission from Kerns *et al.*, 2004.) See also color plate.

were being addressed. ACC blood flow decreased when the task required that internally stored information be suppressed (Deary et al., 1994).

Pregenual anterior cingulate cortex

The ACC is subdivided into a pregenual region (pACC) and a subgenual region (sACC). The pregenual region (pACC) lies anterior to the corpus callosum and includes anterior portions of BA 24, BA 33, and portions of BA 32. The pACC is involved with sensations of emotion and is responsible for the storage of emotional memories. It is activated by internally generated emotions and is important in the retrieval of fear memory (Frankland et al., 2004). For example when stimulated in this area, a patient reported, "I was afraid and my heart started to beat." Bancaud and Talairach (1992) also reported sensations of euphoria, pleasure, and agitation during stimulation of the pACC. It is activated during reward-based decision making (Bush et al., 2002). It is sensitive to pleasant touch in contrast to the midcingulate cortex, which is sensitive to painful touch (Rolls et al., 2003). Bartels and Zeki (2000) found that it was activated by images of individual with whom their subjects were currently romantically involved. Vogt et al. (2003) found that that the pACC was activated when subjects reported experiencing happy emotions whereas the subgenual ACC (sACC) was activated when experiencing sad emotions. However, in another study, the pACC was also activated when subjects were exposed to pain stimuli and the authors suggested it is associated with the "suffering" component of pain

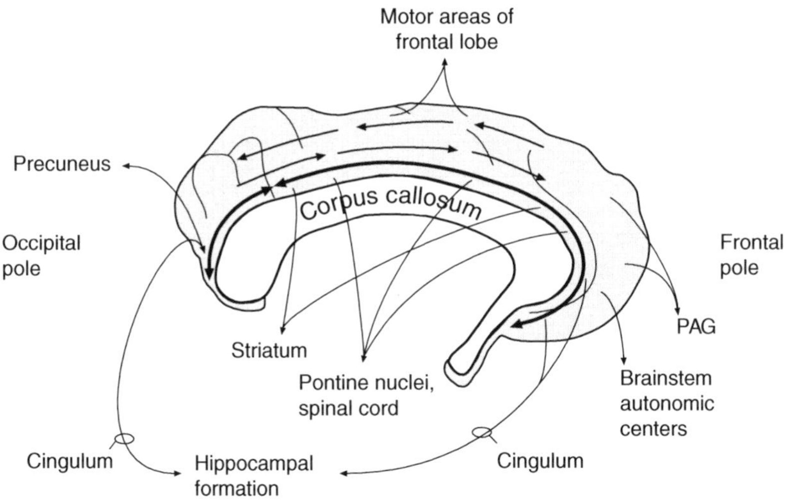

Figure 12.3. Some of the major efferent projections of the cingulate cortex. Fibers to the motor areas of the frontal lobe arise from the skeletomotor control region of the midcingulate cortex. The bold arrows within the cingulate cortex represent connections of the default brain network that includes the subgenual anterior cingulate cortex and retrosplenial cortex. PAG, periaqueductal gray.

(Ploner *et al.*, 2002). pACC has also been implicated in motivational aspects of pain (Sewards and Sewards, 2003) as well as empathy for pain experienced by others (Hein and Singer, 2008).

Subgenual anterior cingulate cortex

The subgenual region of the anterior cingulate cortex (sACC) lies inferior to the genu (knee) of the corpus callosum and consists primarily of BA 25 along with small portions of posterior, inferior BA 12, BA 32, and BA 33. The sACC is recognized as an autonomic control center. It responds to emotions and determines the autonomic expressions of emotion. The sACC has projections to the central nucleus of the amygdala, parabrachial nucleus, and periaqueducal gray, all of which relay signals for the expression of autonomic tone. Direct projections to the solitary nucleus, dorsal vagal nucleus and spinal cord lateral horn provide a route for direct control of expression of emotions in terms of the sympathetic and parasympathetic divisions. Vogt (2005) argues that the sACC is true limbic cortex and not infralimbic as it is sometimes described.

Midcingulate cortex

The midcingulate cortex (MCC) occupies posterior portions of BA 24, BA 32, and BA 33. It consists of the middle third of the cingulate gyrus. Like the pACC it receives input from the amygdala and registers emotional sensations, but instead of contacting autonomic centers it sends projections to motor areas. Reciprocal connections link the MCC with the motor cortex. Projections from the MCC also include fibers to the red

nucleus, putamen, pontine gray, and spinal cord: all motor control centers.

The anterior MCC (aMCC) is involved in error detection (conflict monitoring). It detects conflicts in information processing and signals the occurrence to other areas where motor responses may be made. Botvinick *et al.* (1999) reported that activity increased with high levels of conflict. It is hypothesized that the aMCC determines the most cost-effective option and selects the one option judged to be the most preferred (Assadi *et al.*, 2009).

The posterior MCC (pMCC) contains two motor areas. The pMCC is important in planning skeletomotor reactions to emotional sensations (Durn and Strick, 1991; Morecraft and Van Hoesen, 1992). For example it is activated during aversive movements in anticipation to a learned painful stimulus (Yágüez *et al.*, 2005). However it may initiate cognitive activity that does not necessarily require movement (Bush *et al.*, 2002). Cognitive activity includes anticipation of movement, motor imagery, mismatch detection, and establishing changes in new motor programs. Motor behavior associated with the MCC includes attention to specific external stimuli; including orienting movements of the eyes and head toward a significant stimulus as well as inhibition of attention to less relevant internal and external stimuli. The MCC is involved in obsessive-compulsive disorder (see below).

Earlier studies that describe behaviors seen during stimulation of the ACC may reflect stimulation of the posterior ACC that is now considered MCC. Studies have described simple and complex movements similar to those seen after stimulation of the premotor areas found on the lateral aspect of the frontal lobe (Chapter 6; Luppino *et al.*, 1991). Behavioral changes have also been seen, including primitive gestures such as kneading or pressing the hands together, lip-smacking, and picking at bedclothes. Devinsky *et al.* (1995) found that these movements were modified with sensory stimulation and could be resisted by voluntary efforts of the patients. Connections between the MCC and supplementary cortex may underlie these behaviors. Lesions that interrupt these connections may account for the motor neglect that is sometimes seen after damage to this region.

The MCC makes decisions on the basis of the reward value of the anticipated outcome of a particular motor response. The pMCC is part of the medial pain system that is involved in the affective and/or cognitive dimensions of pain processing. In addition, through its motor centers, the pMCC is responsible for fast orientation and motor withdrawal responses to pain inputs (Frot *et al.*, 2009). The emotional aspect of pain as well as empathy for others who are suffering pain activates the MCC (Vogt, 2005; Hein and Singer, 2008).

Posterior cingulate cortex

The posterior cingulate cortex (PCC) includes BA 23 and BA 31 and is sometimes divided into a dorsal (dPCC) and ventral (vPCC) component. The PCC and adjacent retrosplenial cortex make up the "posterior cingulate area" (Takahashi, 2004). The PCC receives input from the anterior thalamic nucleus and frontal, occipital and posterior parietal cortices. It receives heavy input from the hippocampal formation (Kobayashi and Amaral, 2003). In contrast to the ACC, it receives little if any input from the amygdala. The PCC is strongly linked to saccade circuitry and is involved in visuospatial orientation in response to somatosensory input. In animal studies, PCC neurons were activated when monkeys had to choose by generating saccades between two rewards of similar value but reward certainty differed. Neuron responsiveness

correlated with reward size (McCoy *et al.*, 2003; McCoy and Platt, 2005).

Both the PCC and retrosplenial cortex have connections with the superior temporal sulcus and superior temporal gyrus. These connections may play a role in the localization of sounds (Seltzer and Pandya, 2009).

The PCC is important in successful retrieval of autobiographical memories. Maddock *et al.* (2001) demonstrated that the PCC showed strong activation during successful retrieval of memories elicited by name-cued recall of family members and friends (Figure 12.4). The authors speculated that dysfunction of this area may be involved early in Alzheimer disease related to its strong ties to the hippocampal formation. Simultaneous reduction in blood flow in early Alzheimer disease in both the entorhinal area and PCC provides some evidence in support of the above claim (Hirao *et al.*, 2006).

Cognitive impairment correlates with alterations in activity in the posterior cingulate cortex (Martinez-Bisbal *et al.*, 2004). Elfgren *et al.* (2003) reported that subjects with isolated memory impairment coupled with slight verbal and/or visuospatial impairments showed reduced cerebral blood flow in the posterior cingulate cortex. This group was at high risk for Alzheimer disease. Individuals with mild cognitive impairment are at high risk of developing Alzheimer disease. In another study, subjects who developed Alzheimer disease demonstrated significantly decreased regional cerebral blood flow in the left posterior cingulate cortex two years previously (Huang *et al.*, 2002).

Mouras *et al.* (2003) reported decreased activity in the right PCC when men reported sexual desire in response to viewing sexually stimulating photographs. Parietal areas (attention) and frontal areas (motor preparation and imagery) were also activated. In another study, the PCC also showed deactivation in subjects in response to photographs of individuals with whom they were in love (Bartels and Zeki, 2000).

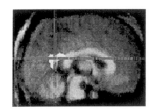 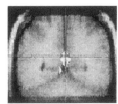 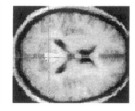

Figure 12.4. Functional magnetic resonance study demonstrates activation of the posterior cingulate gyrus region (including retrosplenial cortex) in assessing the familiarity of a person (faces or voices). (Reproduced with permission from Shah *et al.*, 2001.) See also color plate.

Retrosplenial cortex (RSC)

The retrosplenial cortex (RSC) includes BA 29 and BA 30, which extend around the splenium of the corpus callosum. Most of the RSC is found on the inferior aspect of the cingulate gyrus. The PCC/RSC and BA 23 are adjacent and are reciprocally connected. There are also strong connections between pACC and BA 23, providing an intimate link between the RSC and sACC (Figure 12.3). The PCC and RSC are part of the default brain network (Chapters 4 and 6) (Buckner *et al.*, 2008; Hayden *et al.*, 2009). They are active during the resting, mind-wandering state. Glucose levels in the PPC/RSC area were measured to be about 20% above other brain regions when in the resting state. This network is active during mind-wandering. Memories associated with emotional states stored in the pACC may be released to consciousness by activity in the PCC or RSC. For example, Maddock *et al.* (2003) reported that the PCC/RSC was significantly activated bilaterally when hearing both unpleasant and pleasant words although the strongest activation was observed in the left sACC.

A lesion of the left RSC can produce an amnestic syndrome characterized by anterograde loss of verbal and nonverbal memories accompanied by a mild retrograde amnesia. A lesion of the right RSC results in amnesia for topographical features. Familiar buildings and landscapes are recognized but the positional relationship of two familiar locations is lost. The RSC may play a role in encoding novel locations and their relationships (Takahashi, 2004).

Cingulum

The cingulum is a large bundle of fibers that parallels the arc of the cingulate gyrus (Figures 12.3 and 12.5). The cingulum appears in some publications as the "sagittal bundle of the gyrus fornicatus." It is an association bundle and contains short fibers that interconnect different areas of the cingulate cortex. Long fibers located within the cingulum project to the occipital cortex and to the hippocampus (Figures 12.3 and 12.5). The cingulum also contains fibers that connect the cingulate cortex reciprocally with the prefrontal, temporal, and parietal areas (Figure 12.6).

Nociception (pain)

The MCC is a major component of the medial pain system. The area of the MCC involved in pain lies behind and below the skeletomotor control region (Figure 12.1; NCC, Figure 12.7). Neurons in this region respond to noxious stimuli. The region seems to have no localizing

value since noxious stimuli applied anywhere on the body result in activation of these neurons. This generalized activation coupled with the fact that the MCC receives projections from medially located diffuse thalamic nuclei as opposed to laterally located relay nuclei (Chapter 9, Table 9.1), makes the MCC part of the medial pain system (Vogt *et al.*, 1993). The ACC/MCC appears to be involved in specifying the affective content of the noxious stimulus, selecting a motor response to the stimulus, and with learning associated with the prediction and avoidance of noxious stimuli. It is speculated that the MCC organizes appropriate skeletomotor responses to pain. One response to pain is the inhibition of activity in the prefrontal cortex during noxious stimulation (Devinsky *et al.*, 1995). The MCC projects to the midbrain periaqueductal gray (PAG in Figure 12.3), an area known to regulate pain perception (Chapter 10). These findings are consistent with the data showing that cingulotomy may be effective in otherwise refractory pain.

The MCC is activated by application of noxious stimuli (Casey *et al.*, 1994). Response to noxious heat stimulus has been reported to increase activity in the contralateral MCC in humans (Talbot *et al.*, 1991). Derbyshire *et al.* (1994) found that blood flow increased in the MCC during application of noxious stimuli, while at the same time prefrontal cortex blood flow decreased. A lesion surgically introduced in the anterior cingulum bilaterally is referred to as cingulotomy. Foltz and White (1962) found that patients with chronic pain who had been treated with cingulotomy continued to feel the pain but that the pain did not bother the patient and did not trigger an adverse emotional reaction. In other studies, psychiatric patients who received surgical lesions of the cingulate cortex or cingulum, or both, reported relief from chronic, intractable pain (Ballantine *et al.*, 1967). Many other studies have found mixed results (Cetas *et al.*, 2008).

Social interactions

Social interactions require complex processing of information from a number of sources, including the memory of past events. The ACC appears to play a pivotal role in the generation of socially appropriate behavior. It lies in a position to evaluate the consequences of future behavior by the prefrontal cortex with motor and autonomic responses to ongoing social behavior.

Lesions of the ACC in animals commonly result in reduced aggressivity, diminished shyness, emotional blunting, impaired maternal–infant interactions, and

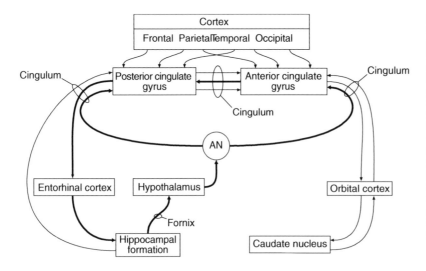

Figure 12.5. An overview of the connections associated with the cingulate gyrus. Papez's circuit is shown with bold lines (compare with Figure 13.8). The cingulum is an association bundle that interconnects one part of the cingulate gyrus with the other as well as with other cortical areas. Many fibers course ventrocaudally in the cingulum to terminate in the entorhinal cortex (right). Others course rostroventrally to terminate in the orbital cortex, caudate nucleus, and other structures (left). The majority of the fibers from the hippocampus to the hypothalamus terminate in the mammillary nucleus. Many cortical connections are reciprocal (see text). AN, anterior nucleus of the thalamus, a major component of the "limbic thalamus."

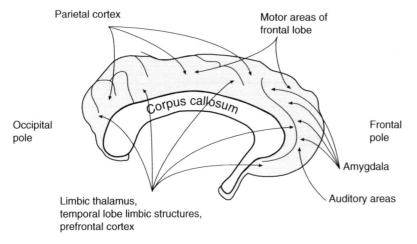

Figure 12.6. Some of the major projections to the cingulate cortex. The area served by the amygdala is restricted to the "affect" portion of the cingulate cortex and does not overlap the area served by the parietal cortex.

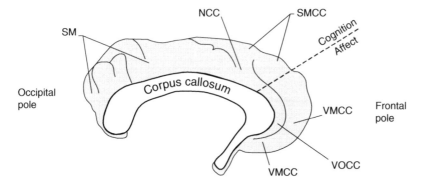

Figure 12.7. The cingulate cortex can be divided functionally into regions that subserve vocalization (VOCC), visceromotor functions (VMCC), skeletomotor functions (SMCC), and nociception (NCC) as well as a posterior region that appears to function in spatial orientation and spatial memory (SM). The anterior cingulate cortex can be divided into regions that serve affect and cognition. The border between these two regions is indicated by the dashed line (after Devinsky et al., 1995).

inappropriate intraspecies social behavior. The fact that aggressive behavior is reduced following bilateral cingulotomy in animals led to the use of this procedure in humans in an attempt to reduce aggression, agitation, psychosis, and compulsive behavior (Devinsky et al., 1995).

Patients with cingulate lesions or with cingulate epilepsy may express impulsivity, apathy, aggressive behavior, psychosis, and sexually deviant behavior as well as obsessions and compulsions. Hypometabolism seen in the ACC of patients with borderline personality disorder is speculated to be related to impulsiveness, a main characteristic of this disorder (De La Fuente *et al.*, 1997). Surgical cingulotomy, which removes cortex in the region of BA 24 and BA 32 and the cingulum, may produce impaired social behavior. In some cases the behavior of patients with cingulate lesions has resulted in institutionalization (Bancaud and Talairach, 1992). The skin conductance of one patient following bilateral cingulate and orbitofrontal cortex surgery showed no response to emotional stimuli (Damasio *et al.*, 1990).

Clinical vignette

The following three clinical vignettes demonstrate the intertwined relationship between neurological and psychiatric aspects of abnormal brain processing, which involves brain regions that are responsible for emotional or cognitive regulation.

Case 1

An 11-year-old girl had been having seizures since 2.5 years. At age 3 she developed obsessive features and by age 8 she was preoccupied with Satan, feared punishment for real and imagined behaviors, and spent long periods of time washing her hands, brushing her teeth, and showering. Depth electroencephalographic (EEG) recording documented seizure onset from the right anterior cingulate region. Surgical destruction of 4 cm of the affected cortex eliminated her seizures and markedly reduced her obsessive-compulsive behaviors during the first 15 postoperative months (Levin and Duchowny, 1991).

Case 2

A 43-year-old man had a long history of medically intractable complex partial seizures. The seizures were stereotyped and characterized by laughter, repetition of the phrase "Oh my God," and bilateral arm extensions followed by repeated touching of the forehead and mouth. The seizures were short (<10 seconds) and were without auras or postictal confusion. The patient was amnestic for the seizure. Eventually he became reclusive and lost his job. Depth EEG recording showed that the seizures originated from the right anterior cingulate region. After resection of this region, the seizures improved and the patient was able to live independently and entered into a romantic relationship (Devinsky *et al.*, 1995).

Case 3

A 42-year-old man similarly had a long history of intractable complex partial seizures. In addition he

Clinical vignette (cont.)

had a history of sociopathic behavior (15 years) that began about 1 year after a mild head injury. During a seizure the patient would exhibit grotesque facial contortions, tongue thrusting, a strangulated yell, and bilateral arm and leg extensions with side-to-side thrashing. This patient similarly had no pre- or postictal problems. Consciousness was preserved unless the seizure generalized. Interictally, the patient was irritable and demonstrated poor impulse control with sexual preoccupation and deviance. Depth EEG recording showed that the seizures stemmed from the right cingulate cortical region. After surgery his family reported that his irritability was diminished and that he exhibited better social conduct. At last follow-up he was employed and married (Devinsky *et al.*, 1995).

Connections of the cingulate cortex

The limbic thalamus provides input to all regions of the cingulate cortex (Figure 12.3; Bentivoglio *et al.*, 1993). The major component of the limbic thalamus is the anterior thalamic nucleus (Chapter 9). The anterior nucleus is actually a nuclear complex that consists of the anterior ventral, anterior medial, and anterior dorsal nuclei. Projections from anterior ventral and anterior dorsal nuclei favor the PCC, whereas the anterior medial nucleus projects to the ACC. The anterior nuclear complex is part of the circuit of Papez and lies between the mammillary body and the cingulate cortex (Figures 12.5 and 13.8; Chapter 13). Although the entire cingulate cortex also receives afferents from the lateral dorsal thalamic nucleus, the lateral dorsal nucleus preferentially targets the PCC. The lateral dorsal nucleus is also part of the limbic thalamus and is a relay nucleus that transfers sensory information and especially visual information from the lateral geniculate body of the thalamus and from the pretectum of the midbrain. The pretectum of the midbrain is an area where vision, touch, and hearing converge. The pretectum–lateral dorsal nucleus connection is therefore a route by which visual, touch (somesthesis), and auditory signals can reach the cingulate cortex.

The ventral anterior nucleus and ventromedial nucleus are part of the motor thalamic region. Projections from both of these thalamic motor nuclei favor the MCC, which contains the skeletomotor region of the cingulate cortex. Midline and intralaminar thalamic nuclei, which are considered "diffuse" nuclei, project to all regions of the cingulate cortex with a preference for the ACC. The midline and intralaminar nuclei are significant structures in the medial pain system and play a role in the affective responses to painful stimuli (Vogt *et al.*, 1993).

The PCC receives a large number of fibers from the parietal lobe, including the primary somesthetic area. It has been suggested that the PCC coordinates activities between the limbic system and the somesthetic cortex (Van Hoesen *et al.*, 1993). Targets of fibers from the PCC are similar to those of the ACC with several exceptions. The PCC has reciprocal connections with the motor cortex, but they are much less extensive than those of the ACC. Both regions of the cingulate project to the neostriatum (caudate nucleus and putamen), but PCC projections favor the caudate nucleus. The caudate is recognized to function in emotionally related behaviors (Chapter 7). Considering the connections with the hippocampus and mammillary bodies, it is not surprising that animal studies have shown that both the PCC and ACC are involved in memory. The inferior portion of the PCC (BA 29) in particular has been implicated in spatial memory (Sutherland and Hoesing, 1993).

Efferent fibers from the cingulate gyrus contribute heavily to the cingulum (Figures 12.3 and 12.5). Many cingulum fibers curve ventrally in a caudal direction to terminate in the entorhinal cortex (Figure 11.2). The cingulum is often depicted in diagrams of Papez's circuit, which emphasize the link between the cingulate gyrus and the hippocampus (Figures 12.5 and 13.8). However, an equally large number of fibers course rostrally in the cingulum to make connections with other brain structures. These fibers also curve ventrally. Many fan out to terminate in the orbital cortex of the frontal lobe. Others continue to arch ventrocaudally to terminate in the striatum, the anterior and mediodorsal nuclei of the thalamus, and the hypothalamus (Chapter 8). This account of the elaborate connections between the cingulate cortex and all areas of the limbic system highlights the important and central role that the cingulate cortex plays in mediating our emotion and cognitive function on one hand and motor response on the other.

Behavioral disorders and neurosurgery

There is no clear-cut syndrome associated with cingulate lesions. Electrical stimulation of human cingulate cortex has been reported to produce a spectrum of behaviors, including speech arrest and involuntary vocalization, as well as autonomic, affective, and psychosensory phenomena (Devinsky and Luciano, 1993).

During the last two decades, highly refined neurosurgical procedures have emerged that can alleviate some of the most recalcitrant psychiatric symptoms [Rapoport and Inoff-Germain (1997)]. Current procedures are usually labeled "functional neurosurgery" and depend on the ability to perform microsurgical procedures guided by stereotactic knowledge. The procedures are very different from the old "lobotomy" in that the surgical lesions made are extremely small and are placed in very specific structures bilaterally. Surgery can be performed under local anesthesia, although general anesthesia is used most often. Such procedures have been developed for the treatment of depression, anxiety, and chronic pain. Four procedures are in current use.

Cingulotomy is the most commonly reported psychosurgical procedure used in the United States and Canada. It has proved effective in the relief of pain, anxiety, obsessive-compulsive disorder, and depression with minimal psychiatric, neurological, or general medical morbidity (Ballantine *et al.*, 1987; Jenike *et al.*, 1991; Cosgrove and Rauch, 1995; Marino and Cosgrove, 1997). A second operation is often necessary six months to a year after the initial procedure. About 75% of depression patients showed partial or substantial improvement (Shields *et al.*, 2008). Bilateral lesions are created that measure approximately 8–10 mm in lateral diameter and extend about 2 cm dorsally from the corpus callosum. The lesion destroys the anterior cingulate gyrus and interrupts the cingulum (Ovsiew and Frim, 1997).

Subcaudate tractotomy, developed in the United Kingdom, is used to treat unresponsive affective disorder (Poynton *et al.*, 1995). Bilateral lesions are placed in the white matter beneath and in front of the head of the caudate nucleus using either small radioactive rods or thermocoagulation. During the weeks after the surgery, patients show a significant but transient performance deficit on recognition memory tests (Kartsounis *et al.*, 1991).

Capsulotomy was developed in Sweden and is sometimes performed in the United States. It is used to treat refractory anxiety disorders including obsessive-compulsive disorder. The lesion produced in the anterior third of the internal capsule is approximately 4 mm wide and 16 mm long (Ovsiew and Frim, 1997).

Limbic leukotomy was developed in the United Kingdom (Figure 12.8). It consists of a subcaudate tractotomy bilaterally accompanied by cingulotomy (Mindus and Jenike, 1992).

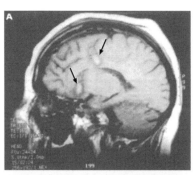

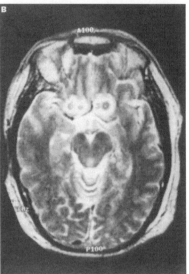

Figure 12.8. Sagittal (A) and low axial (B) magnetic resonance imaging (MRI) of acute limbic leukotomy lesions. The dorsal lesion (A, top arrow) involves the anterior cingulate gyrus in the same location as a cingulotomy. The ventral lesion (A, bottom arrow) is located similarly to those produced in subcaudate tractotomy. (Modified from Ovsiew, F., and Frim, D.M. 1997. Neurosurgery for psychiatric disorders. J. Neurol. Neurosurg. Psychiatry 63:701–705.)

Schizophrenia

A number of studies have revealed abnormalities in the ACC as well as other areas, including the hippocampus and dorsolateral prefrontal cortex in patients with schizophrenia. Reduced total volume (gray and white matter) (Haznedar et al., 2004; Choi et al., 2005) as well as reduced gray matter volume of the ACC (Crespo-Facorro et al., 2000; Job et al., 2003a; Yamasue et al., 2004) have been reported for patients with schizophrenia. Job et al. (2003b) found differences between control and subjects at high risk for schizophrenia as well as first episode patients. The number of interneurons have been reported to be reduced but the number of axon terminals increased

(Benes et al., 1991; Benes, 1996, 1998). The authors speculated that the lost interneurons are GABAergic inhibitory neurons and the axon terminals are from glutamatergic neurons located in the prefrontal cortex (Benes et al., 1991; Benes, 1996, 1998). The concentration of serotonin [5-hydroxytryptamine $(HT)_{1A}$] receptors was increased in BA 24 in schizophrenia patients, whereas the concentration of serotonin (5-$HT_{2A,C}$) receptors was decreased in the same area. These findings correlate with hypofrontality (Gurevich and Joyce, 1997).

The loss in cingulate cortex in schizophrenia is first seen during adolescence compared with frontal cortex loss seen prior to adolescence (Vidal et al., 2006). The white matter tracts in the ACC were also disrupted in early-onset schizophrenia (Kumra et al., 2005; White et al., 2008). Increased activity in the pACC (BA 32) was coincident with decreased activity in the dorsolateral prefrontal cortex leading the authors to suggest a kind of disconnection or connection-disruption syndrome (Glahn et al., 2005).

Schizophrenia patients also demonstrated reduced glucose metabolism in the ACC that correlates with attentional dysfunction seen in these patients (Tamminga et al., 1992; Carter et al., 1997). Both the prefrontal cortex and the ACC are implicated in the psychomotor poverty syndrome of schizophrenia (Liddle et al., 1992). Poverty of movement and catatonia are consistent with a decrease in the motivational aspect of ACC function.

The left ACC along with other structures was activated when schizophrenia patients experienced auditory hallucinations. The PCC was prominently activated when a schizophrenia patient experienced visual hallucinations (Silbersweig et al., 1995).

Schizophrenia patients demonstrate oculomotor abnormalities and use catch-up saccades during pursuit eye movements. The motor region of the MCC projects to the frontal eye fields. The frontal eye field of the prefrontal cortex is well known for its involvement in saccadic (fast) eye movements, but it is also involved in smooth pursuit tracking (MacAvoy et al., 1991).

Depression and bipolar disorder

Reductions in gray matter volume have been reported for the cingulate in patients with major depression (Ballmaier et al., 2004; Pezawas et al., 2005). The sACC is recognized as part of a neural network involved in depression (Seminowicz et al., 2004; Ressler and Mayberg, 2007). Mayberg et al. (1999) found that provoked sadness increased metabolic activity in sACC and insula along with decreases in activity in the pMCC and PCC. Successful drug treatment of the depressed patients resulted in decreased activity in sACC and insula along with increases pMCC and PCC. Successful treatment with vagus nerve stimulation has also been reported to reverse abnormal metabolic activity (Zobel *et al.*, 2005). Other studies have found direct stimulation of the sACC using deep brain stimulation in treatment-resistant depressed patients resulted in improvements in symptoms of depression along with decreased activity in the sACC (Hauptman *et al.*, 2008; Lozano *et al.*, 2008). The changes seen in cingulate gyrus metabolism in depression were linked to changes seen in frontal lobe cortex.

Reductions in gray matter volume are reported for the sACC (Wilke *et al.*, 2004; Houenou *et al.*, 2007) and PCC in bipolar disorder (Lochhead *et al.*, 2004; Farrow, *et al.*, 2005; Kaur *et al.*, 2005) but without neuron loss (Öngür *et al.*, 1998). Glial cell loss was reported (Todtenkopf *et al.*, 2005). There is some evidence that the reduction in gray matter volume increases with the duration of the illness (Farrow *et al.*, 2005; Kaur *et al.*, 2005; Lyoo *et al.*, 2006). Dunn *et al.* (2002) reported that metabolism in the sACC increased during the depressive phase. A decreased response in the ventral pACC to faces (emotional processing) has been reported for euthymic bipolar patients compared with control subjects (Shah *et al.*, 2009). In contrast, tasks designed to elicit emotional responses have been shown to result in greater activation in euthymic bipolar patients in the ACC and PCC (Malhi *et al.*, 2007; Wessa *et al.*, 2007). In other studies, patients with mania had reduced activity in the sACC and increased activity in the PCC in response to images of sad faces. Medicated patients did not exhibit this pattern suggesting that mood stabilizing drugs reverse the abnormal activity (Blumberg *et al.*, 2005; Strakowski *et al.*, 2005).

Obsessive-compulsive disorder

The ACC/MCC and orbitofrontal cortex are intimately connected to the basal ganglia and to each other. The ACC/MCC and orbitofrontal cortex each participate in a loop that runs parallel to each other. The two loops originate in variable areas of the cortex, pass through the head of the caudate nucleus, the anterior nucleus of the thalamus and then to either the ACC/MCC or orbitofrontal cortex (Mega and Cummings, 2001; Middleton and Strick, 2001). There are both direct and indirect pathways through the basal ganglia. The direct pathway is excitatory and the indirect pathway is inhibitory (Chapter 7).

The direct and indirect pathways are in balance in the normal condition. Obsessive thoughts may result from an imbalance between the two pathways with overactivity of the direct pathway (Saxena and Rauch, 2000).

Three areas have been implicated in obsessive-compulsive disorder (OCD): orbitofrontal cortex, ACC/MCC, and the head of the caudate nucleus (Figure 12.9). These areas are hyperactive at rest in OCD, become even more active with symptom provocation, and show less activity at rest following successful treatment with either medication or cognitive-behavioral therapy (Saxena and Rauch, 2000; Whiteside *et al.*, 2004; Maia *et al.*, 2008). It is unknown whether these areas are hyperactive as a consequence of some abnormality elsewhere or reflect attempted inhibition of obsessive thoughts (Shafran and Speckens, 2005; Roth *et al.*, 2007).

ACC/MCC gray matter volume has been found to be greater in children with OCD than in controls (Rosenberg and Keshavan, 1998; Szeszko *et al.*, 2004). In contrast, decreased ACC/MCC gray matter is a consistent finding in adults with OCD (Pujol *et al.*, 2004: Valente *et al.*, 2005; Yoo *et al.*, 2008).

The two main symptoms of OCD are obsessive-compulsive behaviors and anxiety. Anxiety is believed to be mediated through the hippocampus, amygdala, septal nuclei, mammillary bodies (hypothalamus), and anterior thalamic nuclei. The cingulum is a major common pathway. Cingulotomy as well as lesions of the MCC have been used with some success in treatment of resistant OCD. The cingulum contains fibers that project from the ACC/MCC to the orbitofrontal cortex and to the caudate nucleus (Figure 12.5). Psychosurgical lesions limited to the ACC/MCC have resulted in reduced anxiety (Chiocca and Martuza, 1990). Obsessive-compulsive thoughts and sensations are more likely to be mediated through the interaction between the orbitofrontal cortex and the caudate nucleus (Baxter, 1992). It is theorized that a loop connecting the frontal region with the caudate nucleus and passing through the thalamus and back to the frontal area subserves obsessive-compulsive symptoms (Figure 7.9). A lesion that interrupts the caudate-frontal axons (subcaudate tractotomy) is believed to directly decrease obsessive-compulsive symptoms (Martuza *et al.*, 1990).

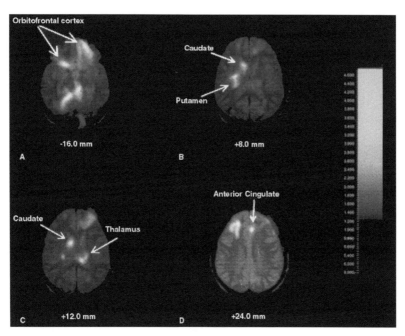

Figure 12.9. Positron emission tomographic omnibus subtraction images of provoked minus resting conditions for all subjects (N = 8; 13 scans per condition) displayed with a "hot iron" scale in units of z score, superimposed over a normal magnetic resonance image transformed to Talairach space, for the purpose of anatomical reference. Patients with obsessive-compulsive disorder were provoked with stimuli tailored to each patient's symptoms. All images are transverse sections parallel to the anterior commissure–posterior commissure plane, shown in conventional neuroimaging orientation (top = anterior, bottom = posterior, right = left, and left = right). Areas of significant activation include the orbitofrontal cortex, caudate nucleus and cingulate cortex. (Reproduced by permission from Rauch, S.L., Jenike, M.A., Alpert, N.M., Baer, L., Breiter, H.C.R., Savage, C.R., and Fischman, A.J. 1994. Regional cerebral blood flow measured during symptom provocation in obsessive-compulsive disorder using oxygen 15–labeled carbon dioxide and positron emission tomography. Arch. Gen. Psychiatry 51:62–70.)

Posttraumatic stress disorder

Posttraumatic stress disorder (PTSD) is character-ized by a state of heightened responsiveness to threat-ening stimuli and/or a state of insufficient inhibitory control over exaggerated threat-sensitivity (Liberzon and Sripada, 2008). It reflects dysregulation of the hypothalamic-pituitary-adrenal axis, the amygdala, medial prefrontal cortex and ACC. Several studies had reported that provocative stimuli (emotional images and negative words) produced increased activation of the ACC, amygdala, and medial prefrontal cortex in subjects with PTSD (Rauch et al., 1996; Lanius et al., 2002; Protopopescu et al., 2005).

Studies have also shown that activity in the amyg-dala increased with symptom severity in response to combat sounds in subjects with PTSD (Liberzon et al., 1999b; Protopopescu et al., 2005). Lanius et al. (2001, 2003) found that activity in the ACC and medial pre-frontal cortex decreased in response to provocative stimuli. The decrease in ACC appears to be specific to PTSD. Others have reported that an emotional com-ponent of the Stroop test (e.g., say the color of the word rape) resulted in slower response times in abuse-related or combat-related PTSD (McNally et al., 1990; Foa et al., 1991). Bremner et al. (2004) showed that this was associated with decreased function of the pACC (BA 24 and BA 32) in abused women with PTSD but not in abused non-PTSD women.

The hypothalamic-pituitary-adrenal axis is affected in PTSD (Liberzon et al., 1999a; Phan et al., 2004). Ottowitz et al. (2004) showed that adrenocorticotropic hormone (ACTH) and cortisol levels during mood induction in subjects with PTSD correlated positively with activity in the ACC, but correlated negatively in control subjects. Activity in the ACC and medial pre-frontal cortex appears to mediate cortisol and sym-pathetic responses to stress (Liberzon and Sripada, 2008).

Akinetic mutism

Akinetic mutism may be seen after bilateral damage to the ACC or to the adjacent supplementary motor cor-tex, or to both. A patient who showed recovery after one month reported that during the period of mutism "she did not talk because she had nothing to say," her mind was "empty," and she "felt no will to reply" (Damasio and Van Hoesen, 1983).

Tourette syndrome

The pathogenesis and the exact anatomical basis of Tourette syndrome (GTS) remain unknown (Chapter 7). It has been suggested that the ACC has a central role in GTS since stimulation of the ACC in animals produces vocalizations. The targets of projections from the ACC include areas involved in vocalization, and dopaminergic hyperactivity is postulated as a primary cause of GTS. In addition, glucose utilization in the ACC of patients with GTS is decreased, and cingulotomy has successfully reduced obsessive-compulsive behaviors in these patients (Devinsky *et al.*, 1995; Anandan *et al.*, 2004). Abnormalities in gray and white matter volumes have been reported in the prefrontal cortex and midbrain (Peterson *et al.*, 2001; Fredericksen *et al.*, 2002; Kates *et al.*, 2002; Garraux *et al.*, 2006).

Decreased gray matter volume in patients with GTS has been reported in the middle (lateral surface) and medial (medial surface) frontal gyri (BA 4, BA 6, and BA 8) and the MCC, along with the left caudate nucleus and left postcentral gyrus (Müller-Vahl *et al.*, 2009). Symptom severity correlated with frontal volume reductions. White matter reductions were also found located deep to the right inferior frontal gyrus and left superior frontal gyrus. The authors hypothesized that abnormalities in the frontal-basal ganglia loops result dysfunction of caudate nucleus. Caudate dysfunction in turn results in disinhibition of the cingulate gyrus.

Cingulate cortex seizures

The description of seizures originating from the cingulate cortex provides strong evidence for the involvement of this region in affective regulation. A number of common features seem to characterize ictal events of cingulate cortex origin. While consciousness may be preserved in spite of bilateral motor involvement, in the majority of patients the level of attention or of consciousness is affected. Automatisms (complex oral, facial, or appendicular movements) occur early in the seizure. Patients may even assume a fetal position, utter brief phrases such as "Oh my God," or exhibit hitting movements (Devinsky *et al.*, 1995).

Interictally, patients with cingulate seizures have been reported to show marked behavioral aberrations such as episodic outbursts or fixed and intermittent psychotic behavior. Patients with cingulate seizures have more paroxysmal aggressive outbursts, greater sociability, and less logorrhea (increased speech) than patients with temporal lobe epilepsy. These behavioral aberrations frequently improve after removal of the abnormal cingulate cortical tissue by cingulectomy (Ledesma and Paniaqua, 1969; So, 1998).

Select bibliography

Bouckoms, A.J. Limbic surgery for pain. In: P.D. Wall, and R.Melzack (eds.) *Textbook of Pain.* (Edinburgh: Churchill Livingstone, 1994.)

Jenike, M.A. Obsessional disorders. *Psychiatric Clinics of North America* (vol. 15). (Philadelphia: Elsevier, 1992).

Rodgers, J.E. *Psychosurgery: Damaging the Brain to Save the Mind.* (New York: Harper Collins, 1992.)

Vogt, B.A. ed. *Cingulate Neurobiology and Disease.* (New York: Oxford University Press, 2009.)

References

Anandan, S., Wigg, C.L., Thomas, C.R., and Coffey, B. 2004. Psychosurgery for self-injurious behavior in Tourette's disorder. *J. Child Adolesc. Psychopharmacol.* **14**:531–538.

Assadi, S.M., Yucel, M., and Pantelis, C. 2009. Dopamine modulates neural networks involved in effort-based decision-making. *Neurosci. Biobehav. Rev.* **33**:383–893.

Ballantine, H.T., Cassidy, W.L., Flanagan, N.B., and Marino, R. Jr. 1967. Stereotaxic anterior cingulotomy for neuropsychiatric illness and intractable pain. *J. Neurosurg.* **26**:488–495.

Ballantine, H.T., Bouckoms, A.J., Thomas, A.K., and Giriunas, I.E. 1987. Treatment of psychiatric illness by stereotactic cingulotomy. *Biol. Psychiatry* **22**:807–819.

Ballmaier, M., Toga, A.W., Blanton, R.E., Sowell, E.R., Lavretsky, H., Peterson, J., Pham, D., and Kumar, A. 2004. Anterior cingulate, gyrus rectus, and orbitofrontal abnormalities in elderly depressed patient: An MRI-based parcellation of the prefrontal cortex. *Am. J. Psychiatry* **161**:99–108.

Bancaud, J., and Talairach, J. 1992. Clinical semiology of frontal lobe seizures. *Adv. Neurol.* **57**:3–58.

Bartels, A., and Zeki, S. 2000. The neural basis of romantic love. *Neuroreport* **11**:3829–3834.

Baxter, L.R. Jr. 1992. Neuroimaging studies of obsessive compulsive disorder. *Psychiatr. Clin. North Am.* **15**: 871–884.

Baxter, L.R., Schwartz, J.M., Mazziotta, J.C., Phelps, M.E., Pahl, J.J., Guze, B.H., and Fairbanks, L. 1988. Cerebral glucose metabolic rates in non-depressed obsessive-compulsives. *Am. J. Psychiatry* **45**:1560–1563.

Benes, F.M. 1996. Excitotoxicity in the development corticolimbic alterations in schizophrenic brain. In: S.J.Watson (ed.) *Biology of Schizophrenia and Affective Disease*. Washington, D.C.: American Psychiatric Press.

Benes, F.M. 1998. Model generation and testing to probe neural circuitry in the cingulate cortex of postmortem schizophrenic brain. *Schizophr. Bull.* **24**:219–230.

Benes, F.M., McSparren, J., Bird, E.D., SanGiovanni, J.P., and Vincent, S.L. 1991. Deficits in small interneurons in prefrontal and cingulate cortices of schizophrenic and schizoaffective patients. *Arch. Gen. Psychiatry* **48**:996–1001.

Bentivoglio, M., Kultas-Ilinsky, K., and Ilinsky, I. 1993. Limbic thalamus: Structure, intrinsic organization, and connections. In: B.A.Vogt, and M.Gabriel (eds.) *Neurobiology of Cingulate Cortex and Limbic Thalamus: A Comprehensive Handbook*. Boston: Birkhauser, pp. 71–122.

Blumberg, H.P., Donegan, N.H., Sanislow, C.A. Collins, S., Lacadie, C., Skudlarski, P., Gueorguieva, R., Fulbright, R.K., McGlashan, T.H., Gore, J.C., and Krystal, J.H. 2005. Preliminary evidence for medication effects on functional abnormalities in the amygdala anterior cingulate in bipolar disorder. *Psychopharmacology* **183**:208–313.

Botvinick, M., Nystrom, L.E., Fissell, K., Carter, C.S., and Cohen, J.D. 1999. Conflict monitoring versus selection-for-action in anterior cingulate cortex. *Nature* **402**: 179–181.

Bremner, J.D., Vermetten, E., Vythilingam, M., Afzal, N., Schmahl, C., Elzinga, B., and Charney, D.S. 2004. Neural correlates of the classic color and emotional Stroop in women with abuse-related posttraumatic stress disorder. *Biol. Psychiatry* **55**:612–620.

Buckner, R.L., Andrews-Hanna, J.R., and Schacter, D.L. 2008. The brain's default network: Anatomy, function, and relevance to disease. *Ann. N. Y. Acad. Sci.* **1124**:1–38.

Bush, G., Vogt, B.A. Holmes, J., Dale, A.M., Greve, D., Jenike, M.A., and Rosen, B.R. 2002. Dorsal anterior cingulate cortex: A role in reward-based decision-making. *Proc. Natl. Acad. Sci. USA.* **99**:523–528.

Carter, C.S., Mintun, M., Nichols, T., and Cohen, J.D. 1997. Anterior cingulate gyrus dysfunction and selective attention deficits in schizophrenia: [15O]H2O PET study during single-trial Stroop task performance. *Am. J. Psychiatry* **154**:1670–1675.

Casey, K.L., Minoshima, S., Berger, K.L., Koeppe, R.A., Morrow, T.J., and Frey, K.A. 1994. Positron emission tomographic analysis of cerebral structures activated specifically by repetitive noxious heat stimuli. *J. Neurophysiol.* **71**:802–807.

Cetas, J.S., Saedi, T., and Burchiel, K.J., 2008. Destructive procedures for the treatment of nonmalignant pain: A structured literature review. *J. Neurosurg.* **109**:389–404.

Chiocca, E.A., and Martuza, R.L. 1990. Neurosurgical therapy of obsessive-compulsive disorder. In: M.A.Jenike, L.Baer, and W.E.Minichiello (eds.) *Obsessive-Compulsive Disorders: Theory and Management*. Littleton, MA: Year Book Medical Publishers.

Choi, J.S., Kang., D.H., Kim, J.J., Ha, T.H., Roh, K.S., Yopun, T., and Kwon, J.S. 2005. Decreased caudal anterior cingulate gyrus volume and positive symptoms in schizophrenia. *Psychiatry Res.* **139**:239–247

Cosgrove, G.R., and Rauch, S.L. 1995. Psychosurgery. *Neurosurg. Clin. North Am.* **6**:167–176.

Crespo-Facorro, B., Kim, J.M., Andreasen, N.C., O' Leary, D.S., and Magnotta, V. 2000. Regional frontal abnormalities in schizophrenia: A quantitative grey matter volume and cortical surface size study. *Biol. Psychiatry* **48**:110–119.

Damasio, A.R., and Van Hoesen, G.W. 1983. Focal lesions of the limbic frontal lobe. In: K.M.Heilman, and P.Satz (eds.) *Neuropsychology of Human Emotion*. New York: Guilford Press.

Damasio, A.R., Tranel, D., and Damasio, H. 1990. Individuals with sociopathic behavior caused by frontal damage fail to respond autonomically to social stimuli. *Behav. Brain Res.* **41**:81–94.

De La Fuente, J.M., Goldman, S., Stanus, E., Vizuete, C., Morlan, I., Bobes, J., and Mendlewicz, J. 1997. Brain glucose metabolism in borderline personality disorder. *J. Psychiatr. Res.* **31**:531–541.

Deary, I.J., Ebmeier, K.P., MacLeod, K.M., Dougall, N., Hepburn, D.A., Grier, B.M., and Goodwin, G.M. 1994. PASAT performance and the pattern of uptake of 99mTc-exametazime in brain estimated with single photon emission tomography. *Biol. Psychol.* **38**: 1–18.

Derbyshire, S.W.G., Jones, A.K.P., Devani, P., Friston, K.J., Feinmann, C., Harris, M., Pearce, S., Watson, J.D., and Frackowiak, R.S. 1994. Cerebral responses to pain in patients with atypical facial pain measured by positron emission tomography. *J. Neurol. Neurosurg. Psychiatry* **57**:1166–1172.

Devinsky, O., and Luciano, D. 1993. The contributions of cingulate cortex to human behavior. In: B.A.Vogt, and M.Gabriel (eds.) *Neurobiology of Cingulate Cortex and Limbic Thalamus: A Comprehensive Handbook*. Boston: Birkhauser, pp. 527–556.

Devinsky, O., Morrell, M.J., and Vogt, B.A. 1995. Contribution of anterior cingulate cortex to behaviour. *Brain* **118**:279–306.

Drevets, W.C., Price, J.L., Simpson, J.R. Jr., Todd, R.D., Reich, T., Vannier, M., and Raichle, M.E. 1997. Subgenual prefrontal cortex abnormalities in mood disorders. *Nature* **386**:824–827.

Dunn, R.T., Kimbrell, T.A., Ketter, T.A., Frye, M.A., Willis, M.W., Luckenbaugh, D.A., and Post, R.M. 2002. Principal components of the Beck depression inventory and regional cerebral metabolism in unipolar and bipolar depression. *Biol. Psychiatry* **51**:387–399.

Durn, R.P., and Strick, P.L. 1991. The origin of corticospinal projections from the premotor areas in the frontal lobe. *J. Neurosci.* **11**:667–689.

Elfgren, C., Gustafson, L, Vestberg, S., Risberg, J., Rosen, I., Ryding, E., and Passant, U. 2003. Subjective experience of memory deficits related to clinical and neuroimaging findings. *Dement. Geriatr. Cogn. Disord.* **16**: 84–92.

Farrow, T.F., Whitford, T.J., Williams, L.M., Gomes, L., and Harris, A.W. 2005. Diagnosis-related regional gray matter loss over two years in first episode schizophrenia and bipolar disorder. *Biol. Psychiatry* **58**:713–723.

Foa, E.B., Feske, U., Murdock, T.B., Kozak, M.J., and McCarthy, P.R. 1991. Processing of threat related information in rape victims. *J. Abnorm. Psychol.* **100**:156–162.

Foltz, E.L., and White, L.E. 1962. Pain "relief" by frontal cingulumotomy. *J. Neurosurg.* **19**:89–100.

Frankland, P.W., Bontempi, B., Talton, I.E., Kaczmarek, L., and Silva, A.J. 2004. The involvement of the anterior cingulate cortex in remote contextual fear memory. *Science* **304**:881–883.

Fredericksen, K.A., Cutting, L.E., Kates, W.R., Mostofsky, S.H., Singer, H.S., Cooper, K.L., Singer, H.S., Cooper, K.L., Lanham, D.C., Denckia, M.B., and Kaufmann, W.E. 2002. Disproportionate increases of white matter in right frontal lobe in Tourette syndrome. *Neurology* **58**:85–89.

Frot, M., Mauguière, F., Magnin, M., and Garcia-Larreal, L. 2009. Parallel processing of nociceptive A- inputs in SII and midcingulate cortex in humans. *J. Neurosci.* **28**:944–952.

Garraux, G., Goldfine, A., Bohlhlter, S., Lerner, A., Hanakawa, T., and Hallett, M. 2006. Increased midbrain gray matter in Tourette's syndrome. *Psychiatry Res.* **59**:381–385.

Glahn, D.C., Ragland, J.D., Abramoff, A., Barrett, J., Laird, A.R., Bearden, C.E., and Velligan, D.I. 2005. Beyond hypofrontality; A quantitative meta-analysis of functional neuroimaging studies of working memory in schizophrenia. *Hum. Brain Mapp.* **25**:60–69.

Grasby, P.M., Firth, C.D., Friston, K.J, Bench, C., Frackowiak, R.S.J., and Dolan, R.J. 1993. Functional mapping of brain areas implicated in auditory-verbal memory function. *Brain* **116**:1–20.

Gurevich, E.V., and Joyce, J.N. 1997. Alterations in the cortical serotonergic system in schizophrenia: A postmortem study. *Biol. Psychiatry* **42**:529–545.

Hauptman, J.S., DeSalles, A.F., Espinoza, R., Sedrak, M., and Ishida, W. 2008. Potential surgical targets for deep brain stimulation in treatment-resistant depression. *Neurosurg. Focus* **25**:1–9.

Hayden, B.Y., Smith, D.V., and Platt, M.L. 2009. Electrophysiological correlates of default-mode processing in macaque posterior cingulate cortex. *Proc. Nat. Acad. Sci. USA.* **106**: 5948–5953.

Haznedar, M.M., Buchsbaum, M.S., Hazlett, E.A., Shihabuddin, L., New, A., and Siever, L.J., 2004. Cingulate gyrus volume and metabolism in the schizophrenia spectrum. *Schizophr. Res.* **712**:249–262.

Hein, G., and Singer, T. 2008. I feel how you feel but not always: The empathic brain and its modulation. *Curr. Opin. Neurobiol.* **18**:153–158.

Hirao, K., Ohnishi, T., Matsuda, H., Nemoto, K., Hirata, Y., Yamashita, F., Asada, T., and Iwamoto, T. 2006. Functional interactions between entorhinal cortex and posterior cingulate cortex at the very early stage of Alzheimer's disease using brain perfusion single-photon emission computed tomography. *Nucl. Med. Commun.* **27**:151–156.

Houenou, J., Wessa, M., Douaud, G., Leboyer, M., Chanraud, S., Perrin, M., Poupon, C., Martinot, J.L., and Paillere-Martinot, M.L. 2007. Increased white matter connectivity in euthymic bipolar patients: Diffusion tensor tractography between the subgenual cingulate and amygdalo-hippocampal complex. *Mol. Psychiatry* **12**:1001–1010.

Huang, C., Whalund, L-O., Svensson, L., Winblad, B., and Julin, P. 2002. Cingulate cortex hypoperfusion predicts Alzheimer's disease in mild cognitive impairment. *BMC Neurol.* **2**:9.

Jenike, M.A., Bear, L., Ballantine, H.T., Martuza, R.L., Tyners, S., Giriunas, I., Buttolph, M.L., and Cassem, N.H. 1991. Cingulotomy for refractory obsessive-compulsive disorder. A long-term follow-up of 33 patients. *Arch. Gen. Psychiatry* **48**:548–554.

Job, D.E., Whalley, H.C., McConnell, S., Glabus, M., Johnstone, E.C., and Lawrie, S.M.2003a. Voxel-based morphometry of grey matter densities in subjects at high risk of schizophrenia. *Schizophr. Res.* **64**:1–13.

Job, D.E., Whalley, H.C., Yates, S.L., Glabus, M., Johnstone, E.C., and Lawrie, S.M. 2003b. Voxel based morphometry of grey matter reductions over time in subjects with schizophrenia. *Schizophr. Res.* **60**(Suppl.):198.

Kartsounis, L.D., Poynton, A., Bridges, P.K., and Bartlett, J.R. 1991. Neuropsychological correlates of stereotactic subcaudate tractotomy. A prospective study. *Brain* **114**:2657–2673.

Kates, W.R., Frederikse, M., Mostofsky, S.H., Folley, B.S., Cooper, K., Mazur-Hopkins, P., Kofman, O., Singer, H.S., Denckia, M.B., Pearlson, G.D., and Kaufmann, W.E. 2002. MRI parcellation of the frontal lobe in boys with attention deficit hyperactivity disorder or Tourette syndrome. *Psychiatry Res.* **116**:63–81.

Kaur, S., Sassi, R.B., Axelson, D., Nicoletti, M., Brambilla, P., Monkul., E.S., Hatch, J.P., Keshavan, M.S., Ryan, N., Birmaher, B., and Soares, J.C., 2005. Cingulate cortex anatomical abnormalities in children and adolescents with bipolar disorder. *Am. J. Psychiatry* **162**:1637–1643.

Kerns, J.G., Cohen, J.D., Macdonald III, A.W., Cho, R.Y. Stenger, V.Q., and Carter, C.S. 2004. Anterior cingulate conflict monitoring and adjustments in control. *Science* **303**:1023–1026.

Kobayashi, Y., and Amaral, D.G. 2003. Macaque monkey retrosplenial cortex: II. Cortical afferents. *J. Comp. Neurol.* **466**:48–79.

Kondo, H., Morishita, M., Osaka, N., Osaka, M., Fukuyama, H., and Shibasaki, H. 2004. Functional roles of the cingulo-frontal network in performance on working memory. *Neuroimage* **21**:2–14.

Kumra, S., Ashtari, M., Cervellione, K.L., Henderson, I., Kester, H., Roofeh, D., Wu, J., Clarke, T., Thaden, E., Kane, J.M., Rhinewine, J., Lencz, T., Diamond, A., Ardekani, B.A., and Szeszko, P.R. 2005. White matter abnormalities in early-onset schizophrenia: A voxel-based diffusion tensor imaging study. *J. Am. Acad. Child Adolesc. Psychiatry* **44**:934–941.

Lanius, R.A., Williamson, P.C., Densmore, M., Boksman, K., Gupta, M.A., Neufeld, R.W., Gati, J.S., and Menon, R.S. 2001. Neural correlates of traumatic memories in posttraumatic stress disorder: A functional MRI investigation. *Am. J. Psychiatry.* **158**:1920–1922.

Lanius, R.A., Williamson, P.C., Boksman, K., Densmore, M. Gupta, M., Neufeld, R.W., Gati, J. A., and Menon, R.S. 2002. Brain activation during script-driven imagery induced dissociative responses in PTSD: A functional magnetic resonance imaging investigation. *Biol. Psychiatry* **52**:305–311.

Lanius, R.A., Williamson, P.C., Hopper, J., Densmore, M., Boksman, K., Gupta, M.A., Neufeld, R.W., Gati, J.S., and Menon, R.S. 2003. Recall of emotional states in posttraumatic stress disorder: An fMRI investigation. *Biol. Psychiatry* **53**:204–210.

Ledesma, J.A., and Paniaqua, J.L. 1969. Circunvolucion del cingulo y agrisividad. *Actas Luso Esp. Neurol. Psiquiatr.* **28**:289–298.

Levin, B., and Duchowny, M. 1991. Childhood obsessive compulsive disorder and cingulate epilepsy. *Biol. Psychiatry* **30**:1049–1055.

Liberzon, I., Taylor, S.F., Amdur, R., Jung, T.D., Chamberlain, K.R., Minoshima, S., Koeppe, R.A., and Fig, L.M. 1999a. Brain activation in PTSD in response to trauma-related stimuli. *Biol. Psychiatry* **45**:817–826.

Liberzon, I., Ableson, J.L., Flagel, S.B., Raz, J., and Young, E.A. 1999b. Neuroendocrine and psychophysiological responses in PTSD: A symptom provocation study. *Neuropsychopharmacology* **21**:40–50

Liberzon, I., and Sripada, C.S. 2008. The functional neuroanatomy of PTSD: A critical review. *Prog. Brain Res.* **167**:151–169.

Liddle, P.F., Friston, K.J., Frith, C.D., Hirsch, S.R., Jones, T., and Frackowiak, R.S.J. 1992. Patterns of cerebral blood flow in schizophrenia. *Br. J. Psychiatry* **160**:179–186.

Lochhead, R.A., Parsey, R.V., Oquendo, M.A., and Mann, J.J. 2004. Regional brain gray matter volume differences in patients with bipolar disorder as assessed by optimized voxel-based morphometry. *Biol. Psychiatry* **55**:1154–1162.

Lozano, A.M., Mayberg, H.S., Giacobbe, P., Harmani, C., Craddock, R.C., and Kennedy, S.K. 2008. Subcallosal cingulate gyrus deep brain stimulation for treatment-resistant depression. *Biol. Psychiatry* **64**:461–467.

Luppino, G., Matelli, M., Camarada, R.M., Gallese, V., and Rizzolatti, G. 1991. Multiple representations of body movements in mesial area 6 and the adjacent cingulate cortex: an intracortical microstimulation study in the macaque monkey. *J. Comp. Neurol.* **311**:463–482.

Lyoo, I.K., Sung, Y.H., Dager, S.R., Friedman, S.D., Lee, J.Y., Kim, S.J., Kim, N., Dunner, D.L., and Renshaw, P.R. 2006. Regional cerebral cortical thinning bipolar disorder. *Bipolar Disord.* **8**:65–74.

MacAvoy, M.G., Bruce, C.J., and Gottlieb, J.P. 1991. Smooth pursuit eye movement representation in the primate frontal eyefield. *Cereb. Cortex* **1**:95–102.

Maddock, R.J., Garrett, A.S., and Buonocore, M.H. 2001. Remembering familiar people: The posterior cingulate cortex and autobiographical memory retrieval. *Neuroscience* **104**:667–676.

Maddock, R.J., Garrett, A.S., and Buonocore, M.H. 2003. Posterior cingulate cortex activation by emotional words: fMRI evidence from a valence decision task. *Hum. Brain Mapp.* **18**:30–41.

Maia, T.V., Cooney, R.E., and Peterson, B.S. 2008. The neural bases of obsessive-compulsive disorder in children and adults. *Dev. Psychopathol.* **20**:1251–1283.

Malhi, G.S., Lagopoulos, J., Owen, A.M., Ivanovski, B., Shnier, R., and Sachdev, P. 2007. Reduced activation to implicit affect induction in euthymic bipolar patients: an fMRI study. *J. Affect. Disord.* **7**:109–122.

Marino, R. Jr., and Cosgrove, G.R. 1997. Neurosurgical treatment of neuropsychiatric illness. *Psychiatr. Clin. North Am.* **20**:933–943.

Martinez-Bisbal, M.C., Arana, E., Marti-Bonmati, L., Molla, E., and Celda, B. 2004. Cognitive impairment: classification by 1H magnetic resonance spectroscopy. *Eur. J. Neurol.* **11**:187–193.

Martuza, R.L., Chiocca, E.A., Jenike, M.A., Giriunas, I.E., and Ballantine, H.T. 1990. Stereotactic radiofrequency thermal cingulotomy for obsessive compulsive disorder. *Neuropsychiatr. Pract. Opin.* **2**:331–335.

Mayberg, H.W., Liotti, M., Brannan, S.K., McGinnis, S., Mahurin, R.K., Jerabek, P.A., Silva, J.A., Tekell, J.L., Martin, C.C., Lancaster, J.L., and Fox, PT. 1999. Reciprocal limbic-cortical function and negative mood: Converging PET findings in depression and normal sadness. *Am. J. Psychiatry* **156**: 675–682.

McCoy, A.N., and Platt, M.L. 2005. Risk-sensitive neurons in macaque posterior cingulate cortex. *Nat. Neurosci.* **8**:1220–1224.

McCoy, A.N., Crowley, J.C., Haghighian, G., Dean, H.L., and Platt, M.L. 2003. Saccade reward signals in posterior cingulate cortex. *Neuron* **40**:1031–1040.

McNally, R.J., Kaspi, R.J., Riemann, B.C., and Zeitlin, S.B. 1990. Selective processing of threat cues in posttraumatic stress disorder. *J. Abnorm. Psychol.* **99**:398–402.

Mega, M.S., and Cummings, J.L. 2001. Frontal subcortical circuits. In: S.Salloway, P.Malloy, and J.D.Duffy (eds.) *The Frontal Lobes and Neuropsychiatric Illness.* Washington, D.C.: American Psychiatric Publishers, pp. 15–32.

Middleton, F.A., and Strick, P.L. 2001. A revised neuroanatomy of frontal-subcortical circuits. In: D.G. Lichter, and J.L.Cummings (eds.) *Frontal-subcortical Circuits in Psychiatric and Neurological Disorders.* New York: Guilford Press.

Mindus, P., and Jenike, M.A. 1992. Neurosurgical treatment of malignant obsessive compulsive disorder. *Psychiatr. Clin. North Am.* **15**:921–938.

Morecraft, R.J., and Van Hoesen, G.W. 1992. Cingulate input to the primary and supplementary motor cortices in the rhesus monkey: Evidence for somatotopy in areas 24c and 23c. *J. Comp. Neurol.* **322**:471–489.

Mouras, H., Stoleru, S., Bittoun, J., Glutron, D., Pelegrini-Issac, M., Paradis, A-L., and BurnonY. 2003. Brain processing of visual sexual stimuli in healthy men: a functional magnetic resonance imaging study. *Neuroimage* **20**:855–869.

Müller-Vahl, K., Kaufmann, J., Grosskreutz, J., Dengler, R., Emrich, H.M., and Peschel, T. 2009. Prefrontal and anterior cingulate cortex abnormalities in Tourette syndrome: Evidence from voxel-based morphometry and magnetization transfer imaging. *BMC Neurosci.* **10**:47–60.

Öngür, D., Drevets., W.C., and Price, J.L. 1998. Glial reduction in the subgenual prefrontal cortex in mood disorders. *Proc. Natl. Acad. Sci. USA.* **95**:13290–13295.

Ottowitz, W.E., Dougherty, D.D., Sirota, A., Niaura, R., Rauch, S.L., and Brown, W.A. 2004. Neural and endocrine correlates of sadness in women. Implications for neural network regulation of HPA activity. *J. Neuropsychiatry Clin. Neurosci.* **16**:446–455.

Ovsiew, F., and Frim, D.M. 1997. Neurosurgery for psychiatric disorders. *J. Neurol. Neurosurg. Psychiatry* **63**:701–705.

Peterson, B.S., Staib, L., Scahill, L., Zhang, H. Anderson, C., Leckman, J.F., Cohen, D.J., Gore, J.C., Albert, J., and Webster, R. 2001. Regional brain and ventricular volumes in Tourette syndrome. *Arch. Gen. Psychiatry* **58**:427–440.

Pezawas, L., Meyer-Lindenberg, A., Drabant, E.M., Verchinski, B.A., Munoz, K.E., Kolachan, B.S., Egan, M.F., Mattay, V.S., Ahmad R Hariri, A.R., and Weinberger, D.R. 2005. 5-HTTLPR polymorphism impacts human cingulate-amygdala interactions: a genetic susceptibility mechanism for depression. *Nat. Neurosci.* **8**:828–834.

Phan, K.L., Taylor, S.F., Welsh, R.C., Ho., S.H., Britton, J.C., and Liberzon, I. 2004. Neural correlates of individual ratings of emotional salience: A trial-related fMRI study. *Neuroimage* **21**:768–780.

Ploner, M., Gross, J., Timmermann, L., and Schnitzler, A. 2002. Cortical representation of first and second pain sensation in humans. *Proc. Natl. Acad. Sci. USA.* **99**:12444–12448.

Polli, F.E., Barton, J.J.S., Cain, M.S., Thakkar, K.N., Rauch, S.L., and Manoach, D.S. 2005. Rostral and dorsal anterior cingulate cortex make dissociable contributions during antisaccade error commission. *Proc. Natl. Acad. Sci. USA.* **102**:157000–157005.

Poynton, A.M., Kartsounis, L.D., and Bridges, P.K. 1995. A prospective clinical study of stereotactic subcaudate tractotomy. *Psychol. Med.* **25**:763–770.

Protopopescu, X., Pan, H., Tuescher, O., Cloitre, M., Goldstein, M., Engelien, W., Epstein, J., Yang, Y., Gorman, J., Ledoux, J., Sibersweig, D., and Stern, E. 2005. Differential time courses and specificity of amygdala activity in posttraumatic stress disorder subjects and normal control subjects. *Biol. Psychiatry* **57**:464–473.

Pujol., J., Soriano-Mas, C., Alonso, P., Cardoner, N., Menchon, J.M., Deus, J., and Vallejo, J. 2004. Mapping structural brain alterations in obsessive-compulsive disorder. *Arch. Gen. Psychiatry* **61**:720–730.

Raichle, M.E., Fiez, J.A., Videen, T.O., MacLeod, A-M.K., Pardo, J.V., Fox, P.T., and Petersen, S.E. 1994. Practice-related changes in human brain functional anatomy during nonmotor learning. *Cereb. Cortex* **4**:8–26.

Rapoport, J.L., and Inoff-Germain, G. 1997. Medical and surgical treatment of obsessive-compulsive disorder. *Neurol. Clin. North Am.* **15**:421–428.

Rauch, S.L., Jenike, M.A., Alpert, N.M., Baer, L., Breiter, H.C.R., Savage, C.R., and Fischman, A.J. 1994. Regional cerebral blood flow measured during symptom provocation in obsessive-compulsive disorder using oxygen 15–labeled carbon dioxide and positron emission tomography. *Arch. Gen. Psychiatry* **51**:62–70.

Rauch, S.L. Van Der Kolk, B.A., Fisler, R.E., Alpert, N.M., Orr, S.P., Savage, C.R., Fioschman, A.J., Jenike, M.A., and Pitman, R.K. 1996. A symptom provocation study of posttraumatic stress disorder using positron emission tomography and script-driven imagery. *Arch. Gen. Psychiatry* 53:380–387.

Ressler, K.J., and Mayberg, H.S. 2007. Targeting abnormal neural circuits in mood and anxiety disorders: from the laboratory to the clinic. *Nat. Neurosci.* **10**:1116–1124.

Rolls, E.T., O'Doherty, J., Kringelbach, M.L., Francis, S., Bowtell, R., and McGlone, F. 2003. Representations of pleasant and painful touch in the human orbitofrontal and cingulate cortices. *Cereb. Cortex* **13**:308–317.

Rosenberg, D.R., and Keshavan, M.S. 1998. A.E. Bennett Research Award: Toward a neurodevelopmental model of obsessive-compulsive disorder. *Biol. Psychiatry* 43:623–1640.

Roth, R.M., Saykin, A.J., Flashman, L.A., Pixley, H.S., West, J.D., and Mamourian, A.C. 2007. Event-related functional magnetic resonance imaging of response inhibition in obsessive-compulsive disorder. *J. Child Adolesc. Psychopharmacol.* 13(Suppl. 1):S31–S38.

Saxena, S., and Rauch, S.L. 2000. Functional neuroimaging and the neuroanatomy of obsessive-compulsive disorder. *Psychiatr. Clin. North Am.* 23:563 –586.

Seltzer, B., and Pandya, D.N., 2009. Posterior cingulate and retrosplenial cortex connections of the caudal superior temporal region in the rhesus monkey. *Exp. Brain Res.* 195:1432–1106.

Seminowicz, D.A., Mayberg, H.S., McIntosh, A.R., Goldapple, K., Kennedy, S., Segal, Z., and Rafi-Tarib, S. 2004. Limbic–frontal circuitry in major depression: a path modeling metanalysis. *Neuroimage* 22:409–418.

Sewards, T.V., and Sewards, M.A. 2003. Representations of motivational drives in mesial cortex, medial thalamus, hypothalamus and midbrain. *Brain Res. Bull.* 61:25–49.

Shafran, R., and Speckens, A. 2005. Reply to Rosenberg *et al.* Biological versus psychological approaches to OCD: War or peace? In: J.S.Abramowitz, and A.C.Houts (eds.) *Concepts and Controversies in Obsessive-Compulsive Disorder*. New York: Springer, pp. 255–260.

Shah, M.P., Wang, F., Kalmar, J.H., Chepenik, L.G., Tie, K., Pittman, B., Jones, M.M., Constable, R.T., Gelernter, J., and Blumberg, H.P. 2009. Role of variation in the serotonin transporter protein gene (SLC6A4) in trait disturbances in the ventral anterior cingulate in bipolar disorder. *Neuropsychopharmacology* 24:1301–1310.

Shah, N.J., Marshall, J.C., Zafiris, O., Schwab, A., Zilles, K., Markowitsch, H.J., and Fink, G.R. 2001. The neural correlates of person familiarity. A functional magnetic resonance imaging study with clinical implications. *Brain* 124:804–815.

Shields, D.C., Asaad, W., Eskandar, E., Jain, F., Cosgrove, G.R, Flaherty, A., Cassem, E.H., Price, B.H., Rauch, S.L., and Dougherty, D. 2008. Prospective assessment of stereotactic ablative surgery for intractable major depression. *Biol. Psychiatry* **64**:449–454.

Silbersweig, D.A., Stern, E., Frith, C., Cahill, C., Holmes, A., Grootoonk, S., Seaward, J., McKenna, P., Chua, S.E., and Schnorr, L. 1995. A functional neuroanatomy of hallucinations in schizophrenia. *Nature* **378**:176–799.

So, N.K. 1998. Mesial frontal epilepsy. *Epilepsia* **39**(Suppl. 4):S49–61.

Strakowski, S.M., Adler, C.M., Holland, S.K., Mills, N.P., DelBello, M.P., and Eliassen, J.C. 2005. Abnormal fMRI brain activation in euthymic bipolar disorder patients during a counting Stroop interference task. *Am. J. Psychiatry* **162**:1697–1705.

Sutherland, R.J., and Hoesing, J.M. 1993. Posterior cingulate cortex and spatial memory: A microlimnology analysis. In: B.A.Vogt, and M.Gabriel (eds.) *Neurobiology of Cingulate Cortex and Limbic Thalamus: A Comprehensive Handbook*. Boston:Birkhauser, pp. 461–477.

Szeszko, P.R., MacMillan, S., McMeniman, M., Chen, S., Baribault, K., Lim, K.O., Ivey, J., Rose, M., Banerjee, S.P., Bhandari, R., Moore, G.J., and Rosenberg, D.R. 2004. Brain structural abnormalities in psychotropic drug-naïve pediatric patients with obsessive-compulsive disorder. *Am. J. Psychiatry.* **161**:1049–1056.

Takahashi, T. 2004. Symptomatology of retrosplenial cortex damage: comparison between lesions in the right and left hemisphere. *Adv. Neurol. Sci.* **48**:649–656.

Talbot, J.D., Marrett, S., Evans, A.C., Meyer, E., Bushnell, M.C., and Duncan, G.H. 1991. Multiple representations of pain in human cerebral cortex. *Science* **251**:1355–1358.

Tamminga, C.A., Thaker, G.K., Buchanan, R., Kirkpatric, B., Alphs, G.D., Chase, T.N., and Carpenter, W.T. 1992. Limbic system abnormalities identified in schizophrenia using positron emission tomography with fluorodeoxyglucose and neocortical alterations with deficit syndrome. *Arch. Gen. Psychiatry* **49**:522–530.

Taylor, S.F., Bartis, B., Fitzgerald, K.D., Welsh, R.C., Abelson, J.L., Liberzon, I., Himle, J.A., and Gehring, W.J. 2006. Medial frontal cortex activity and loss-related responses to errors. *J. Neurosci.* **26**:4063–4070.

Todtenkopf, M.S., Vincent, S.L., and Benes, F.M. 2005. A cross-study meta-analysis and three-dimensional comparison of cell counting in the anterior cingulate cortex of schizophrenic and bipolar brain. *Schizophr. Res* **73**:79–89.

Valente, A.A. Jr., Miguel, E.C., Castro., C.C., Amaro, E. Jr., Duran, F.L., Buchpiguel, C.A., Chitnis, X., McGuire, P.K., and Busatto, G.F. 2005. Regional gray matter abnormalities in obsessive-compulsive disorder: A voxel-based morphometry study. *Biol. Psychiatry* **58**:479–487.

Van Hoesen, G.W., Morecraft, R.J., and Vogt, B.A. 1993. Connections of the monkey cingulate cortex. In: B.A. Vogt, and M.Gabriel (eds.) *Neurobiology of Cingulate Cortex and Limbic Thalamus: A Comprehensive Handbook*. Boston: Birkhauser, pp. 249–286.

Vidal, C.N., Rapoport, J.L., Hayashi, K.M., Geaga, J.A., Sui, Y., McLemore, L.E., Alaghband, Y., Giedd, J.N., Gochman, P., Blumenthal, J., Gogtay, N., Nicolson, R., Toga, A.W., and Thompson, P.M. 2006. Dynamically spreading frontal and cingulate deficits mapped in adolescents with schizophrenia. *Arch. Gen. Psychiatry* **63**:25–34.

Vogt, B.A. 2005. Pain and emotion interactions in subregions of the cingulate gyrus. *Nat. Rev. Neurosci.* **6**:533–544.

Vogt, B.A., Sikes, R.W., and Vogt, L.J. 1993. Anterior cingulate cortex and the medial pain system. In: B.A. Vogt, and M.Gabriel (eds.) *Neurobiology of Cingulate Cortex and Limbic Thalamus: A Comprehensive Handbook*. Boston: Birkhauser, pp. 313–344.

Vogt, B.A., Berger, G.R., and Derbyshire, S.W.J. 2003. Structural and functional dichotomy of human midcingulate cortex. *Eur. J. Neurosci.* **18**:3134–3144.

Wessa, M., Houenou, J., Paillere-Martinot, M.L., Berthoz, S., Artiges, E., Leboyer, M., and Martinot, J.L. 2007. Fronto-striatal overactivation in euthymic bipolar patients during an emotional go/nogo task. *Am. J. Psychiatry* **164**:638–646.

White, T., Nelson, M., and Lim, K.O. 2008. Diffusion tensor imaging in psychiatric disorders. *Top. Magn. Reson. Imaging* **19**:97–109.

Whiteside, S.P., Port, J.D., and Abramowitz, J.S. 2004. A meta-analysis of functional neuroimaging in obsessive-compulsive disorder. *Psychiatry Res.* **132**:69–79.

Wilke, M., Kowatch, R.A., DelBello, M.P., Mills, N.P., and Holland, S.K. 2004. Voxel-based morphometry in adolescents with bipolar disorder: First results. *Psychiatry Res.* **131**:57–69.

Yágüez, L., Coen, S., Gregory, L.J., Amaro, E. Jr, Altman, C., Brammer, M.J., Bullmore, E.T., Williams, S.C.R., and Aziz, Q. 2005. Brain response to visceral aversive conditioning: A functional magnetic resonance imaging study. *Gastroenterology* **128**:1819–1829.

Yamasue, H., Iwanami, A., Hirayasu, Y., Yamada, H., Abe, O., Kuroki, N., Fukuda, R., Tsujii, K., Aoki, S., Ohtomo, K., Kato, N., and Kasai, K. 2004. Localized volume reduction in prefrontal, temporolimbic, and paralimbic regions in schizophrenia: An MRI parcellation study. *Psychiatry Res.* **131**:195–207.

Yoo, S.Y., Roh, M.S., Choi, J.S., Kang do, H., Ha, T.H., Lee, J.M., Kim, I.Y., Kim, S.I., and Kwon, J.S. 2008. Voxel-based morphometry study of gray matter abnormalities in obsessive-compulsive disorder. *J. Korean Med. Sci.* **23**:24–30.

Zobel, A., Joe, A., Freymann, N., Clusmann, H., Schramm, J., Reinhardt, M., Biersack, H.J., Maier, W., and Broich, K. 2005. Changes in regional cerebral blood flow by therapeutic vagus nerve stimulation in depression: an exploratory approach. *Psychiatry Res.* **139**:165–179.

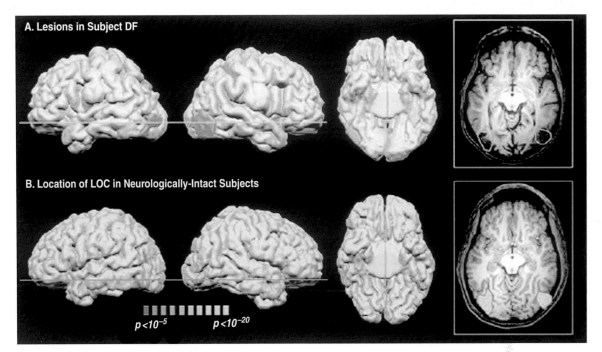

Figure 4.3. A, B. The ventral visual stream lesions in a patient with visual agnosia (subject DF) are compared with the expected region (lateral occipital complex) for object recognition. A. Lesions in subject DF. Her lesions were traced on slices that indicated tissue damage and rendered on the pial surface in pale blue (see color plate). Lateral views of the left and right hemispheres are shown, as is a ventral view of the underside of the brain. B. The expected location of the lateral occipital complex based on functional magnetic resonance imaging date from seven neurologically intact participants. The activation of the slice is shown in orange in panel A in the color plate for comparison with the lesions in patient DF's brain. (Reproduced with permission from Oxford University Press from James *et al.*, 2003.)

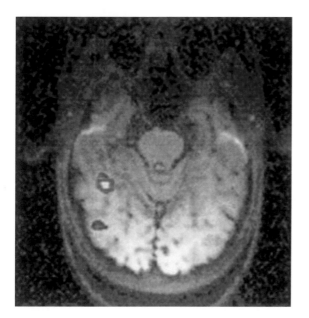

Figure 5.5. This functional magnetic resonance image shows activation of the "fusiform face area" responsive to human faces. The right hemisphere appears on the left. The brain images at the left show (in color in the color plate) the voxels that produced a significantly higher magnetic resonance signal intensity during the epochs containing faces than during those containing objects. These significance images are overlaid on a T1-weighted anatomical image of the same slice. In each image, the region of interest is shown outlined in green. (Reproduced with permission from Kanwisher *et al.*, 1997.)

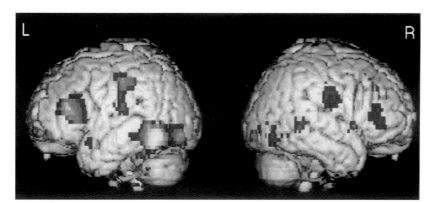

Figure 6.5. Functional magnetic resonance images demonstrating greater activation to words than to consonant letter strings during a nonlinguistic visual feature detection task. The images illustrate a left hemisphere language network for reading, probably including temporal-occipital visual word form and lexical regions, an inferior parietal phonological encoding region, and Broca's area in the inferior frontal lobe. The right hemisphere also participates but to a much smaller degree than the left hemisphere. See also color plate. (Reproduced with permission from Price *et al.*, 1998.)

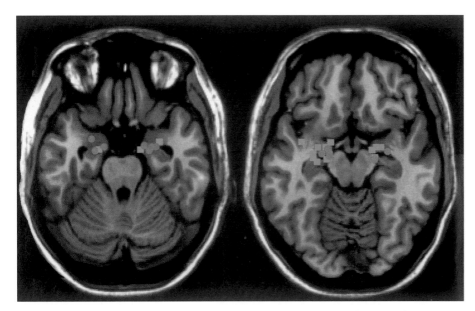

Figure 11.7. Functional magnetic resonance imaging demonstrates activation of both the left and right amygdalae when processing facial expressions of fright (green – see color plate) as well as during conditioned fear (red). Expressions of fright produce activity more in the left side of the upper amygdala than in the right side, whereas the response to conditioned fear is more evenly distributed. (Reproduced with permission from Vass, 2004.)

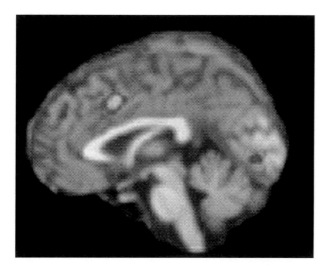

Figure 12.2. Functional magnetic resonance study demonstrates activation of the anterior cingulate gyrus region in the monitoring of conflict (incongruent trials). (Reproduced with permission from Kerns *et al.*, 2004.)

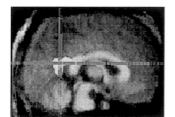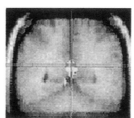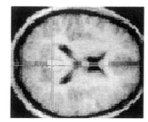

Figure 12.4. Functional magnetic resonance study demonstrates activation of the posterior cingulate gyrus region (including retrosplenial cortex) in assessing the familiarity of a person (faces or voices). (Reproduced with permission from Shah *et al.*, 2001.)

Chapter

13

Limbic system: Overview

Introduction

The term limbic lobe was used by the French physician, Paul Broca, to designate the structures on the limbus or margin of the neocortex. These structures lie in a C-shaped arc on the medial and basilar surfaces of the cerebral hemispheres that surround the lateral ventricles (Figure 13.1). Broca defined the limbic lobe as the parahippocampal and cingulate gyri (*le grand lobe limbique*). In addition to the limbic cortex, a number of subcortical structures can be added that make up what is today considered the limbic system. The subcortical structures include the hippocampus, the amygdala and the septal nuclei. Depending on the author, the list of limbic structures can be expanded to include portions of the hypothalamus and thalamus, the habenula, the raphe nuclei, the ventral tegmental nucleus, the nucleus accumbens, the basal nucleus (of Meynert), the posterior frontal orbital cortex, and others (Trimble, 1991; Van Hoesen *et al.*, 1996).

The limbic system works in collaboration with other brain systems. Therefore, a more complete theory of the function of the limbic system can be developed only in tandem with a more complete understanding of the entire brain. The limbic system provides the animal with a means of coping with the environment and with other members of the species found in that environment. More basic parts of the system are concerned with primal activities (i.e., food and sex), while others are related to feelings and emotions. More sophisticated parts of the system combine the external and internal inputs into one whole reality. This chapter attempts to present an overview of the limbic system.

Imaging studies show that the localization of pathological functioning in schizophrenia is predominantly in the anterior cingulate and hippocampal/parahippocampal cortices (Tamminga, 1998). The limbic cortices are a major target of dopaminergic fibers, and dopamine has been implicated in schizophrenia (Chapter 3). In addition, the highest concentration of *N*-methyl-D-aspartic acid (NMDA)-sensitive glutamate receptors is found in the hippocampus and anterior cingulate cortex. Glutamate also has been implicated in schizophrenia (Tamminga, 1998).

Anatomy

The basic anatomical components of the limbic system include:

- Cortical structures:
  - Parahippocampal gyrus.
  - Cingulate gyrus.

- Subcortical structures:
  - Hippocampal formation.
  - Amygdala.
  - Septal nuclei.

Structures that are closely linked with the limbic system include:

- Olfactory system.
- Sensory association cortices.
- Hypothalamus.
- Nucleus accumbens.
- Orbital prefrontal cortex.

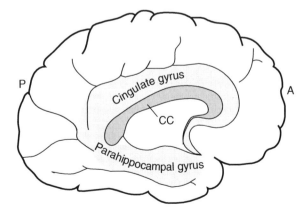

Figure 13.1. The limbic lobe consists of the parahippocampal gyrus and cingulate gyrus, which form an arch around the corpus callosum (see Figure 12.1). A, anterior; P, posterior; CC, corpus callosum.

The limbic system is the anatomical substrate of behaviors including social behaviors that assure the survival of the individual and of the species. Social interaction in many species continues to rely on the importance of olfactory cues. Olfactory cues are of lesser importance to humans but the emotions and behaviors controlled by the limbic system remain critical for human survival. The complex interconnections that allow the limbic system to perform its many functions can be simplified into two subsystems. The hippocampus and septal nuclei make up one subsystem; the hippocampal formation is associated with memory. The second subsystem revolves around the amygdala and is involved with the assignment of anxiety to sensory stimuli. A brief discussion of the olfactory system is followed by an overall view of the interactions of limbic structures and their interactions.

Olfactory structures

The olfactory system plays an important role in limbic function in many animals. The olfactory stria is made up of fibers that arise from the olfactory bulb and terminate in limbic structures (Figure 13.2; no. 1 and 2, Figure 13.3). The targets of these olfactory fibers include prepyriform and pyriform areas, the entorhinal cortex, and the underlying amygdala (Figures 11.1 and 13.2). For many years these connections led authors to assume that the limbic system processed olfactory cues.

Olfactory connections with the limbic structures account for the emotional aspects of olfaction. The olfactory cues are vital to many animals for appropriate social interaction and for affiliative behavior. Olfactory cues, however, are relatively unimportant to humans.

Hippocampal formation and related structures

Parahippocampal gyrus

The rostral parahippocampal gyrus includes portions of the pyriform lobe and receives primary olfactory information. The caudal part of the parahippocampal gyrus is represented by the entorhinal cortex (Figures 11.2 and 13.2). The primary source of input into the entorhinal cortex is the multimodal association areas of the cortex. The entorhinal cortex represents the port of entry into the hippocampal formation (Chapter 11).

Hippocampal formation

The hippocampal formation consists of the hippocampus proper along with the dentate gyrus and the subiculum (Figure 11.3). Sensory signals are directed toward the hippocampus by way of relays in the entorhinal cortex and the dentate gyrus (Figures 11.3 and 13.4). In addition to information arriving from the entorhinal cortex, there is input from the hypothalamus, the septal nuclei, and the amygdala.

Outgoing projections from the hippocampal formation are represented by the axons of the pyramidal neurons of the hippocampus as well as axons from the subiculum. These axons are distributed largely through the fornix (no. 2, Figure 13.5). The fornix projects to the septal nuclei, to the ventromedial hypothalamus and to the mammillary bodies of the hypothalamus (no. 20, Figure 13.5). The fibers of the fornix that terminate in the septal nuclei make up the precommissural fornix (no. 14, Figure 13.5). The fibers from the hippocampus to the septal nuclei contribute to the "septohippocampal axis," which is especially important to nonprimate mammals. Other fibers project directly to the amygdala (Canteras and Swanson, 1992).

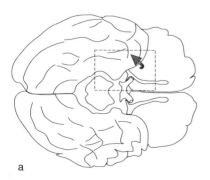

a

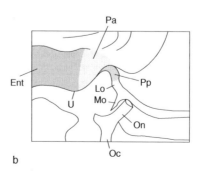

b

Figure 13.2. The ventromedial temporal lobe is rolled back (arrow) and enlarged to show the components of the pyriform lobe (see Figure 5.2). These components include the prepyriform area (Pp), the periamygdaloid area (Pa) and the entorhinal area (Ent). Other structures include the lateral olfactory stria (Lo), medial olfactory stria (Mo), uncus (U), optic nerve (On), and optic chiasm (Oc).

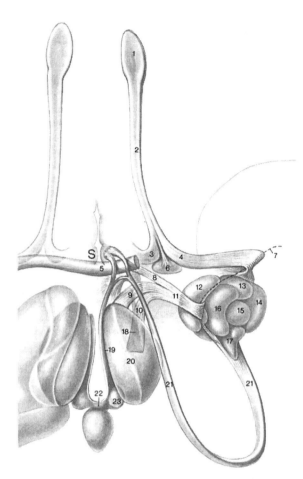

Figure 13.3. Dorsal view of some of the connections of the amygdala. 1–4, olfactory structures; 5, anterior commissure; 6, olfactory tubercle; 7, limen insulae; 8, diagonal band (of Broca); 9, inferior thalamic peduncle; 10, medial telencephalic fasciculus; 11, ventral amygdalofugal pathway; 12–17, amygdala; 18, lateral hypothalamic area; 19–20, nucleus and stria medullaris; 21, stria terminalis; 22, habenular commissure; 23, habenular nuclei; S, septal nuclei. (Modified with permission from Nieuwenhuys, R., Voogd, J., and Van Huijzen, C. 1988. The Human Nervous System. New York: Springer-Verlag.)

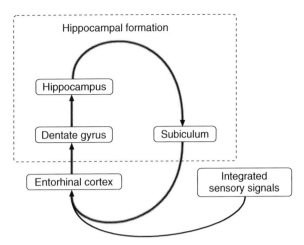

Figure 13.4. The hippocampal formation consists of the dentate gyrus, the subiculum, and the hippocampus proper. Sensory signals enter the hippocampal formation by way of the entorhinal cortex. A feedback loop exists between the hippocampus and the entorhinal cortex. This circuit facilitates the memory function of the hippocampus.

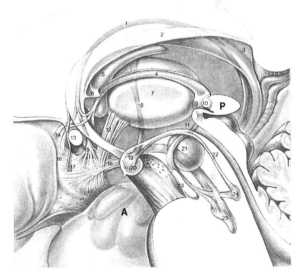

Figure 13.5. Limbic system structures located close to the midline. 1, stria terminalis; 2–3, fornix and commissure; 4, stria medullaris; 6, medial thalamic nuclei; 8, mammillothalamic tract; 9, habenular nuclei; 10, habenular commissure; 11, habenulointerpeduncular tract; 12, inferior thalamic peduncle; 13, anterior commissure; 14, precommissural fornix; 15, stria terminalis; 17, lamina terminalis; 20, mammillary body; 21, red nucleus; 22, mammillotegmental tract; 23, interpeduncular nucleus; 24, dorsal tegmental nucleus; 25, central superior nucleus (raphe); A, amygdala; P, pineal. (Modified with permission from Nieuwenhuys, R., Voogd, J., and Van Huijzen, C. 1988. The Human Nervous System. New York: Springer-Verlag.)

Septal nuclei and nucleus accumbens

The septum pellucidum is a thin, membranous midline structure that separates the left and right lateral ventricles (Figure 7.1). The space between the two leaflets of the septum pellucidum is called the cavum septum pellucidum. The cavum is seen during fetal development but normally disappears during infancy. The nuclei that make up the septal complex are situated below the corpus callosum and just in front of the anterior commissure. The lateral septal nucleus lies on the lateral aspect of the base of the septum pellucidum (Figure 7.1). Just below and slightly medial to the lateral septal nucleus is

the medial septal nucleus. Both of these nuclei are relatively small. The nucleus of the diagonal band of Broca is included as part of the septal nuclear complex. All

Case 1

A 35-year-old patient with a history of treatment-resistant schizophrenia since age 21 was readmitted for an acute exacerbation. The patient had a significant formal thought disorder with loosening of association and tangential speech. Neurological examination revealed subtle dysmetria and dysdiadochokinesia of the left arm. A computed tomographic scan revealed a large, cyst-like structure interposed between the bodies of the lateral ventricles (Wolf *et al.*, 1994). Agenesis of the septum pellucidum has been described in some cases of chronic psychosis but much less frequently than agenesis of the cavum septum pellucidum. Direct pathways from the cerebellum to the septum may be related to the dysmetria (Heath *et al.*, 1978).

Case 2

A 31-year-old male patient presented with a long history of chronic paranoid schizophrenia that was unresponsive to treatment. He had a history of enuresis and febrile seizures between the ages of 2 and 4 and was reported to be notably awkward at sports as a child. He also had developed polydipsia after the onset of psychosis. On examination he demonstrated difficulty with tandem walking. He had a total IQ score of 120 with a 136 for verbal and 95 for performance. Magnetic resonance imaging revealed the absence of the septum pellucidum and marked dilation of the lateral ventricles (Wolf *et al.*, 1994). Lesions of dysgenesis of the septal region may have cognitive or emotional manifestations, or both, given the region's key role in the limbic system.

of these nuclei are important sources of acetylcholine (Gaykema *et al.*, 1990).

The nucleus accumbens lies immediately lateral to the septal nuclei. It is generally considered to be part of the corpus striatum (Chapter 7). Nucleus accumbens consists of a core and more medially located shell. Separate functions have been assigned to each (Ito *et al.*, 2004).

Amygdala

The many nuclei of the amygdala are summarized in Chapter 11 (12–17, Figure 13.3). Overall, the amygdala has access to integrated sensory information from higher-order cortical areas. The sensory information that reaches the amygdala provides details that help identify the object rather than determine its location (Amaral *et al.*, 1992). Auditory signals may arrive directly from the medial geniculate body (Norita and Kawamura,

1980). Dopaminergic fibers arrive from the ventral tegmental area (Figure 10.2). Other connections link the amygdala directly with the orbital cortex of the frontal lobe (Figure 13.6). The extended amygdala consists of a corridor of cells that extend forward from the amygdala to the nucleus accumbens (Alheid and Heimer, 1996). In addition, a special relationship exists between the amygdala and the hippocampal formation (Figure 13.7). There are direct fibers between these two limbic structures as well as an indirect link from the amygdala back to the hippocampal formation by way of the entorhinal cortex (Figures 11.3, 13.6, and 13.7).

One group of fibers that leaves the amygdala makes up the stria terminalis, which arches dorsally and terminates in the hypothalamus, thalamus, and nucleus accumbens (21, Figure 13.3; 1, Figure 13.5). A second contingent of fibers projects ventrally from the

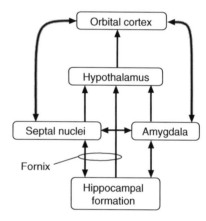

Figure 13.6. The amygdala and septal nuclei both interact directly with the orbital cortex. Hippocampal input to the orbital cortex is by way of the hypothalamus.

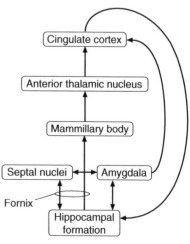

Figure 13.7. The amygdala projects to the cingulate gyrus via the stria terminalis and the ventral amygdalofugal pathway. The septal nuclei and amygdala interact with the hippocampus and the circuit of Papez.

amygdala to the septal nuclei, the nucleus accumbens, and the orbital cortex as well as to the hypothalamus and thalamus (no. 8–11, Figure 13.3; Gloor, 1997).

Behavioral considerations

The limbic system has extensive connections within itself and with almost all other areas of the brain. Most of the data supporting such circuitry come from animal work. It should be noted that although much of the limbic circuitry has been identified, the specific contributions of each circuit to our emotional and cognitive behaviors are not yet fully known.

The loop formed by the hippocampus, fornix, and mammillary bodies, mammillothalamic tract, anterior thalamic nuclei, cingulate gyrus, and projections back to the hippocampus form the circuit of Papez (Figures 12.3 and 13.8). Papez (1937) described this circuit as the substrate of "a harmonious mechanism which may elaborate the functions of central emotions."

Two functional divisions of the limbic system have been suggested (Mega *et al.*, 1997). An older paleocortical division has the amygdala and orbital prefrontal cortex at its center. The newer archicortical division has the hippocampus and cingulate cortex at its center. The older division functions in the integration of affect, drive, and object association, while the newer division functions in explicit sensory processing, encoding, and attentional control. The authors suggest that the distinction between the orbital prefrontal/amygdala division (emotional associations and appetitive drives) and the hippocampal/cingulate division (mnemonic and attentional processes) can further our interpretation of limbic system disorders. They further suggest that psychiatric disorders can be reinterpreted within a brain-based framework of limbic dysfunction and divided into three general groups: decreased (e.g., depression, Kluver–Bucy), increased (e.g., mania, obsessive-compulsive disorder), and dysfunctional (e.g., psychosis) limbic syndromes.

Hippocampal formation and related structures

The hippocampal formation is of primary importance in the storage and in the recall of new information in the form of declarative memory (Chapter 11). Declarative memory is based on configural learning in both space and time. Nondeclarative memory (e.g., motor skills, habits, emotions) is independent of the hippocampus (Squire, 1992). The hippocampal formation retains new

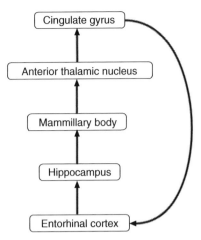

Figure 13.8. The classic circuit of Papez provides feedback to the hippocampus by way of the cingulate gyrus (compare with Figure 12.3). The fornix connects the hippocampus with the mammillary body. The mammillothalamic tract ascends to the anterior thalamic nucleus. The cingulum contains the efferents from the cingulate gyrus to the entorhinal cortex.

information for only a short time. The long-term storage of new information is dependent on neocortical areas and may be coincident with the same sensory association areas that first supplied the information to the hippocampal formation. Feedback signals from the hippocampus to sensory association areas may be important in the consolidation of new memory. The hippocampal–entorhinal circuit provides a feedback pathway and is hypothesized to be a reinforcement circuit that lowers the threshold of the neurons of the entorhinal cortex in order to more quickly recognize a pattern of sensory signals (Figure 13.4; Buzsaki *et al.*, 1990).

Memory is believed to reflect a conceptual cognitive map that is inherent to the hippocampal formation and possibly to the hippocampus itself (Jarrard, 1993). Verbal and contextual memory may have developed from mechanisms already in place in the hippocampal formation. The mapping concept has been extended by some authors to include linguistic and semantic relationships (Gloor, 1997).

Bilateral damage to the hippocampal formation has a devastating effect on the ability to store and recall new information. Even minor damage to the hippocampus can produce significant and lasting memory impairments (Zola-Morgan and Squire, 1993). Left temporal lobe damage affects verbal learning, whereas right temporal lobe damage affects nonverbal learning.

Projections from the hippocampal formation make up the fornix, and many of the fibers of the fornix terminate in the septal nuclei and in the mammillary bodies (nos. 2 and 20, Figure 13.5; S, Figure 13.3; Figures 13.6 and 13.7). Lesions of the fornix are reported to produce amnesia (Von Cramon and Schuri, 1992). Lesions seen in the mammillary bodies in Korsakoff syndrome also correlate with amnesia (Kopelman, 1995). Damage to other related structures including the medial thalamus (Chapter 9) can also produce amnesia.

The theta rhythm is an electroencephalographic (EEG) pattern ranging from 4 Hz to 12 Hz that has been recorded from the hippocampus of rodents and rabbits during certain behavioral conditions (Vanderwolf, 1988). It has been speculated that the theta rhythm is important in arousal and in the creation of a spatial map that is conducive to learning. Surprisingly the theta rhythm appears to be absent in primates and humans (Huh *et al.*, 1990).

Septal nuclei and nucleus accumbens

The septal nuclei have been implicated in memory (S, Figure 13.3). They, along with the basal nucleus (of Meynert) are cholinergic nuclei and exhibit degeneration in Alzheimer disease (Arendt *et al.*, 1983; Coyle *et al.*, 1983). Lesions in humans that include the septal area can produce memory loss along with hyperemotionality (Bondi *et al.*, 1993).

A cavity in the septum pellucidum (cavum septum pellucidum) of varying size has been reported to occur in up to 85% of the population (Figure 13.9; Nopoulos *et al.*, 1996, 1997). The presence or absence of a cavum septum pellucidum does not differentiate between control and psychiatric patients. However, a significant number of moderate to large (grade 3–4) cavum septi pellucidi were found only in schizophrenia (Shioiri *et al.*, 1996) and in patients with affective disorder and schizotypal personality disorder (Kwon *et al.*, 1998). The closure of the cavum is influenced developmentally by the enlargement of the corpus callosum and hippocampus. The large cavum may reflect the relatively small size of the corpus callosum and hippocampus during the developmental period when the cavum normally closes. This is consistent with the unconfirmed speculation that the severity of cavum septum pellucidum enlargement may correlate with childhood-onset schizophrenia (Nopoulos *et al.*, 1998; Takahashi, *et al.*, 2008).

The nucleus accumbens is well recognized as a reward center of the brain (Figures 7.1 and 13.10). It is associated with locomotor activity and reinforcing actions of psychostimulants and other drugs of abuse. The action of mood-elevating drugs is believed

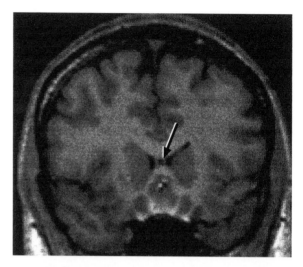

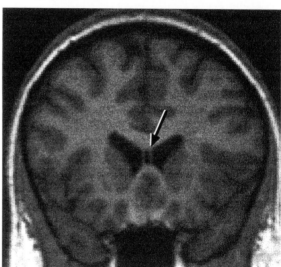

Figure 13.9. A cavum septum pellucidum is found in both normal and schizophrenia populations; however, it is consistently larger in schizophrenia. The cavum septum pellucidum in normal individuals is rated "small" (top arrow) when seen on up to two contiguous magnetic resonance (MR) 1.5 mm coronal slices. The cavum septum pellucidum is rated "large" when seen on at least four contiguous MR 1.5 mm coronal slices (bottom arrow). (Modified with permission from Nopoulos, P., Swayze, V., Flaum, M., Ehrhardt, J.C., Yuh, W.T., and Andreasen, N.C. 1997. Cavum septi pellucidi in normals and patients with schizophrenia as detected by magnetic resonance imaging. Biol. Psychiatry 41:1102–1108.)

to coincide with dopamine release in the nucleus accumbens (Self and Nestler, 1995). Peoples *et al.* (2004) showed that neurons of nucleus accumbens increased activity with the onset of cocaine administration. In contrast, drugs that block the dopamine receptor sites result in an increase in alcohol consumption in rats (Dyr *et al.*, 1993). Components of drug withdrawal correlate

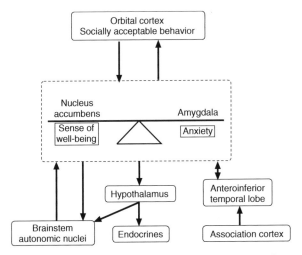

Figure 13.10. A speculative overall scheme of the elements of the limbic system suggests that a balance normally exists between the septal nuclei (contentment) and the amygdala (anxiety). Incoming sensations are identified by cortical association areas and are labeled with a degree of familiarity by the anterior inferior temporal lobe, including the hippocampus. The orbital cortex serves as a reservoir of past experience with social situations. The assignment of emotion by the septal–amygdala complex is influenced by the current autonomic state. The septal–amygdala complex effects emotional responses via the hypothalamus and brainstem autonomic centers.

with a decrease in dopamine release and an increase in acetylcholine release in the nucleus accumbens (Rossetti *et al.*, 1992). Anxiety coincident with drug withdrawal may be due to an increase in activity in the amygdala subsequent to a decrease in dopamine from the ventral tegmental area (Pilotte and Sharpe, 1996). A decrease in dopamine in the amygdala and hippocampus is hypothesized to produce anxiety or cravings, or both, for substances that provide temporary relief by releasing dopamine (Blum *et al.*, 1996).

The shell of the nucleus accumbens is an important target for psychoactive drugs. The shell appears to strengthen stimulus-reward associations in response to dopamine. Addictive drugs increase dopamine in the extracellular space in the accumbens shell rather than the core in both rats and humans (Di Chiara, 2002). The bed nucleus of the stria terminalis, part of the extended amygdala, is also sensitive to psychoactive drugs. Caffeine is a nonaddictive drug and does not increase dopamine in the shell (Acquas *et al.*, 2002; Ikemoto, 2003). Food rewards (e.g., chocolate) also produce dopamine release in the accumbens shell (Bassareo *et al.*, 2002; Di Chiara and Bassareo, 2007). Less activation was seen for both in the core. Release of dopamine in the shell is instrumental in learning the association

between drugs and the stimuli that predict their availability (Di Chiara, 1998). This learning is described as pathological because it does not undergo habituation as does the food-associated learning (Bassareo *et al.*, 2003; Everitt and Robbins, 2005). The core is believed to operate in conjunction with the prefrontal cortex to provide motivation to seek out a reward and convert the motivation to action (Di Chiara, 1999).

Zubieta *et al.* (2002) found that women showed reduced activation of the μ-opioid system in the accumbens nucleus ipsilateral to a pain stimulus when compared with men. Theoretically this reduction would allow more efficient pain transmission and is consistent with studies that found that women show higher perceptual responses to pain (Fillingham and Maixner, 1995; Coghill *et al.*, 1999). Women are also diagnosed more frequently with persistent pain conditions (Unruh, 1996).

Amygdala and related structures

New incoming sensory signals arriving at the sensory association cortices are made available simultaneously to the amygdala and the hippocampus. The hippocampus recalls specific facets of the sensory experience and links them with details of past events, especially with regard to visual signals. It has been suggested that sensory information reaches the amygdala by two routes. One route is direct via the thalamus and supports a quick, primitive emotional response. The second route is indirect via the cortex and results in a slower, more cognitive response (Kandel and Kupfermann, 1995).

Once the stimulus arrives in the amygdala it is recognized and an affective dimension is attached to the stimulus. Evidence suggests that the amygdala represents the central fear system and that it is critical in the acquisition and expression of conditioned fear as well as anxiety (Davis, 1992). The appropriate emotional significance is attached if the current event occurs in the context of a previously learned psychoaffective atmosphere related to social events and other forms of affiliative behavior. The amygdala responds by activating three sets of connections. First, the amygdala recruits appropriate autonomic and endocrine responses through its connections with the hypothalamus and brainstem. Second, the amygdala sends signals back to the hippocampus to reaffirm the emotional significance of the signals that have simultaneously entered the hippocampus. Finally both the hippocampus and the amygdala project signals back to the sensory association cortices, where, with time, the memory of the event is probably created. The next time the same constellation of sensory signals arrives at the sensory association cortex the learned emotional response will be elicited more efficiently. If, in the future, less than the entire set of sensory signals is experienced, the amygdala-hippocampus axis may be triggered to respond with the same emotions (Kesner, 1992).

Connections between the amygdala and the orbital prefrontal cortex are important in formulating reactions to socially significant stimuli and for controlling aggressive behavior (De Bruin, 1990). In some cases a minimal set of stimuli may be able to reactivate a vague recollection of a past experience without the specifics of that experience, producing the sense of *déjà vu* (Gloor, 1997). Connections with the posterior cingulate gyrus have been implicated to be important in the conscious appreciation of anxiety (McGuire *et al.*, 1994); however, others believe that the prefrontal cortex is of particular importance in the appreciation of emotions generated in the amygdala (Kandel and Kupfermann, 1995).

Kluver and Bucy (1939) showed that a bilateral lesion of the anterior temporal lobe produced a marked change in the behavior of the normally aggressive rhesus monkey. Lesioned animals were remarkably tame. Fear and aggression were lost. When released in the wild the monkeys showed no aggressive response when attacked by strangers. They were aloof of the social group and lost all social status. Although in the laboratory they exhibited abnormal sexual behavior with greatly increased autoerotic homosexual or heterosexual activity, they engaged in no sexual behavior in the wild. Mothers lost interest in their infants. Oral behavior was exaggerated and they examined everything orally. They became indiscriminate in their dietary preferences. They ate previously rejected foods and ate nonfood items including feces. They exhibited hypermetamorphosis, which is a tendency to attend to and to react to every visual stimulus. At the same time they exhibited visual agnosia. These behaviors make up the Kluver–Bucy syndrome.

Other behavioral considerations

Kluver–Bucy syndrome

The complete Kluver–Bucy syndrome is seldom seen in humans (Yilmaz *et al.*, 2008; Kile *et al.*, 2009). Humans with bilateral temporal lobe damage who are described as exhibiting the Kluver–Bucy syndrome are very placid and are indiscriminate in dietary preferences. They tend to examine all objects orally, and several have

died from stuffing their mouths with inedible objects (e.g., Styrofoam cups, surgical gauze, toilet paper, etc.; Mendez and Foti, 1997). Hypersexuality is rare; however, inappropriate sexual commentary is common (Trimble *et al.*, 1997).

Temporal lobe epilepsy

A full-blown temporal lobe seizure is often preceded by an aura indicating limbic involvement. The aura may include olfactory hallucinations, visceral sensations, fear, *dèjá vu*, and motor automatisms. Behavioral disorders may be seen in the interictal period (Trimble *et al.*, 1997). These disorders include depression, schizophreniform psychosis, and an interictal behavior syndrome that consists of affective disturbances and long-term personality changes. Delusions may appear several years after the onset of seizures.

A subset of these patients present with the Gastaut–Geschwind syndrome, which consists of a constellation of behaviors that include hyperreligiosity, hypergraphia, exaggerated philosophical concerns, sexual dysfunction, and irritability. This syndrome has been subdivided into three subgroups of behavior (Bear, 1986). The first is an alteration of physiological drives including sexual behavior, aggression, and fear. The second is a preoccupation with religious, moral, and philosophical concepts. Finally, the patient is unable to terminate an idea, often during a conversation, and to move on to another topic.

Patients with temporal lobe epilepsy may exhibit hyperemotionality and increased aggression. Thirty percent of psychiatric patients with intermittent violent outbursts have temporal lobe epilepsy (Elliot, 1992). Projections from the temporolimbic area to the brainstem periaqueductal gray and raphe nuclei (Figures 10.2 and 11.5) may account for the decreased levels of serotonin reported to be associated with violent behavior and suicide (Marazziti and Conti, 1991).

Hallucinations and delusions are associated with limbic dysfunction that involves both superficial and deep structures of the temporal lobe (Elliott *et al.*, 2009). The delusions are often of the paranoid type and are seen in approximately 10% of patients with temporal lobe epilepsy. Delusions are more often seen if the left temporal lobe is involved, whereas the presence of auditory or visual hallucinations correlates with right temporal lobe epilepsy. Recruitment of the frontal lobe may be required together with temporal lobe activity to produce a delusion (Trimble *et al.*, 1997).

Other behavioral considerations

George *et al.* (1995) showed that episodes of transient sadness experienced by a group of healthy women activated bilateral limbic and paralimbic structures as measured by relative blood flow. In contrast, transient happiness corresponded with no regions of increased activity but did correspond with widespread reductions in blood flow, especially in the right prefrontal and bilateral temporoparietal regions.

Intravenous procaine activates limbic structures in animals; in humans, it evokes emotional and psychosensory experiences, including dysphoria, euphoria, fear, and hallucinations. Procaine-induced auditory hallucinations correlate with superior temporal activation. Procaine-induced visual hallucinations correlate with left mesial occipital lobe and amygdala activation coupled with right anterior cingulate and lateral frontal lobe activation (Ketter *et al.*, 1996). An increase in brain activity bilaterally following procaine injection has been reported in limbic areas, including the parahippocampal gyri, insula, and anterior cingulate cortex (Servan-Schreiber and Perlstein, 1997). Videotape stimuli have been shown to increase blood flow in the amygdala and anterior cingulate gyrus of recovering cocaine addicts when compared with lifelong abstainers (Childress *et al.*, 1999).

Select bibliography

Aggleton, J.P. ed. *The Amygdala. A Functional Analysis*, (2nd ed.). (Oxford UK: Oxford University Press, 2000.)

Andersen, P., Morris, R., Amaral, D., Bliss, T., and O'Keefe, J. eds. *The Hippocampus Book*. (New York: Oxford University Press, 2007.)

Gloor, P. *The Temporal Lobe and Limbic System*. (New York: Oxford University Press, 1997.)

LeDoux, J. *The Emotional Brain*. (New York: Simon & Schuster, 1996.)

Rolls, E.T. *The Brain and Emotion*. (New York: Oxford University Press, 1999.)

Salloway, S., Malloy, P., and Cummings, J.L. eds. *The Neuropsychiatry of Limbic and Subcortical Disorders*. (Washington D.C.: American Psychiatric Press, 1997.)

Whalen, P.J., and Phelps, E.A. eds. *The Human Amygdala*. (New York: Guilford Press, 2009.)

References

Acquas, E., Tanda, G., and Di Chiara, G. 2002. Differential effects of caffeine on dopamine and acetylcholine transmission in brain areas of drug-naïve and caffeine-pretreated rats. *Neuropsychopharmacology* 27:182–193.

Alheid, G.F., and Heimer, L. 1996. Theories of basal forebrain organization and the "emotional motor system." In: G.Holstege, R.Bandler, and C.B.Saper (eds.) *The Emotional Motor System*. Amsterdam: Elsevier, pp. 461–484.

Amaral, D.G., Price, J.L., Pitkanen, A., and Carmichael, S.T. 1992. Anatomical organization of the primate amygdaloid complex. In: J.P.Aggleton (ed.) *The Amygdala: Neurobiological Aspects of Emotion, Memory, and Mental Dysfunction*. New York: Wiley-Liss, pp. 1–66.

Arendt, T., Bigl, V., Arendt, A., and Tennstedt, A. 1983. Loss of neurons in the nucleus basalis of Meynert in Alzheimer's disease, paralysis agitans and Korsakoff's disease. *Acta Neuropathol.* **61**:101–108.

Bassareo, V., De Luca, M.A., and Di Chiara, G. 2002. Differential expression of motivational stimulus properties by dopamine in nucleus accumbens shell versus core and prefrontal cortex. *J. Neurosci.* **22**:4709–4719.

Bassareo, V., De Luca, M.A., Aresu, M., Aste, A., Ariu, T., and Di Chiara, G. 2003. Differential adaptive properties of accumbens shell dopamine responses to ethanol as a drug and as a motivational stimulus. *Eur. J. Neurosci.* **17**:1465–1472.

Bear, D. 1986. Behavioural changes in temporal lobe epilepsy: Conflict, confusion, challenge. In: M.R. Trimble, and T.G.Bolwig (eds.) *Aspects of Epilepsy and Psychiatry*. Chichester, England: Wiley, pp. 19–30.

Blum, K., Cull, J.G., Braverman, E.R., and Comings, D.E. 1996. Reward deficiency syndrome. *Am. Sci.* **84**:132–145.

Bondi, M.W., Kaszniak, A.W., Rapcsak, S.Z., and Butters, M. 1993. Implicit and explicit memory following anterior communicating artery aneurysm rupture. *Brain Cogn.* **22**:213–229.

Buzsaki, G., Chen, L.S., and Gage, F.H. 1990. Spatial organization of physiological activity in the hippocampus regions: Relevance to memory formation. In: J.Storm-Mathisen, R.Zimmer, and O.Ottersen (eds.) *Understanding the Brain Through the Hippocampus. Prog. Brain Res.* **83**:257–268.

Canteras, N.S., and Swanson, L.W. 1992. Projections of the ventral subiculum to the amygdala, septum, and hypothalamus: An PHAL anterograde tract-tracing study in the rat. *J. Comp. Neurol.* **324**:180–194.

Childress, A.R., Mozley, P.D., McElgin, W., Fitzgerald, J., Reivich, M., and O'Brien, C.P. 1999. Limbic activation during cue-induced cocaine craving. *Am. J. Psychiatry* **156**:11–18.

Coghill, R., Sang, C., Maisog,J., and Iadarola, M. 1999. Pain intensity processing within the human brain: a bilateral, distributed mechanism. *J. Neurophysiol.* **82**:1934–1943.

Coyle, J.T., Price, D.L., and DeLong, M.R. 1983. Alzheimer's disease: A disorder of cortical cholinergic innervation. *Science* **219**:1184–1190.

Davis, M. 1992. The role of the amygdala in fear and anxiety. *Annu. Rev. Neurosci.* **15**:353–375.

De Bruin, J.P.C. 1990. Social behaviour and the prefrontal cortex. In: H.B.M.Uylings, C.G.VanEden, J.P.C. DeGruin, M.A.Corner, and M.G.P.Feenstra (eds.) *The Prefrontal Cortex: Its Structure, Function and Pathology. Prog. Brain Res.* **85**:485–497.

Di Chiara, G. 1998. A motivational learning hypothesis of the role of mesolimbic dopamine in compulsive drug use. *J. Psychopharmacol.* **12**:54–67.

Di Chiara, G. 1999. Drug addiction as dopamine-dependent associative learning disorder. *Eur. J. Pharmacology* **375**:13–30.

Di Chiara, G. 2002. Nucleus accumbens shell and core dopamine: Differential role in behavior and addiction. *Behav. Brain Res.* **137**:75–114.

Di Chiara, G., and Bassareo, V. 2007. Reward system and addiction: What dopamine does and doesn't do. *Curr. Opin. Pharmacol.* **7**:69–76.

Dyr, W., McBride, W.J., Lumeng, T.K., and Murphy, J.M. 1993. Effects of D1 and D2 dopamine receptor agents on ethanol consumption in the high-alcohol-drinking (HAD) line of rats. *Alcohol* **10**:207–212.

Elliot, B., Joyce, E., and Shorvon, S., 2009. Delusions, illusions and hallucinations in epilepsy: 1. Elementary phenomena. Epilepsy Res. **85**:162–171.

Elliot, F.A. 1992. Violence: The neurological contribution: An overview. *Arch. Neurol.* **49**:595–603.

Everitt, B.J., and Robbins, T.W. 2005. Neural systems of reinforcement for drug addiction: From actions to habits to compulsion. *Nat. Neurosci.* **8**:1481–1489.

Fillingham, R., and Maixner, W. 1995. Gender differences in the responses to noxious stimuli. *PRN Forum* **4**: 209–221.

Gaykema, R.P.A., Luiten, P.G.M., Nyakas, C., and Traber, J. 1990. Cortical projection patterns of the medial septum-diagonal band complex. *J. Comp. Neurol.* **293**:103–124.

George, M.S., Ketter, T.A., Parekh, P.I., Horwitz, B., Herscovitch, P., and Post, R.M. 1995. Brain activity during transient sadness and happiness in healthy women. *Am. J. Psychiatry* **152**:341–351.

Gloor, P. 1997. *The Temporal Lobe and Limbic System*. New York: Oxford University Press.

Heath, R., Dempsy, C., Fontana, C., and Myers, W. 1978. Cerebellar stimulation: Effects on septal region, hippocampus, and amygdala of cats and rats. *Biol. Psychiatry* **13**:501–529.

Huh, K., Meador, K.J., Lee, G.P., Loring, D.W., Murrow, A.M., King, D.W., Gallagher, B.B., Smith, J.R., and

Flanigin, H.F. 1990. Human hippocampal EEG: Effects of behavioral activation. *Neurology* **40**:1177–1181.

Ikemoto, S. 2003. Involvement of the olfactory tubercle in cocaine reward: Intracranial self-administration studies. *J. Neurosci.* **23**:9305–9311.

Ito, R., Tobbins, T.W., and Everitt, B.J. 2004. Differential control over cocaine-seeking behavior by nucleus accumbens core and shell. *Nat. Neurosci.* **7**:389–397.

Jarrard, L.E. 1993. On the role of the hippocampus in learning and memory in the rat. *Behav. Neural. Biol.* **60**:9–26.

Kandel, E., and Kupfermann, I. 1995. Emotional states. In: E.R.Kandel, J.H.Schwartz, and T.M.Jessell (eds.) *Essentials of Neural Science and Behavior*. Norwalk, CT: Appleton & Lange, pp. 595–612.

Kesner, R.P. 1992. Learning and memory in rats with an emphasis on the role of the amygdala. In: J.Aggleton (ed.) *The Amygdala*. New York: Wiley, pp. 379–400.

Ketter, T.A., Andreaseon, P.J., George, M.S., Lee, C., Gill, D.S., Parekh, P.I., Willis, M.W., Herscovitch, P., and Post, R.M. 1996. Anterior paralimbic mediation of procaine-induced emotional and psychosensory experiences. *Arch. Gen. Psychiatry* **53**:59–69.

Kile, S.J., Ellis, W.G., Olichney, J.M., Farias, S., and DeCarli, C. 2009. Alzheimer abnormalities of the amygdala with Kluver-Bucy syndrome symptoms: An amygdaloid variant of Alzheimer disease. *Arch. Neurol.* **66**:125–129.

Kluver, H., and Bucy, P.C. 1939. Preliminary analysis of functions of the temporal lobe in monkeys. *Arch. Neurol. Psychiatry* **42**:979–1000.

Kopelman, M.D. 1995. The Korsakoff syndrome. *Br. J. Psychiatry* **166**:154–173.

Kwon, J.S., Shenton, M.E., Hirayasu, Y., Salisbury, D.F., Fischer, I.A., Dickey, C.C., Yurgelun-Todd, D., Tohen, M., Kikinis, R., Jolesz, F.A., and McCarley, R.W. 1998. MRI study of cavum septi pellucidi in schizophrenia, affective disorder, and schizotypal personality disorder. *Am. J. Psychiatry* **155**:509–515.

Marazziti, D., and Conti, L. 1991. Aggression, hyperactivity, and platelet IMI-binding. *Acta Psychiatr. Scand.* **84**:209–211.

McGuire, P.K., Bench, C.J., Frith, C.D., Marks, I.M., Frackowiak, R.S.J., and Dolan, R.J. 1994. Functional anatomy of obsessive-compulsive phenomena. *Br. J. Psychiatry* **164**:459–468.

Mega, M.S., Cummings, J.C., Salloway, S., and Malloy, P. 1997. The limbic system: An anatomic, phylogenetic, and clinical perspective. *J. Neuropsychiatry Clin. Neurosci.* **9**:315–330.

Mendez, M.F., and Foti, D. 1997. Lethal hyperoral behavior from the Kluver–Bucy syndrome. *J. Neurol. Neurosurg. Psychiatry* **62**:293–294.

Nopoulos, P., Swayze, V., and Andreasen, N.C. 1996. Pattern of brain morphology in patients with schizophrenia and large cavum septi pellucidi. *J. Neuropsychiatry Clin. Neurosci.* **8**:147–152.

Nopoulos, P., Swayze, V., Flaum, M., Ehrhardt, J.C., Yuh, W.T., and Andreasen, N.C. 1997. Cavum septi pellucidi in normals and patients with schizophrenia as detected by magnetic resonance imaging. *Biol. Psychiatry* **41**:1102–1108.

Nopoulos, P.C., Giedd, J.N., Andreasen, N.C., and Rapoport, J.L. 1998. Frequency and severity of enlarged cavum septi pellucidi in childhood-onset schizophrenia. *Am. J. Psychiatry* **155**:1074–1079.

Norita, M., and Kawamura, K. 1980. Subcortical afferents to monkey amygdala: An HRP study. *Brain Res.* **190**:225–230.

Papez, J.W. 1937. A proposed mechanism of emotion. *Arch. Neurol. Psychiatry* **38**:725–743.

Peoples, L., Lynch, K.G., Lesnock, J., and Gangdhar, N. 2004. Accumbal neural response during the initiation and maintenance of intravenous cocaine self-administration. *J. Neurophysiol.* **91**:314–323.

Pilotte, N.S., and Sharpe, L.G. 1996. Cocaine withdrawal alters regulatory elements of dopamine neurons. In: M.D.Majewska (ed.) *Neurotoxicity and Neuropathology Associated with Cocaine Abuse.* Rockville, MD: National Institutes of Health, pp. 193–202.

Rossetti, Z.L., Hmaidan, Y., and Gessa, G.L. 1992. Marked inhibition of mesolimbic dopamine release: A common feature of ethanol, morphine, cocaine and amphetamine abstinence in rats. *Eur. J. Pharmacol.* **221**:227–234.

Self, D.W., and Nestler, E.J. 1995. Molecular mechanisms of drug reinforcement and addiction. *Annu. Rev. Neurosci.* **18**:463–495.

Servan-Schreiber, D., and Perlstein, W.M. 1997. Pharmacologic activation of limbic structures and neuroimaging studies of emotions. *J. Clin. Psychiatry* **58**(Suppl. 16):13–15.

Shioiri, T., Oshitani, Y., Kato, T., Murashita, J., Hamakawa, H., Inubushi, T., Nagata, T., and Takahashi, S. 1996. Prevalence of cavum septum pellucidum detected by MRI in patients with bipolar disorder, major depression and schizophrenia. *Psychol. Med.* **26**:431–434.

Squire, L.R. 1992. Memory and the hippocampus: A synthesis from findings with rats, monkeys, and humans. *Psychol. Rev.* **99**:195–231.

Takahashi, T., Yung, A.R., Yücel, M., Wood, S., Phillips, L., Harding, I.H., Soulsby, B., McGorry, P.D., Suzuki, M., Velakoulis, D., and Pantelis, C., 2008. Prevalence of large cavum septi pellucidi in ultra high-risk individuals and patients with psychotic disorders. *Schizophr. Res.* **105**:236–244.

Tamminga, C.A. 1998. Schizophrenia and glutamatergic transmission. *Crit. Rev. Neurobiol.* **12**:21–36.

Trimble, M.R. 1991. *The Psychoses of Epilepsy.* New York: Raven Press.

Trimble, M.R., Mendez, M.F., and Cummings, J.L. 1997. Neuropsychiatric symptoms from the temporolimbic lobes. *J. Neuropsychiatry Clin. Neurosci.* **9**:429–438.

Unruh, A. 1996. Gender variations in clinical pain experience. *Pain* **65**:123–167.

Van Hoesen, G.W., Morecraft, R.J., and Semendeferi, K. 1996. Functional neuroanatomy of the limbic system and prefrontal cortex. In: B.S.Fogel, R.B.Schiffer, and S.M.Rao (eds.) *Neuropsychiatry.* Baltimore: Williams & Wilkins, pp. 113–143.

Vanderwolf, C.H. 1988. Cerebral activity and behavior: Control by central cholinergic and serotonergic systems. *Int. Rev. Neurobiol.* **30**:225–340.

Von Cramon, D.Y., and Schuri, U. 1992. The septo-hippocampal pathways and their relevance to human memory: A case report. *Cortex* **28**:411–422.

Wolf, S.S., Hyde, T.M., and Weinberger, D.R. 1994. Malformations of the septum pellucidum: Two distinctive cases in association with schizophrenia. *J. Psychiatry Neurosci.* **19**:140–144.

Yilmaz, C., Cemek, F., Guven, A.S., Caksen, H., Atas, B., and Tuncer, O. 2008. A child with incomplete Kluver-Bucy syndrome developed during acute encephalitis. *J. Emerg. Med.* **35**:210–211.

Zola-Morgan, S.M., and Squire, L.R. 1993. Neuroanatomy of memory. *Annu. Rev. Neurosci.* **16**:547–563.

Zubieta, J-K., Smith, Y.R., Bueller, J.A., Xu, Y., Kilbourn, M.R., Jewett, D.M., Meyer, C.R., Koeppe, R.A., and Stohler, C.S. 2002. μ-Opioid receptor-mediated antinociceptive responses differ in men and women. *J. Neurosci.* **22**:5100–5107.

Interhemispheric connections and laterality

Introduction

A hallmark of human brain function is cerebral lateralization and specialization. This specialization necessitates an efficient interhemispheric communication system. No other mammal possesses the degree of localization of function seen in the human. Only the human brain has the intellectual and computational capabilities necessary to study how neural systems both generate and respond to the intense information demands of the environment.

At first glance the anatomical brain appears largely symmetrical. More careful analysis reveals "typical counterclockwise hemispheric torque," which is reflected in the fact that the left parieto-occipital region is wider and extends further posteriorly than the right. On the right side the frontal lobe is larger than the left and extends further anteriorly (Glicksohn and Myslobodsky, 1993). This difference is called petalia (Hadziselimovic and Cus, 1966). Fiber bundles interconnect the left and right sides. It must be assumed that these bundles play a role in the behavioral specializations that are reflected in the laterality of behavior.

Cerebral blood flow is greater on the right than on the left in infants. Left parietal dominance emerges at about 2.5 years concordant with the onset of right-handedness and improved motor skills. Cerebral blood flow dominance shifts from right to left during the third year of life (Chiron *et al.*, 1997).

Speech has long been recognized to be localized in the left (dominant) hemisphere. The right hemisphere has been hypothesized to be specialized in emotional and visuospatial functions that are important in survival of the species (Geschwind and Galaburda, 1985). Norepinephrinergic and serotonergic pathways project more heavily to the right hemisphere (Robinson, 1985).

Interhemispheric communication

Corpus callosum

The corpus callosum is larger in the human than in any other mammal. It is a broad thick plate of fibers that reciprocally interconnects broad regions of the corresponding lobes of the cortex of the left and right side (Figures 14.1, 14.2, and 14.3). The fibers of the corpus callosum make up the floor of the longitudinal cerebral fissure, form most of the roof of the lateral ventricle, and fan out in a massive callosal radiation as they distribute to various cortical regions.

The corpus callosum can be divided into a series of function-specific channels (Zaidel *et al.*, 1990), which are as follows.

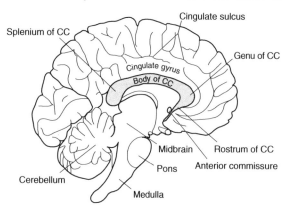

Figure 14.1. The corpus callosum (CC) consists of the rostrum, genu, body, and splenium. It forms the floor of the longitudinal cerebral fissure and lies below the cingulate gyrus.

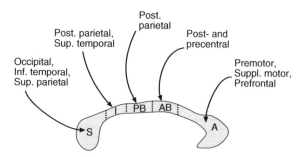

Figure 14.2. Cortical areas whose fibers contribute to each subdivision are indicated. The corpus callosum can be divided approximately in half by the junction of the anterior midbody (AB) and the posterior midbody (PB). The anterior third includes the rostrum, genu, and anterior body (A). The splenium (S) accounts for about the posterior fifth of the corpus callosum. I, isthmus.

Frontal pole

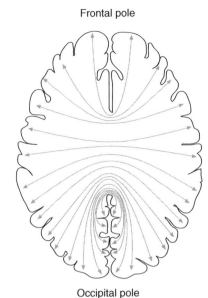

Figure 14.3.
Diagrammatic horizontal section of the brain shows the corpus callosum interconnecting the cortex on each side.

Occipital pole

- Rostrum, genu, and anterior body (Figures 14.1 and 14.2): These make up the anterior third of the corpus callosum. These anterior channels contain interconnecting fibers from the prefrontal, premotor, supplementary, and possibly anteroinferior parietal cortex. Anterior callosal channels are important for the interhemispheric transfer of control signals.
- Anterior midbody: The anterior midbody contains fibers that interconnect the precentral and postcentral gyri and possibly the midtemporal cortex. This channel is particularly important because it interconnects the primary motor cortex of the right and left sides.
- Posterior midbody: The posterior midbody interconnects the postcentral gyrus, the posterior parietal cortex, and possibly the midtemporal cortex. The two midbody channels coordinate motor activity across the midline.
- Isthmus: The isthmus interconnects the posterior parietal and superior temporal cortices, including the auditory cortex.
- Splenium: The splenium contains fibers that interconnect the inferior and ventral temporal cortices as well as the visual cortex of the occipital lobe. The more posterior channels interconnect sensory signals such as visual, auditory, and touch. The anterior corpus callosum is organized topographically but the splenium contains fibers that represent all sensory areas including

olfaction. A lesion sparing the splenium often results in minimal loss of function (Berlucchi, 2004).

The corpus callosum has been divided into seven regions for research purposes by Giedd *et al.* (1994, after Witelson, 1989). The maximum length was taken between the most anterior and posterior points and divided into half, thirds and a posterior fifth. A final perpendicular line was drawn through the anterior convexity of the anterior callosum.

The between-hemisphere corticocortical pathways and within-hemisphere corticocortical pathways have a common embryological origin (Trevarthen, 1990). Many of the fibers are unmyelinated, indicating that interhemisphere information transfer is relatively slow. In addition to providing communication between the left and right hemispheres, many of the neurons that give rise to the callosal fibers also give rise to within-hemisphere collateral fibers. Wherever the callosal fibers terminate in the contralateral hemisphere, the collateral fibers end in the homologous region of the ipsilateral hemisphere. These are referred to as symmetrical heterotopic connections and are common in association regions of the cortex (Liederman, 1995).

The corpus callosum provides a channel for communication between the two hemispheres. It serves three categories of tasks. First, callosal relay tasks are those tasks that can be performed by only one hemisphere. The corpus callosum allows stimuli to be relayed from one hemisphere to the other where the task can be performed. Second, it provides for coordination of direct access tasks, which are tasks that can be performed by either hemisphere. Third, it provides for transfer of signals for tasks that require the interaction of both hemispheres (Zaidel, 1995).

Some investigators speculate that maturation of the corpus callosum is a prerequisite to the finalization of hemispheric specialization. In humans, completion of callosal myelination approximately coincides with puberty. The splenium tends to contain more fibers in females than males, although there is significant overlap in the number of fibers between sexes. The midsagittal area of the corpus callosum is significantly larger in the female rat than in the male. Early postnatal exposure to cocaine abolishes this sexual dimorphism (Ojima *et al.*, 1996).

Disconnection of the hemispheres ("split brain") in an adult produces few disturbances of ordinary daily behavior, temperament, or intellect. Visual signals reach both sides of the cortex by way of fibers that cross in the optic chiasm and auditory signals that cross in the brainstem. Special tests that project sensory signals to either the left or right side have been performed (Gazzaniga, 2005). Results indicate that identical signals presented to the opposite cortex may sometimes produce conflicting emotional responses.

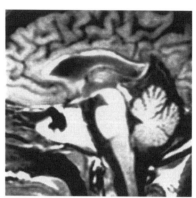

Figure 14.4. The patient's magnetic resonance image (T1-weighted, midsagittal view) revealed marked thinning of the corpus callosum as a result of demyelination. (Reprinted with permission from Mendez, 1995.)

Clinical vignette

A 38-year-old right-handed woman developed a personality change over a two-month period. She became progressively apathetic and disengaged. On examination, she had prominent psychomotor slowing, pallor of the left optic disk, left central facial nerve weakness, gait instability, sensory loss on the left side of her body, and upper motor neuron signs. Magnetic resonance imaging disclosed multiple subcortical and periventricular lesions and pronounced atrophy of the corpus callosum (Figure 14.4). An eventual frontal brain biopsy confirmed the presence of advanced multiple sclerosis. The patient's neuropsychological evaluation disclosed an interhemispheric disconnection syndrome from demyelination of her corpus callosum. She could formulate and write sentences with her right hand but not with her left. She could draw and copy figures with her left hand but not with her right. The spatial elements of her constructions were worse with her right hand than with her left hand. She had greater trouble naming items placed out-of-sight in her left hand as compared with her right hand. With her left hand, the patient had difficulty saluting, mimicking the use of a toothbrush, flipping a coin, pretending to comb her hair, and other praxis tasks. Finally, on a tachistoscopic task, the patient could not read any of the items presented in her left hemifield.

The presence of a number of small tracts interconnecting the left and right temporal lobes allows abnormal ongoing epileptic activity to be transmitted between the two lobes without necessarily involving the much larger corpus callosum. Since the corpus callosum is not involved, generalization of the epileptic activity may not occur. In such cases, the patient may be able to maintain some contact with the environment while at the same time experiencing a complex partial seizure. This should not be taken as evidence that the seizure is of psychogenic origin (pseudoseizure).

Signs and symptoms of complete callosal damage may include left ideomotor apraxia, right or bilateral construction apraxia, left agraphia, left tactile anomia, left alien hand sign, impaired bimanual coordination, alexia in the left visual field, anomia for objects felt with the left hand, and left visual anomia. Obvious symptoms usually appear only after large callosal lesions (Peru *et al.*, 2003). Certain lesions involving the corpus callosum, or association areas of the cortex that give rise to commissural fibers, produce disturbances of brain functions collectively known as disconnection syndromes. Split-brain patients may be slow to respond. Once one hemisphere is activated, it may be very difficult for the split-brain patient to activate the inactivated hemisphere. In such a situation, Sperry (1962) has questioned whether consciousness may have been shifted entirely to the active hemisphere. A common sequela of callosectomy is neglect. There is a significant tendency to neglect left-sided targets, and it is argued that this is due to underactivation of the nondominant hemisphere (Liederman, 1995). Mutism following callosal section is an extreme example of such an imbalance. Mutism is more common if speech is centered in one hemisphere and control of the dominant hand in the opposite hemisphere. The role of the corpus callosum in conscious awareness and cognitively determined behavior continues to be the subject of much research.

A role for the corpus callosum in the pathogenesis of schizophrenia has been suggested (Crow, 1997). Nasrallah (1985) proposed a mechanism for schizophrenia signs and symptoms based on a body of evidence pointing to a disturbance of interhemispheric integration. Velek *et al.* (1988) reported a case of congenital agenesis of the corpus callosum that presented with strong features of first-rank Schneiderian symptoms. The posterior subregions and the body of the corpus callosum have been found to be significantly smaller in individuals with autism (Piven *et al.*, 1997), and lack of normal asymmetry is also reported in schizophrenia (Crow, 1990, 1997).

A reduction in the total midsagittal corpus callosum area along with a reduction in the overall center-line length has been reported in adults with Tourette syndrome (Peterson *et al.*, 1994). In contrast, another study found that the anterior corpus callosum was significantly larger in children with Tourette syndrome but significantly smaller in children with attention-deficit hyperactivity disorder (Baumgardner *et al.*, 1996). The corpus callosum is thinner and the white matter is less dense in children with attention-deficit hyperactivity disorder and bipolar disorder (Caetano *et al.*, 2008; Hamilton *et al.*, 2008; Luders *et al.*, 2009). Seidman *et al.* (2005) found that the posterior region was more affected, and several other studies found that that medial and posterior regions were also affected in posttraumatic stress disorder and borderline personality disorder (Villarreal *et al.*, 2004; Rusch *et al.*, 2007; Jackowski *et al.*, 2009). Alterations in the size of the corpus callosum may reflect alterations in the cortical areas served by the corpus callosum.

A rather intriguing disorder called alien hand sign can develop with a lesion that involves the region of the anterior corpus callosum (Chapter 6). Reportedly there is a feeling of loss of voluntary control over the nondominant hand (Brion and Jednyak, 1972). A feeling of estrangement for the nondominant hand (*la main étrangère*) is reported. Other features include a tendency for the arm to drift off and assume odd postures, especially when the eyes are closed or when there is intermanual conflict or competition. Indeed, studies of patients in whom the corpus callosum has been sectioned have led to the notion that these individuals function with two independent minds, the left under the control of consciousness and the right largely functioning unconsciously and automatically (Bogen, 1993).

Anterior commissure

The anterior commissure is a small compact bundle that crosses the midline rostral to the fornix (Figures 14.1, 14.5, and 14.6). This commissure consists of two divisions that are not distinguishable on gross examination: a small anterior division that interconnects olfactory structures on either side, and a large posterior division that connects the anterior, middle, and inferotemporal regions.

The role of the anterior commissure remains unresolved (Zaidel, 1995). Prenatal stress in rats disrupts sexual differentiation and sexual behavior. The anterior division of the anterior commissure is sexually

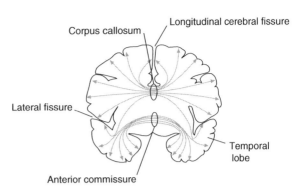

Figure 14.5. Diagrammatic coronal view of the brain shows the corpus callosum dorsal to the anterior commissure. The anterior commissure interconnects anterior portions of the temporal cortex on each side.

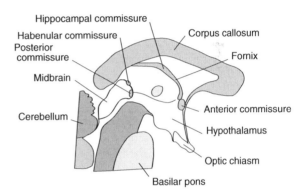

Figure 14.6. Diagrammatic midline view of the brain shows five commissures: the corpus callosum, the anterior commissure, the posterior commissure, the hippocampal commissure, and the habenular commissure. The corpus callosum is shown divided into the seven regions described by Giedd *et al.* (1994).

dimorphic in rats, and prenatal stress eliminates the male–female difference (Jones *et al.*, 1997). The number of axons in the anterior commissure is 17% greater in mice with a hereditary absence of the corpus callosum. However, the regions of the brain served by the axons remain the same (Livy *et al.*, 1997). It is hypothesized that the larger anterior commissure seen in females provides for better intercommunication between the two amygdalae and predisposes females to be more emotionally intelligent and socially sensitive (Joseph, 1993).

Hippocampal commissure

The hippocampal commissure (fornical commissure or psalterium) consists of fibers that originate in the hippocampus and cross the midline beneath the splenium of the corpus callosum (Figure 14.6). This commissure interconnects the hippocampus of both sides and is poorly developed in the human.

Supraoptic commissure

The small supraoptic commissure lies dorsal to the optic chiasm (Figure 14.6). It consists of several bundles of fine fibers that cross the midline. Included among these bundles is the hypothalamic commissure, which fans out into the lateral preoptic-hypothalamic area. A ventrally located bundle (ventral supraoptic decussation) is thought to arise from the reticular formation of the rostral pons and ascends in association with fibers of the medial longitudinal fasciculus. A dorsally located bundle (dorsal supraoptic decussation) may interconnect parts of the basal ganglia.

Papez (1937) believed that these decussations linked the thalamus with the hypothalamus and suggested that they played a role in emotions and in emotional expression.

Habenular commissure

The habenular commissure lies immediately beneath the pineal and is a small commissure whose fibers originate from the stria medullaris (Figure 14.6). Some of these fibers link the habenula with the superior colliculus. Other fibers within the habenular commissure interconnect the amygdala and the hippocampus of the two sides. The function of this commissure is not known.

Posterior commissure

The posterior commissure lies at the junction of the midbrain and diencephalon (Figure 14.6). It contains fibers that join the pretectal nuclei as well as fibers that interconnect oculomotor control nuclei located in the periaqueductal gray of the midbrain. These fibers are important in the pupillary reflex and in lid and vertical eye movements (Yun *et al.*, 1995; Kokkoroyannis *et al.*, 1996).

Hemispheric specialization

The anatomical projection of fibers to primary regions of the cortex is generally equally distributed between the hemispheres. In contrast, control of many complex functions is markedly asymmetrical. It is possible that complex functions can be more efficiently executed in a restricted unilateral site, while relying on transcortical fibers to interconnect with the contralateral hemisphere. Some asymmetry may be localized to specific lobes of the cerebral cortex and is discussed below.

Asymmetries that involve the entire hemisphere are presented in this section.

Left hemisphere

Language is the first area of behavior for which hemispheric dominance was demonstrated. The left hemisphere is dominant for linguistic functions in approximately 98% of individuals. The left hemisphere is specialized for the manipulation of numbers in the process of calculation.

Roughly 90% of the population is right-handed. In these people the left hemisphere is specialized for fine motor control. Most left-handed people, however, have their speech centers located in the left hemisphere.

The supratemporal plane (planum temporale), a region generally included in Wernicke's area, is larger on the left side of the brain in 65% of individuals. The right planum is larger in only about 10% of brains (Geschwind and Levitsky, 1968). This asymmetry is speculated to play a role in the left hemispheric language superiority.

The left cerebral hemisphere of right-handers is believed to be specialized for tool use. The network responsible for this function favors the inferior parietal lobule and the middle frontal gyrus. A second network that controls hand-to-target interaction lies slightly superiorly in the intraparietal and dorsal premotor areas and operates contralateral to the hand being used at the time (Johnson and Grafton, 2003).

Clinical vignette

A 76-year-old right-handed man developed environmental disorientation after a stroke. He had difficulty finding his way in the hospital and in his neighborhood. He had special problems with corridors, public bathrooms, and theaters. At one point, he could not get out of a public bathroom because he could not find the exit. He was able to read a map, draw an accurate floor plan of his house, and give verbal directions of familiar routes, yet he quickly got lost when taken out on familiar routes. This patient had a relatively isolated environmental disorientation, or topographagnosia, from a stroke involving the parahippocampal place area located in the right hemisphere. His neurological examination was otherwise remarkable only for a visual field deficit in his upper left quadrant. Magnetic resonance imaging confirmed the presence of an infarction involving the right posterior-inferior temporal and occipital lobes (Figure 14.7).

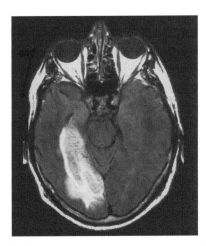

Figure 14.7. The patient's magnetic resonance image (fluid attenuated inversion recovery [FLAIR], horizontal view) revealed a posterior circulation stroke in the right medial occipitotemporal region extending to the presumed parahippocampal place area. (Reprinted with permission from Mendez and Cherrier, 2003.)

Right hemisphere

Complex nonlinguistic perceptual skills, facial recognition, and spatial distribution of attention are centered in the right hemisphere. Patients with right hemisphere lesions, especially in the posterior areas, have a much greater impairment in complex visuospatial tasks than do those with equivalent left-sided lesions. The identification of faces is a most complex perceptual task that is also of great biological importance (Chapter 5, see Fusiform gyrus and fusiform face area). Under certain circumstances either hemisphere can recognize faces. However, the right hemisphere is specialized in face recognition (Sergent, 1995; Mandal and Ambady, 2004). Recent works point to the fact that the right hemisphere is also specialized for determining the distribution of attention within the extrapersonal space. This leads to marked contralateral neglect after right hemispheric injury. Contralateral neglect is seldom seen after the occurrence of a left hemisphere lesion.

The right hemisphere is more important than the left both in experiencing and in expressing emotions. It contains records of prototypic facial emotional representations. These records are innate and appear to be localized to the temporal lobe (Heilman and Bowers, 1996). Limbic and temporal association areas were more activated on the right during sexual arousal in men (Stoléru et al., 1999).

Lesions in the right temporoparietal area can produce receptive aprosodia, disrupting the patient's ability to understand, name, or discriminate emotional expressions. Patients with right hemisphere stroke can be impaired at recognizing facial displays. Right hemisphere lesions may impair the patient's ability to determine if two faces, previously unknown to the patient, are the same or different people. Patients with right hemisphere lesions are impaired at determining the emotional content of verbal descriptions (Blonder et al., 1991a).

Patients with left hemisphere lesions tend to be agitated, anxious, and depressed ("catastrophic reaction"), whereas those with right hemisphere lesions tend to be indifferent to their predicament or may even be mildly euphoric. The patient's inability to express emotion may contribute to the appearance of indifference. Deficits in the display of emotional expressions are associated with right frontal lesions similar to lesions that cause Broca's aphasia on the left hemisphere. A deficit in the expression of emotion is termed expressive aprosodia. Patients with right hemisphere lesions are less emotionally expressive (Blonder et al., 1991b).

Frontal hemisphere activation is asymmetrical in patients with panic disorder. Right frontal activation appears to represent acute activation of avoidance-withdrawal and is associated with negative emotions (Wiedemann et al., 1999).

Lobular specializations

Occipitoparietal lobe

A lesion of the inferiomedial aspect of the left occipitotemporal lobe below the splenium of the corpus callosum can produce color agnosia. Affected individuals can sort colors according to hue but cannot name colors. These individuals usually also have right homonymous hemianopia and alexia.

A lesion of the right occipitotemporal region can produce prosopagnosia, although this disorder is more frequently seen after the occurrence of a bilateral lesion. The patient with prosopagnosia is unable to recognize familiar faces, often including his or her own face.

A large lesion of the parietal lobe can produce sensory neglect in the contralateral hemifield. The right lobe plays a greater role in controlling attention and contains a map of both visual fields, and therefore sensory neglect is more often seen after the occurrence of a right-sided parietal lesion. A lesion in the right parietal lobe can produce confusion and disorientation for place. A patient with a large left-sided parietal lesion involving the supramarginal gyrus may react inappropriately to painful stimuli. Patients who demonstrate construction apraxia after a parietal lobe lesion may differ in their ability to draw based on the side of the lesion. With a right-sided parietal lesion, the drawing maintains its complexity, but the left side of the drawing is missing. With a left-sided lesion, the drawing is symmetrical, but details are missing and it is drawn slowly. Gerstmann syndrome is seen following a left-sided parietal (angular gyrus) lesion (Chapter 4).

Temporal lobe

Both visual and auditory responses can result from stimulation of the temporal lobe; however, these responses are seen more often when the right temporal lobe is stimulated (Gloor, 1990). Cell densities in the left hippocampus were found to be greater than in the right hippocampus of men. The left planum temporale is larger in females than in males, but the asymmetry seen in the planum temporale in males is not present in females. No differences were seen between sexes or between hemispheres for the primary auditory area (Heschl's gyrus) (Kulynych et al., 1994). Asymmetries in women are less apparent in both the planum temporale and the hippocampus (Zaidel et al., 1994).

Patients with lesions of the temporal lobe that affect audition have difficulty distinguishing words if the lesion is on the left and difficulty distinguishing non-verbal sounds, including music, if the lesion is on the right. Left temporal lobe lesions that affect memory involve the loss of language-related information. Right temporal lesions affect the memory of musical melodies and of geometrical shapes.

Lesions of the left posterior superior temporal gyrus including Brodmann's area (BA) 22 produce receptive aphasia (Wernicke's). Comprehension of verbal language is primarily affected. If the lesion extends into the inferior parietal lobe, reading may also be affected. In some left-handed individuals, the left hemisphere may be dominant for comprehension whereas the right hemisphere is dominant for the production of speech.

Patients with epileptogenic foci localized to the left temporal lobe tend to be paranoid and to exhibit schizophrenia-like and antisocial behavior. Patients with right-sided temporal foci tend to show emotional extremes, manic-depressive symptoms, and denial (Sherwin et al., 1982; Bear, 1986). Exceptions have been reported in which patients with right-sided foci present with thought disturbances (Sherwin, 1982).

A lesion of the right posterior temporoparietal area can produce aprosodia in which patients are unable to appreciate the emotional content of speech based on pitch and intonation, although they comprehend the semantic meaning. In contrast, a person with Wernicke's aphasia will not understand the meaning of the words but will react to the emotion (e.g., anger) expressed by the speaker.

Volume of the left temporal lobe is reduced in schizophrenia (Turetsky et al., 1994), and the left lateral fissure is larger (Rubin et al., 1993). Reite et al. (1997) reported that male schizophrenia patients demonstrated a smaller superior temporal gyrus than that of male control subjects, and female schizophrenia patients demonstrated less laterality than did female controls. The left temporal lobe exhibits higher metabolic activity than the right. Whether there is a left hypometabolism or a right hypermetabolism when compared with controls remains an open question (Gur et al., 1995).

Surgical removal of portions of the temporal lobe is sometimes effective in the treatment of epilepsy. It is essential to determine the hemisphere that is dominant for language and speech before surgery. The lateral portion of the temporal lobe, which contains the receptive speech area, is served by the middle cerebral artery (Figure 2.5). The Wada test can be used in this situation to determine laterality. In this test, short-acting barbiturates are injected into the internal carotid artery. Aphasia is induced when the barbiturate perfuses the dominant hemisphere. More recently, the use of transcranial magnetic stimulation (TMS) has been proposed as a less invasive procedure to determine language and speech dominance (George, 2003).

Frontal lobe

The pars opercularis (Broca's region) is larger in the left than in the right frontal lobe (Geschwind and Galaburda, 1985). Folds surrounding the lateral fissure appear earlier on the right than on the left side (Simonds and Scheibel, 1989).

The left frontal region is proposed to be responsible for approach behavior, including planning, intention, and self-regulation. The right frontal region is responsible for withdrawal (Davidson, 1995). Ten-month-old infants who cry frequently show more right frontal activation (Fox and Davidson, 1988). Davidson (1995) found that children at 38 months of age who spent more time proximal to their mother in a novel situation were inhibited and showed greater right frontal activation than uninhibited children.

A lesion of the opercular portion of the inferior frontal gyrus (BA 44 and BA 45) on the left side produces expressive aphasia (Broca's aphasia). Comprehension of speech is intact but speech production is reduced. The individual with expressive aphasia speaks slowly and with effort.

A lesion of the right premotor area (BA 6 and BA 8) of the frontal lobe can produce hemiakinesia, in which the patient cannot look toward and has difficulty reaching into the opposite hemifield. Hemiakinesia produced by a left premotor area lesion is seen less frequently, and when it appears it is less pronounced. The right hemisphere mediates attention to both hemifields, whereas the left directs attention only to the right hemifield (Knight, 1984).

Patients with a lesion of the left hemisphere tend to be anxious, tearful, depressed and abusive. Patients with right-sided lesions may be inappropriately cheerful. The degree of emotional involvement, irrespective of side of involvement, is greater if the lesion is closer to the frontal pole. Activation of the left frontal lobe in normal individuals correlates with heightened approach-related positive affect, whereas activation of the right frontal lobe correlates with withdrawal-related negative affect (Wheeler et al., 1993). Patients with unipolar depression exhibit hypometabolism in the left anterolateral prefrontal cortex (George et al., 1993). It is suggested that frontal lobe emotional asymmetry may reflect subcortical asymmetries such as catecholamine asymmetries in the amygdala and thalamus (Jacobs and Snyder, 1996). The normal frontal lobe asymmetry is reversed in autistic subjects (Nowell et al., 1990).

Subcortical regions

The lenticular nucleus (globus pallidus and putamen) is normally larger on the left than on the right. This asymmetry in the lenticular nucleus is missing in children and adults with Tourette syndrome (Yank et al., 1995). Changes seen in caudate nucleus glucose metabolism following treatment for obsessive-compulsive disorder indicate greater dysfunction on the right side in this disorder (Baxter et al., 1990). Patients with Parkinson disease who have symptoms that primarily reflect a left-sided lesion are more depressed (Starkstein et al., 1990). The depression may be the result of disruption of connections between the basal ganglia and the frontal cortex (Mayberg, 1992).

Activation of the right side has been seen during the recall of painful memories in patients with posttraumatic stress disorder (Figure 11.8) (Rauch et al., 1996). Right-sided activation was not seen during recall of neutral memories. The authors suggested that the results reflected activation of the right amygdala. The patients also showed deactivation of Broca's area. The authors stated that this may reflect the difficulty these patients have in cognitively reconstructing their traumatic experience.

Select bibliography

Brazis, P.W., Masdeu, J.C., and Biller, J. *Localization in Clinical Neurology*. (Boston: Little, Brown, 1990.)

Davidson, R.J., and Hugdahl, K. (eds.) *Brain Asymmetry (electronic resource)*. (Cambridge, MA: MIT Press, 2003.)

Nass, R.D., and Gazzaniga, M.S. Cerebral lateralization and specialization in human central nervous system. In: N.Plum, F.Plum, and V.B.Mountcastle (eds.) *Handbook of Physiology – The Nervous System V*. (Bethesda, MD: American Physiological Society, 1987.)

Toga, A.W., and Thompson, P.M. Mapping brain asymmetry. *Nature Reviews. Neuroscience*, 2003; **4**:37–48.

Trimble, M.R. *Biological Psychiatry*. (New York: Wiley, 1988.)

References

Baumgardner, T.L., Singer, H.S., Denckla, M.B., Rubin, M.A., Abrams, M.T., Colli, M.J., and Reiss, A.L. 1996. Corpus callosum morphology in children with Tourette syndrome and attention deficit hyperactivity disorder. *Neurology* **47**:477–482.

Baxter, L.R., Schwartz, J.M., Guze, B.H., Bergman, K., and Szuba, M.P. 1990. Neuroimaging in obsessive-compulsive disorder: Seeking the mediating neuroanatomy. In: M.A.Jenike, L.Baer, and W.E.Minichiello (eds.) *Obsessive-Compulsive Disorders: Theory and Management*. Littleton, MA: Year Book Medical Publishers.

Bear, D. 1986. Hemispheric asymmetries in emotional function: a reflection of lateral specialization in cortical-limbic connections. In: B.K.Doane, and K.E.Livingston (eds.) *The Limbic System: Functional Organization and Clinical Disorders*. New York: Raven Press, pp. 29–42.

Berlucchi, G. 2004. Some effects of cortical and callosal damage on conscious and unconscious processing of visual information and other sensory inputs. *Prog. Brain Res.* **144**:79–93.

Blonder, L.X., Bowers, D., and Heilman, K.M. 1991a. The role of the right hemisphere on emotional communication. *Brain* **114**:1115–1127.

Blonder, L.X., Burns, A., Bowers, D., Moore, R., and Heilman, K.1991b. Right hemisphere expressivity during natural conversation. *J. Clin. Exp. Neuropsychol.* **13**:85.

Bogen, J.E. 1993. The callosal syndromes. In: K.M. Heilman, and E.Valenstein (eds.) *Clinical Neuropsychology* (3rd ed.). New York: Oxford University Press, pp. 337–407.

Brion, S., and Jednyak, C.P. 1972. Troubles du transfert interhemispherique. *Rev. Neurol.* **126**:257–266.

Caetano, S.C., Silveira, C.M., Kaur, S., Nicoletti, M., Hatch, J.P., Brambilla, P., Sassi, R., Axelson, D., Keshavan, M.S., Ryan, N.D., Birmaher, B., and Soares, J.C. 2008. Abnormal corpus callosum myelination in pediatric bipolar patients. *J. Affect. Disord.* **108**:297–301.

Chiron, C., Jambaque, I, Nabbout, R., Lounes, R., Syrota, A., and Dulac, O. 1997. The right brain hemisphere is dominant in human infants. *Brain* **120**:1057–1065.

Crow, T.J. 1990. Temporal lobe asymmetries as the key to the etiology of schizophrenia. *Schizophr. Bull.* **16**:433–443.

Crow, T.J. 1997. Temporolimbic or transcallosal connections: Where is the primary lesion in schizophrenia and what is its nature? *Schizophr. Bull.* **23**:521–523.

Davidson, R.J. 1995. Cerebral asymmetry, emotion, and affective style. In: R.J.Davidson and K.Hugdahl (eds.) *Brain Asymmetry*. Cambridge, MA: MIT Press, pp. 361–387.

Fox, N.A., and Davidson, R.J. 1988 Taste-elicited changes in facial signs of emotion and the asymmetry of brain electrical activity in human newborns. *Neuropsychology* **24**:417–422.

Gazzaniga, M.S. 2005. Forty-five years of split-brain research and still going strong. *Nat. Rev. Neurosci.* **6**:653–659.

George, M.S. 2003. Stimulating the brain. *Sci. Am.* **289**:66–73.

George, M.S., Ketter, T.A., and Post, R.M. 1993. SPECT and PET imaging in mood disorders. *J. Clin. Psychiatry* **54**(Suppl. 11):6–13.

Geschwind, N., and Levitsky, W. 1968. Human brain: Left-right asymmetries in temporal speech region. *Science* **161**:186–187.

Geschwind, N., and Galaburda, A.M. 1985. Cerebral lateralization. *Arch. Neurol.* **42**:428–459.

Giedd, J.N., Castellanos, F.X., Casey, B.J., Kozuch, P., King, A.C., Hamburger, S.D., and Rapoport, J.L. 1994. Quantitative morphology of the corpus callosum in attention deficit hyperactivity disorder. *Am. J. Psychiatry* **151**:665–669.

Glicksohn, J., and Myslobodsky, M.S. 1993. The presentation of patterns of structural brain asymmetry in normal individuals. *Neuropsychologia* **31**:145–159.

Gloor, P. 1990. Experimental phenomena of temporal lobe epilepsy: Facts and hypotheses. *Brain* **113**:1673–1694.

Gur, R.E., Mozley, P.D., Resnick, S.M., Mozley, L.H., Shtasel, D.L., Gallacher, F., Arnold, S.E., Karp, J.S., Alavi, A., Reivich, M., and Gur, R.C. 1995. Resting cerebral glucose metabolism in first-episode and previously treated patients with schizophrenia relates to clinical features. *Arch. Gen. Psychiatry* **52**:657–667.

Hadziselimovic, H., and Cus, M. 1966. The appearance of internal structures of the brain in relation to configuration of the human skull. *Acta Anat.* **63**:289–299.

Hamilton, L.S., Levitt, J.G., O' Neill, J., Alger, J.R., Luders, E., Phillips, O.R., Caplan, R., Toga, A.W., McCracken, J., and Narr, K.L. 2008. Reduced white matter integrity in attention-deficit hyperactivity disorder. *Neuroreport* **19**:1705–1708.

Heilman, K.M., and Bowers, D. 1996. Emotional disorders associated with hemispheric dysfunction. In: B.S.Fogel, R.B.Schiffer, and S.M.Rao (eds.) *Neuropsychology*. Baltimore: Williams & Wilkins, pp. 401–406.

Jackowski, A.P., de Araújo, C.M., de Lacerda, A.L.T., Mari, J.J., and Kaufman, J. 2009. Neurostructural imaging findings in children with post-traumatic stress disorder: Brief review. *Psychiatry Clin. Neurosci.* **63**:1–8.

Jacobs, G.D., and Snyder, D. 1996. Frontal brain asymmetry predicts affective style in men. *Behav. Neurosci.* **110**:3–6.

Johnson, S.H., and Grafton, S.T. 2003. From "acting on" to "acting with": the functional anatomy of object-oriented action schemata. *Prog. Brain Res.* **142**:127–139.

Jones, H.E., Ruscio, M.A., Keyser, L.A., Gonzalez, C., Billack, B., Rowe, R., Hancock, C., Lambert, K.G., and Kinsley, C.H. 1997. Prenatal stress alters the size of the rostral anterior commissure in rats. *Brain Res. Bull.* **42**:341–346.

Joseph, R. 1993. *The Naked Neuron: Evolution and the Languages of the Body and Brain*. New York: Plenum.

Knight, R.T. 1984. Decreased response to novel stimuli after prefrontal lesions in man. *Electroencephalogr. Clin. Neurophysiol.* **59**:9.

Kokkoroyannis, T., Scudder, C.A., Balaban, C.D., Highstein, S.M., and Moschovakis, A.K. 1996. Anatomy and physiology of the primate interstitial nucleus of Cajal I. Efferent projections. *J. Neurophysiol.* **75**:725–739.

Kulynych, J.J., Vladar, K., Jones, D.W., and Weinberger, D.R. 1994. Gender differences in the normal lateralization of the supratemporal cortex: MRI surface-rendering morphometry of Heschl's gyrus and the planum temporale. *Cereb. Cortex* **4**:107–118.

Liederman, J. 1995. A reinterpretation of the split-brain syndrome: Implications for the function of corticocortical fibers. In: R.J.Davidson, and K.Hugdahl (eds.) *Brain Asymmetry*. Cambridge, MA: MIT Press, pp. 451–490.

Livy, D.J., Schalomon, P.M., Roy, M., Zacharias, M.C., Pimenta, J., Lent, R., and Wahlsten, D. 1997. Increased axon number in the anterior commissure of mice lacking a corpus callosum. *Exp. Neurol.* **146**:491–501.

Luders, E., Narr, K.L., Hamilton, L.S., Phillips, O.R., Thompson, P.M., Valle, J.S., Del' Homme, M., Strickland, T., McCracken, J.T., Toga, A.W., and Levitt, J.G. 2009. Decreased callosal thickness in attention-deficit/hyperactivity disorder. *Biol. Psychiatry* **65**:84–88.

Mandal, M.K., and Ambady, N. 2004. Laterality of facial expressions of emotion: universal and culture-specific influences. *Behav. Neurol.* **15**:23–34.

Mayberg, H.S. 1992. Neuroimaging studies of depression in neurological disease. In: S.E.Starkstein, and R.G.Robinson (eds.) *Depression in Neurologic Disease.* Baltimore: Johns Hopkins University Press.

Mendez, M.F. 1995. The neuropsychiatry of multiple sclerosis. *Int. J. Psychiatry Med.* **25**:123–135.

Mendez, M.F., and Cherrier, M.M. 2003. Agnosia for scenes in topographagnosia. Neuropsychologia **41**:1387–1395.

Nasrallah, H.A. 1985. The unintegrated right cerebral hemispheric consciousness as alien intruder: A possible mechanism for Schneiderian delusions in schizophrenia. *Compr. Psychiatry* **26**:273–282.

Nowell, M.A., Hackmery, D.B., Muraki, A.S., and Coleman, M. 1990. Varied MR appearance of autism: Fifty three pediatric patients having full autistic syndrome. *Magn. Reson. Imaging* **8**:811–816.

Ojima, E., Abiru, H., and Fukui, Y. 1996. Effects of cocaine on the rat cerebral commissure. *Int. J. Develop. Neurosci.* **14**:649–654.

Papez, J.W. 1937. A proposed mechanism of emotion. *Arch. Neurol. Psychiat.* **38**:725–743.

Peterson, B.S., Leckman, J.F., and Duncan, J. 1994. Corpus callosum morphology from MR images in Tourette's syndrome. *Psychiatry Res.* **55**:85–99.

Piven, J., Bailey, J., Ranson, B.J., and Arndt, S. 1997. An MRI study of the corpus callosum in autism. *Am. J. Psychiatry* **154**:1051–1056.

Peru, A., Beltramello, A., Moro, V., Sattibaldi, L., and Berlucchi, G. 2003. Temporal and permanent signs of interhemispheric disconnection after traumatic brain injury. *Neuropsychologia* **41**:634–643.

Rauch, S.L., van der Kolk, B.A., Fisler, R.E., Alpert, N.M., Orr, S.P., Savage, C.R., Fischman, A.J., Jenike, M.A., and Pitman, R.K. 1996. A symptom provocation study of posttraumatic stress disorder using positron emission tomography and script-driven imagery. *Arch. Gen. Psychiatry* **53**:380–387.

Reite, M., Sheeder, J., Teale, P., Adams, M., Richardson, D., Simon, J., Jones, R.H., and Rojas, D.C. 1997. Magnetic source imaging evidence of sex differences in cerebral lateralization in schizophrenia. *Arch. Gen. Psychiatry* **54**:433–440.

Robinson, R.G. 1985. Lateralized behavioral and neurochemical consequences of unilateral brain injury in rats. In: S.D.Glick (ed.) *Cerebral Lateralization in Nonhuman Species.* New York: Academic Press, pp. 135–156.

Rubin, P., Karle, A., Moller-Madsen, S., Hertel, C., Povlsen, U.J., Noring, U., and Hemingsen, R. 1993. Computerised tomography in newly diagnosed schizophrenia and schizophreniform disorder: A controlled blind study. *Br. J. Psychiatry* **163**: 604–612.

Rusch, N., Luders, E., Lieb, K., Zahn, R., Ebert, D., Thompson, P.M., Toga, A.W., and van Elst, L.T. 2007. Corpus callosum abnormalities in women with borderline personality disorder and comorbid attention-deficit hyperactivity disorder. *J. Psychiatry Neurosci.* **32**:417–422.

Seidman, L.J., Valera, E.M., and Makris, N. 2005. Structural brain imaging of attention-deficit/hyperactivity disorder. *Biol. Psychiatry* **57**:1263–1272.

Sergent, J. 1995. Hemispheric contribution to face processing: Patterns of convergence and divergence. In: R.J.Davidson, and K.Hugdahl (eds.) *Brain Asymmetry.* Cambridge, MA: MIT Press, pp. 157–181.

Sherwin, I. 1982. The effect of the location of an epileptogenic lesion on the occurrence of psychosis in epilepsy. In: W.Koella, and M.R.Trimble (eds.) *Temporal Lobe Epilepsy, Mania, and Schizophrenia and the Limbic System.* Basel: Karger, pp. 81–97.

Sherwin, I., Peron-Magnan, P., Bancaud, J., Bonis, A., and Talairach, J. 1982. Prevalence of psychosis in epilepsy as a function of the laterality of the epileptogenic lesion. *Arch. Neurol.* **39**:621–625.

Simonds, R.J., and Scheibel, A.B. 1989. The postnatal development of the motor speech area: A preliminary study. *Brain Lang.* **37**:42–58.

Sperry, R. 1962. Some general aspects of interhemispheric integration. In: V.B.Mountcastle (ed.) *Interhemispheric Relations and Cerebral Dominance.* Baltimore: Johns Hopkins, Press, pp. 43–49.

Starkstein, S.E., Cohen, B.S., Fedoroff, P., Parikh, R.M., Price, T.R., and Robinson, R.G. 1990. Relationship between anxiety disorders and depressive disorders in patients with cerebrovascular injury. *Arch. Gen. Psychiatry* **47**:246–251.

Stoléru, S., Grégoire, M-C., Gérard, D., Decety, J., Lafarge, E., Cinotti, L., Lavenne, F., LeBars, D., Vernet-Maury, E., Rada, H., Collet, C., Mazoyer, B., Forest, M.G., Magnin, F., Spira, A., and Comar, D. 1999. Neuroanatomical correlates of visually evoked sexual arousal in human males. *Arch. Sex. Behav.* **28**:1–21.

Trevarthen, C. 1990. Growth and eduction in the hemispheres. In: C.Trevarthen (ed.) *Brain Circuits and Functions of the Mind.* Cambridge, England: Cambridge University Press, pp. 334–363.

Turetsky, B.I., Cowell, P.E., Gur, R.C., Grossman, R.I., and Gur, R.E. 1994. *Frontal and temporal lobe brain volumes in schizophrenia: Relationship to symptomatology and clinical subtype. Presented at the 49th Annual Meeting for the Society for Biological Psychiatry: May 21, 1994.* Philadelphia, PA.

Velek, M., White, L.E., Williams, J.P., Stafford, R.L., and Marco, L.A. 1988. Psychosis in a case of corpus callosum agenesis. *Alabama Med.* **58**:27–29.

Villarreal, G., Hamilton, D.A., Graham, D.P., Driscoll, I., Qualls, C., Petropoulos, H., and Brooks, W.M. 2004. Reduced area of the corpus callosum in posttraumatic stress disorder. *Psychiatry Res.* **131**:227–235.

Wheeler, R.E., Davidson, R.J., and Tomarken, A.J. 1993. Frontal brain asymmetry and emotional reactivity: A biological substrate of affective style. *Psychophysiology* **30**:82–89.

Wiedemann, G., Pauli, P., Dengler, W., Lutzenberger, W., Birbaumer, N., and Buchkremer, G. 1999. Frontal brain asymmetry as a biological substrate of emotions in patients with panic disorders. *Arch. Gen. Psychiatry* **56**:78–84.

Witelson, S.F. 1989. Hand and sex differences in the isthmus and genu of the human corpus callosum. *Brain* **112**:799–835.

Yank, M., Yazgan, B.P., Wexler, B.E., and Leckman, J.F. 1995. Behavioral laterality in individuals with Gilles de la Tourette Syndrome and basal ganglia alterations: A preliminary report. *Biol. Psychiatry* **38**:386–390.

Yun, S., Shoumura, K., Ichinohe, N., Hirama, H., and Amayasu, H. 1995. Functional and anatomical fiber analysis of the posterior commissure (PC) in the cat: Evidence for PC fibers of which stimulation elicits non-oculosympathetic pupillary dilation. *J. Hinforschung* **36**:29–50.

Zaidel, D.W., Esiri, M.M., and Oxbury, J.M. 1994. Sex-related asymmetries in the morphology of the left and right hippocampi? *J. Neurol.* **241**:620–623.

Zaidel, E. 1995. Interhemispheric transfer in the split brain: Long-term status following complete cerebral commissurotomy. In: R.J.Davidson, and K.Hugdahl (eds.) *Brain Asymmetry.* Cambridge, MA: MIT Press, pp. 491–532.

Zaidel, E., Clarke, J., and Suyenobu, B. 1990. Hemispheric independence: A paradigm case for cognitive neuroscience. In: A.B.Scheibel, and A.F.Wechsler (eds.) *Neurobiology of Higher Cognitive Function.* New York: Guilford Press, pp. 297–362.

Index